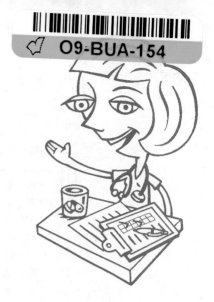

Pediatric Nursing Demystified

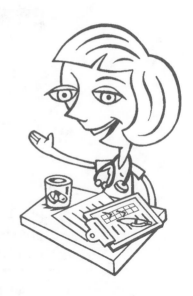

Pediatric Nursing Demystified

Joyce Y. Johnson, RN, PhD

Dean and Professor
College of Sciences and Health Professions
Albany State University
Albany, Georgia

James Keogh, RN

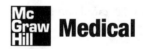 Medical

New York Chicago San Francisco Lisbon London
Madrid Mexico City Milan New Delhi San Juan
Seoul Singapore Sydney Toronto

Pediatric Nursing Demystified

Copyright © 2010 by The McGraw-Hill Companies, Inc. All rights reserved. Printed in the United States of America. Except as permitted under the United States Copyright Act of 1976, no part of this publication may be reproduced or distributed in any form or by any means, or stored in a data base or retrieval system, without the prior written permission of the publisher.

1 2 3 4 5 6 7 8 9 0   DOC/DOC   14 13 12 11 10 9

ISBN 978-0-07-160915-9   618.92
MHID 0-07-160915-6

This book was set in Times Roman by Glyph International.
The editors were Joe Morita and Regina Y. Brown.
The production supervisor was Phil Galea.
Project management was provided by Gita Raman, Glyph International.
Cover design art directed by Margaret Webster-Shapiro.
The cover designer was Lance Lekander.
RR Donnelley was printer and binder.

This book is printed on acid-free paper.

CIP data is on file with the Library of Congress.

McGraw-Hill books are available at special quantity discounts to use as premiums and sales promotions, or for use in corporate training programs. To contact a representative please e-mail us at bulksales@mcgraw-hill.com.

This book is dedicated to my mother Dorothy C. Young who has always been an inspiration to me, to my husband Larry and to Virginia and Larry Jr. who are the wind beneath my wings.

Joyce Y. Johnson

This book is dedicated to Anne, Sandy, Joanne, Amber-Leigh Christine, Shawn, and Eric, without whose help and support this book could not have been written.

James Keogh

We dedicate this book to our students who are the reason we teach and write. Much success in your nursing careers!

Authors

CONTENTS

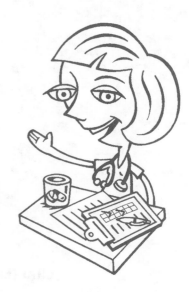

PREFACE

Pediatric Nursing Demystified offers a detailed overview of the essential concepts involved in the nursing care of the pediatric client. The major conditions seen in the pediatric population are highlighted along with the associated nursing care.

Because the client is a child or adolescent, nursing care involves a family-centered process. Chapter 1 discusses family dynamics and community resources. Chapter 2 focuses on growth and development stages from infancy through adolescence with an emphasis on the impact of developmental stage on the care being provided to a client. Concepts of growth and development related to the pediatric client that informs nursing care and communications with this population and their family members are discussed. Major theories are summarized, and the key aspects that relate to care of the pediatric client are highlighted. Chapter 3 follows with a review of health assessment with a focus on the pediatric client. Part II includes 12 chapters that address individual pediatric conditions with a systematic review of illnesses and conditions encountered in the pediatric population.

Pediatric Nursing Demystified is an easy-to-understand presentation of concepts and focuses on the information that students need most to deal with the common conditions that face pediatric clients. This review focuses on the most critical information in pediatric nursing by discussing the underlying factors involved in maintaining or restoring the health and well-being of the pediatric client and family and those factors that threaten that well-being. *Pediatric Nursing Demystified* contains clear language and helpful features to guide the student through application of concepts to real-life situations.

The features of the book are organized as follows:

- ◗ Each detailed chapter contains learning objectives.
- ◗ Key words are identified for the content area.
- ◗ A brief overview of the topic is provided.
- ◗ Content is divided into:
  - • A brief review of anatomy and physiology
  - • Discussion of what went wrong that resulted in the condition
  - • Signs and symptoms

- Test results
- Treatment
- Nursing intervention

- Illustrations are provided to aid memory and understanding of the condition.
- Diagrams and tables are provided to summarize important details.
- Routine checkups are provided to briefly test understanding gained after a portion of the information is presented.
- A conclusion summarizes the content presented.
- A Final Checkup is provided with NCLEX-style questions to test the knowledge gained from the chapter.
- A comprehensive exam that includes NCLEX-style questions that cover content presented throughout *Pediatric Nursing Demystified* appears at the end of the book.

Pediatric Nursing Demystified is a nursing student's best friend in the study for course exams and the NCLEX.

ACKNOWLEDGMENTS

We would like to thank Joe Morita for his direction and tremendous support in the development of this project.

Thank you to Edna Boyd Davis for her contributions to this project.

Thank you to Clemmie Riggins for her assistance in the preparation of the manuscript.

PART I

Roles and Relationships

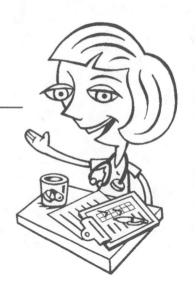

CHAPTER 1

Families and Communities

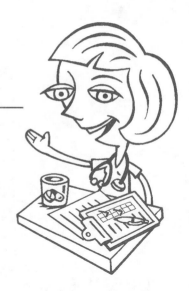

Learning Objectives

At the end of the chapter, the student will be able to

1 Describe the impact of family dynamics on the nursing care of the pediatric client.

2 Distinguish the types of families in a community.

3 Contrast the health-related concerns resulting from families and communities at varied socioeconomic levels.

4 Indicate appropriate nursing approaches to address family and community concerns related to care of the pediatric client.

5 Discuss ethnic-cultural influences on family and community dynamics.

6 Determine appropriate nursing implications of ethnic-cultural concepts.

KEY WORDS

Assimilated	Nuclear family
Cohabitation family	Reconstituted/Binuclear family
Ethnocentric	Sibling
Extended family	Stereotyping
Gay/lesbian family	Subculture
High-risk population	

OVERVIEW

1 The family and community provide the foundation for the growth and development of a pediatric client. Health promotion, maintenance, and restoration activities can be supported or hindered by family dynamics and the presence or absence of family and community support resources. Challenges presented by family or community distress can severely limit a child's successful progression through the developmental stages of life. Understanding the basic concepts of family and community dynamics helps the nurse to provide comprehensive care to the pediatric client and family.

◐ Foundational concepts
- Family-centered nursing recognizes family support as a needed constant in a child's life.
- The family, in addition to the child, is supported throughout the health-care experience.
- Collaboration with family is facilitated throughout hospital, community, and home care.
- Family advocacy includes enabling families to build on current strengths and helping them maintain a sense of control over their lives.
- Separation of the child from the family should be kept at a minimum to reduce psychological distress.
- In the home setting, the nurse is a visitor and should respect the authority of the family.
- Community support resources are crucial for families with a child with special needs—developmental delay, sensory deficits (blindness, deafness, etc.).

◐ Roles and relationships
- Family members often play more than one role in the family system. Family roles:
  ○ Include but are not restricted to parent (mother, father, stepmother, stepfather, foster parent), child, sibling, provider, homemaker, or caregiver.

- ○ Vary depending on type and structure of family, including number and age of members and ethnic-cultural background.
- ○ May change as a result of the illness or the changes in the needs of a child. Illness can cause stress in a family, and that stress can in turn increase the distress of the child.

TYPES OF FAMILIES

2 Types of families may be described in different ways, and needs may vary based on family composition and function. The type of family a child belongs to may include

- **Nuclear family:** Husband (usually the provider), wife (usually homemaker although frequently works also), and child/children.
- **Reconstituted/binuclear/blended family:** Child or children and one parent in one home and another parent in a different home. A stepparent and step-siblings may be present in one or both homes, reconstituting two families into one and resulting in two blended nuclear families.
- **Cohabitation family:** A man and woman who live together with a child or children without being married.
- **Single-parent family:** A man or woman living with one or more children.
- **Gay/lesbian family:** Two men or two women who live together as parents to one or more biological or adopted children.
- **Extended family:** Multigenerational groups consisting of parents and children with other relatives (i.e., grandparents, aunts, uncles, cousins, grandchildren).

NURSING IMPLICATIONS

- Perform a family assessment to determine the presence or absence of support for the child during and after hospitalization.
- Identify and collaborate with key individuals within the family unit to promote restoration and maintenance of health after the child is discharged home.
- Plan activities to minimize separation of child from family.
- Involve parents and family in care activities to promote learning for after-discharge care.
- Assess the home environment and determine the presence of contributing factors to pediatric illness and risk factors for additional physical or psychological health problems.
- Collaborate with family members to minimize risk factors and prepare the home environment to meet the needs of the pediatric client and ensure follow-up after discharge.

○ Develop an action plan that addresses the needs of the pediatric client and family from admission through discharge back into the community and home setting.

Nursing alert **When possible, determine who has legal custodial rights and can make decisions regarding the child *before* critical decisions must be made.**

SOCIAL AND ECONOMIC FACTORS

❸ Social factors such as living environment and community relationships, in addition to economic factors such as poverty, unemployment, or homelessness, can impact the health of a child and family because of limited access to clean water, food, shelter, or health. Some groups are considered **high-risk populations,** groups of people at higher risk for illness than the general population, due to social, economic, or cultural factors. Be aware of these key social factors:

○ Poverty may limit access to healthy food leading to nutritional deficits.
○ Lack of access to health care decreases health promotion and maintenance and contributes to late diagnosis of illness and delayed treatment.
○ Unemployment contributes to poverty and possible homelessness, increasing exposure to overcrowded shelters, dangerous situations, and illness.
○ High-risk behaviors such as unprotected sex, drugs, and reckless driving can lead to unwanted pregnancy, infections, addiction, and injury.
○ Teen pregnancy can result in poor prenatal care, premature birth, and birth defects as well as poor parenting, leading to physiologic and psychological damage to the pediatric client.
○ Family disruption due to factors such as drug or alcohol abuse, mental illness, domestic violence, or divorce can destabilize the child's life, leading to distress.
○ Community instability because of gang activity, crime, violence, high unemployment, and poverty can result in decreased available health resources.

❹ NURSING IMPLICATIONS

○ Perform community assessment to identify contributing factors to pediatric illness and risk factors for additional health problems.
○ Address community resource needs prior to discharge; follow up in community or home setting after discharge.
○ Work collaboratively with community agencies to provide comprehensive care to the pediatric client and family and facilitate follow-up assessment and evaluations.

ROUTINE CHECKUP 1

1. Ben, age 6, lives with his father and his father's male partner. What type of family does Ben have?
   a. Nuclear
   b. Binuclear
   c. Gay
   d. Blended

Answer:

2. Explain why poverty might place family members at risk for health problems.

Answer:

DIVERSITY ISSUES

Diversity commonly relates to ethnic-cultural differences found in persons of varied races or religious beliefs. Knowledge of practices that are acceptable or preferred and those that are forbidden allows the nurse to plan care that is appropriate according to the client's ethnic and cultural background. The most effective process for determining appropriate care is to ask the client, family, or significant other about preferences and taboos. Many cultural preferences and rituals do not conflict with medical care or pose harm to the client; however, some natural supplements may interact with medications or diet. Support of cultural norms can result in increased client and family comfort and decreased anxiety.

5 Consider these principles when providing care to clients of varied ethnic or cultural origin:

- Cultural norms are communicated from generation to generation.
- Clients from families that have first- or second-generation members who emigrated from a different culture are more likely to adhere to cultural rituals, whereas clients born in the United States or coming to the country early in childhood may be fully assimilated (acculturated) having adopted American customs, cultural norms, behaviors, and attitudes.
- A **subculture** is a group within a culture that has different beliefs and values from that deemed typical for the culture; the nurse should note individualized preferences.

- ○ **Stereotyping** is categorizing a group of people together, usually by race, rather than respecting individual characteristics.
- ○ In some cultures, females should not be addressed directly but through the dominant male family member.
- ○ Some cultures are matriarchal with the oldest female family member accepted as the decision maker.
- ○ Older family members in some cultures are respected as the decision makers for the family.
- ○ Children in some cultures are not allowed to communicate directly with nonfamily members without family presence and permission.
- ○ It is unacceptable to touch a child without permission, and some parts of the body, such as the head, should not be touched, if avoidable.
- ○ Photographs should not be taken without first consulting with client and family.
- ○ **Ethnocentric** behavior (belief that one's own culture is best) can block communication with client and family by decreasing trust and comfort.
- ○ Communication in the native tongue may be needed for full understanding of client concerns.

NURSING IMPLICATIONS

6 Consider the following concepts when providing care to clients from different ethnic-cultural groups.

Communication

- ○ Assess the family dynamics and consult with family member (or the client if older child or adolescent) to determine preferences relative to communication and the decision-making process between nurse and family members.
- ○ Monitor your own behavior and avoid imposing cultural preferences on the client.
- ○ Provide an interpreter or use technology to assist in translation of concerns voiced in native tongue.

Physical Touch

- ○ Determine taboos related to physical contact, and if possible avoid unacceptable touching by asking the client or family to move body part as you examine them.
- ○ When unacceptable touching is needed, explain the purpose and minimize contact as much as possible.
- ○ If cross-gender touch is forbidden and you are the nurse of the opposite gender assigned to provide care, enlist a same-gender assistant to provide physical care as you manage the care.

Diet and Rituals

- ○ Ask the client and family about preferences because not all individuals from a cultural group practice the same rituals.
- ○ Determine food preferences and relay information to dietician to promote offering of appropriate meal choices.
- ○ Instruct family regarding dietary restrictions secondary to medical condition and if desired allow them to supply desired foods if otherwise unavailable.
- ○ Instruct family to notify you regarding any foods or supplements provided to the client to avoid harmful drug–substance interaction.
- ○ Consult family prior to removal of jewelry, bedside structures, or ointments from the client or the room to avoid disruption of religious or cultural ritual for luck or well-being.

ROUTINE CHECKUP 2

1. The basic concepts of family and community dynamics include which of the following?
   a. Family support as a needed constant
   b. Family roles restricted to mother and father
   c. Family advocacy that enables families to maintain a sense of control
   d. a and c only

Answer:

2. If a client is experiencing an underarm rash and touching the arm of a child by nonfamily member is forbidden in the culture, how would you examine the child? What explanation would you need to provide about touching that is required for proper assessment?

Answer:

_____

_____

CONCLUSION

Factors related to family and community can positively or negatively impact the care of the pediatric client. You should deliver family-centered care to ensure that support systems are maximized and not disrupted so the client receives needed support throughout the illness and the return to the home and community. Note these key points:

◐ Assessment of family and community provides the nurse with a full picture of risks that threaten and benefits that are available to promote the health of the pediatric client.

◐ Collaboration with community resources is key to a successful transition from hospital to the home or community setting, particularly for children with special needs.

◐ Cultural and ethnic preferences should be considered and accommodated when possible.

◐ The nurse should not impose cultural norms and preferences on the clients.

 FINAL CHECKUP

1. Felecia's mother has no family to support her during her child's illness. The nurse would speak with the social worker about services to support which type of family?
   a. Nuclear
   b. Single parent
   c. Extended
   d. Reconstituted

2. What type of community assessment should be done to determine if Dawn, a 5-year-old who is blind after a recent accident, should be discharged home?
   a. Home
   b. Neighborhood
   c. School
   d. All of the above

3. Ifehi is a 12-year-old from Brazil. Her mother asked for a female nurse because unmarried females in their culture cannot be touched by males who are not family members. How should the nurse respond?
   a. Tell the mother that Ifehi has to request a female nurse because she is an adolescent.
   b. Inform the physician of the request and wait for an order to schedule female nurses for Ifehi.
   c. Introduce the male staff nurses so that Ifehi and her mother can become accustomed to them.
   d. Adjust the assignments as much as possible to provide female nurses to care for Ifehi.

4. **What cultural religious ceremony could be accommodated without monitoring by the nurse?**
   a. Drinking of herbal teas by the client several times a day to restore balance
   b. Rubbing of a chemical ointment on the head and torso to drive away spirits
   c. Keeping a statue of the mystical god of health on the client's bedside table
   d. Cooling the room temperature to block hot illnesses from the body

5. **Which of the following factors can be hindered or supported by the presence or absence of community support services?**
   a. Health promotion
   b. Pediatric growth and development
   c. Health restoration activities
   d. All of the above

6. **The basic concepts of family and community dynamics include which of the following?**
   a. Family support as a needed constant
   b. Family roles restricted to mother and father
   c. Family advocacy that enables families to maintain a sense of control
   d. a and c only

7. **Which example represents a reconstituted family?**
   a. Judy and her mother and father live in Kansas in the fall and Paris in the summer.
   b. Peter and his mother live in one house, and his father and stepmother live across town.
   c. Angela and her two fathers live in an apartment attached to her grandparents' home.
   d. b and c only.

8. **Sally says she lives with her two mothers and her brothers. Her family is probably classified as which of the following?**
   a. Cohabited family
   b. Lesbian family
   c. Family
   d. None of the above

9. **Papa Estavez wants to take Emilio back to Mexico for treatment that he believes will be more beneficial. This attitude is a possible example of which of the following?**
   a. The need to bring in a translator
   b. Ethnocentric behavior
   c. Acculturated behavior
   d. Subcultural behavior

10. Nurses should be aware of which factors when assessing clients of a different ethnic or cultural group from their own?
a. Communication dynamics
b. Dietary restrictions
c. Religious rituals and taboos
d. All of the above

ANSWERS

Routine checkup 1
1. c.
2. Poverty could lead to poor nutrition, malnourishment, possible homelessness, exposure to overcrowded shelters, dangerous situations, decreased access to medical services, and illness due to lack of health maintenance activities such as immunizations or dental treatments.

Routine checkup 2
1. d.
2. Ask the child to hold the arm up so it can be examined or have a family member position the arm. All touch will be limited to the site and the duration needed to examine the affected and surrounding area for treatment purposes only.

Final checkup

1. b	2. d	3. d	4. c
5. d	6. d	7. b	8. b
9. b	10. d		

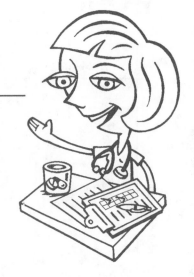

CHAPTER 2

Growth and Development

Learning Objectives

At the end of the chapter, the reader will be able to

1 Discuss types of growth and development.

2 Recognize the characteristics common to each developmental stage.

3 Discuss categories of development cited by two theorists.

4 Discuss the common causes of pediatric injury and death for each developmental stage.

5 Explain appropriate adaptations to nursing measures to provide age-appropriate care.

 KEY WORDS

Biological age	Enuresis
Chronological age	Psychological age
Dyslexia	Social age

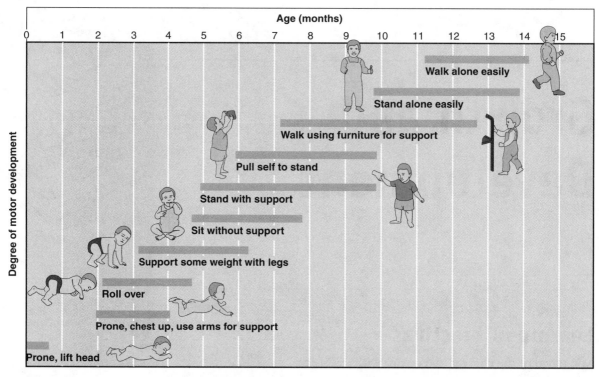

FIGURE 2-1

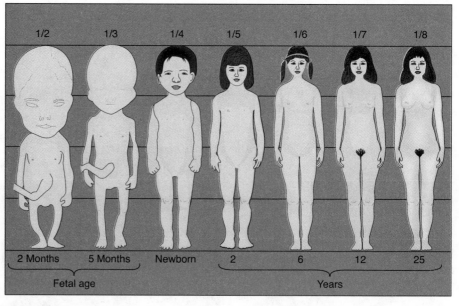

FIGURE 2-2

OVERVIEW

Every developmental stage comes with a particular set of challenges and accomplishments. Care of the client in a particular stage of development requires an understanding of the particular physical and psychosocial reactions that typically takes place with the client in that stage. Although concepts are stated as being typical for an age group, the nurse should be flexible and expect that some clients may overlap developmental stages. The nurse must recognize the presence of expected developmental characteristics or signs of developmental delays that may result from prolonged or chronic illness when planning age-appropriate care for the client and family.

THEORETICAL FOUNDATIONS FOR GROWTH AND DEVELOPMENT

1 Growth and development can be categorized from various perspectives: physical, language, cognitive, social, and emotional. All areas must be assessed and progression in each area supported. **Biological age** refers to child's age based on biological health and functional capabilities, whereas **chronological age** is the number of years that have elapsed since birth. **Social age** refers to the social roles and expectations related to the child's age, and **psychological age** is the adaptive capacities compared to another child of the same chronological age. Developmental stages and ages may overlap depending on the reference used. Psychosocial theorists Freud, Erikson, and Piaget propose behaviors that may be anticipated as a child develops.

2 NEWBORN/INFANT

Age range: birth to 12 months (up to 24 months)

Physical Milestones

- Makes jerky, quivering arm thrusts
- Brings hands within range of eyes and mouth
- Moves head from side to side while lying on stomach
- Head flops backward if unsupported
- Keeps hands in tight fists
- Strong reflex movements
- Progresses from five to eight feedings per day to three meals and two snacks by 12 months
- Progresses from sleeping 20 hours per day to 12 hours and two naps by 12 months

Sensory Milestones

- Focuses 8 to 12 inches (20.3 to 30.4 cm) away
- Eyes wander and occasionally cross
- Prefers black-and-white or high-contrast patterns

- Prefers the human face to all other patterns
- Hearing is fully mature; recognizes some sounds
- May turn toward familiar sounds and voices
- Prefers sweet smells; avoids bitter or acidic smells
- Prefers soft to coarse sensations
- Dislikes rough or abrupt handling

Social Milestones

- Birth to 1 month: helpless and dependent; eye contact, but minimal social interaction; sleeps extensively
- Up to 3 months: smile and fixates on faces
- Three to 6 months: distinguishes and smiles at certain, prefers familiar people; enjoys peek-a-boo
- Six to 12 months: responds to name, gives and takes objects, understands simple commands

Emotional Growth

- Birth to 1 month: demonstrates general tension
- After 1 month: delight or distress shown
- After 6 months: attachment to mother with some separation anxiety
- Six to 12 months: may demonstrate stranger anxiety; shows curiosity by 12 months

Language Development

Progresses from

- Cries, grunts at birth to coos in 3 months
- Babbling, making most vowels and about half of the consonants up to 6 months
- Saying one or two words, imitating sounds, and responding to simple commands at 12 months

④ CONDITIONS AND CONCERNS COMMON TO DEVELOPMENTAL STAGE

Signs of Possible Developmental Delays (if noted in weeks 2 to 4 or later)

- Poor sucking reflex; slow nursing or bottle feeding.
- Absent or minimal blink reflex to bright light.
- Doesn't focus and track (follow) a nearby object that is moving side to side.
- Moves arms and legs minimally and infrequently; appears stiff.
- Limb movement is floppy or excessively loose.

Chronological Age Range	Developmental Theory	Stage or Phase	Defining Characteristics	Key Impact on Nursing Care
Birth to 18 months	Sigmund Freud Personality Id, ego, superego Psychoanalytical	Oral stage	Pleasure centers on mouth	Encourage self-feeding, avoid foreign object ingestion
First year	Eric Erikson Life-span stages Psychoanalytical	Trust vs. mistrust	Dependence on significant other for comfort and support to build trust	Support bonding and maintenance of family relationships
Birth to 2 years	Jean Piaget Social/cognitive	Sensorimotor stage	Coordinates sensory experiences with physical action	Plan tactile experiences and colorful materials, to stimulate senses

TABLE 2–1 • Developmental Characteristics: Birth to 24 Months

- Lower jaw trembling is noted constantly, even when not crying or excited.
- Response to loud sounds is absent or minimal.

Signs of Poor Parent–Child Bonding

- Parent touches child minimally (i.e., only when feeding or providing care).
- Minimal eye contact noted between parent and child (unless culture related).
- Possible signs of abuse noted: bruising, poor hygiene, malnourishment.
- Infant older than 6 months of age shows minimal attachment to parent.

Potential Illness or Injury

- Congenital conditions (see maternal-child text) may manifest through developmental delays or distress.
- Respiratory distress may be noted secondary to decreased surfactant or as in later months due to airway obstruction, particularly due to foreign body insertion.
- Accidents and falls (after 4 months) may occur due to unanticipated mobility and unsecured elevated surface or insufficient hold on body part.
- Infection risk factor due to immature immune system.
- Hypothermia due to diminished temperature control.
- Malnutrition secondary to poverty or failure to thrive.

⑤ NURSING IMPLICATIONS

- Note presence or absence of age-appropriate responses during each interaction with infant and parent; report and fully assess any signs of developmental delay.
- If visual fixation and following are not present by 4 months, refer for evaluation of sight.
- Observe parent–child interaction and note signs of minimal or absent bonding that might require nursing intervention; report possible signs of abuse.
- Support infant–parent/caregiver bond by having caregiver serve as a source of comfort for infant during procedures.
- Avoid placing caregiver as participant in painful or distressing care procedures.
- Provide bottle, cup, then finger foods, as appropriate, to encourage progressive independence in feeding as ability to feed self increases.
- Remove small objects from infant's reach because curiosity places infant in danger of blockages due to small objects being obtained and inserted, swallowed, or inhaled.
- Note and report respiratory distress or difficulty swallowing immediately because these may be a sign of obstructed airway or blocked esophagus.
- Keep infants dressed and covered to avoid exposure to drafts and cold environment.
- Exercise caution and close supervision as mobility increases to avoid injury from falls and traffic accidents (upon return to home).
- Monitor length and weight to detect malnutrition and plan diets with adequate fat, carbohydrate and protein; watch for other signs of protein-calorie deficiency (marasmus or kwashiorkor).
- Remove all poisons from infant's reach and teach family poison control measures.

EARLY CHILDHOOD (PRESCHOOL)

Marked by increasing self-sufficiency and preparation for school.
Age range: 2 to 5 years (up to 6 years)

Physical Milestones

- Slower, more stable physical growth noted.
- Weight gain of 5 pounds per year and 2- to 3-inch height gain may be noted.
- More slender body build than noted with toddler with erect posture.
- Organ systems adapt to stress to a moderate degree.

- Bones and muscles still immature, requiring nutrition and exercise for adequate development.
- Well-established walking, jumping, and climbing skills noted.
- Eye-hand and muscle coordination demonstrated.
- Progressive development of fine motor skills; refined drawing and writing skills noted.

Sensory Milestones

- Bladder control gained; potty training done.
- Brain is 90% developed by age 5 with minimal major changes in senses.

Social Milestones

- Separation anxiety is overcome as child easily relates to unfamiliar persons.
- Parental security and reassurance is sought even as child ventures to preschool.
- Security is gained from familiar object such as a toy, blanket, or picture.
- Learning sense of right and wrong and correct behavior to avoid punishment; conscience development noted.
- Play is associative without rigid rules; group play is noted; mutual play with adult fosters development.
- Imitation of observed behavior through dolls or imaginary activity such as tea party builds social skills and role understanding.
- Body image development noted; may fear injury or mutilation by medical procedures.
- Sexual identity develops with building of self-concept; modesty is present.
- Alert to attitudes of others about gender roles and appropriate play for boys or girls.
- Sexual exploration more pronounced with questions about body and reproduction.
- Attention span is short, so, to avoid boredom, limit craft projects to one per year of age.

Emotional Growth

- Experience many emotions during one day
- Increased use of emotion language and understanding of emotions noted
- Begin understanding of causes and consequences of emotions
- Growing ability to conform emotions to social standards (fewer tantrums)

Language Development

- Vocabulary development increases dramatically; names of objects, including body parts, animals, and familiar locations are learned.

TABLE 2–2 • Developmental Characteristics: Infancy to Early Childhood 3				
Chronological Age Range	Developmental Theory	Stage or Phase	Defining Characteristics	Key Impact on Nursing Care
18 months to 3 years		Anal stage	Pleasure focuses on the anus	Explain to family and teach child hygiene
1 to 3 years	Erikson Life-span stages Psychoanalytical	Autonomy vs. shame and doubt	Mastering physical environment; building self-esteem	Support bonding and family relationships
2 to 7 years	Piaget Social/cognitive	Preoperational stage	Represents the world with words and images; symbolic thinking	Plan experiences like drawing and writing for expressing ideas
3 to 6 years	Freud Id, ego, superego Psychoanalytical	Phallic stage	Pleasure focuses on the genitals	Explain to family and teach child hygiene
3 to 5 years	Erikson Life-span stages Psychoanalytical	Initiative vs. guilt	Initiates activities, begins to develop conscience; developing sexual identity	Monitor activities and protect from injury and accidental poisoning; encourage questioning
2 to 7 years	Piaget Social/cognitive	Preoperational stage (continued)	Coordinates sensory experiences with physical action	Plan tactile experiences and colorful materials, to stimulate senses

- Language is a primary method of communication and socializing; mutual play with adult encourages language development.
- Continuous questioning may be noted with persistence until answer is provided.
- Toys that talk or play music are preferred.
- Brief sentences (telegraphic speech) are common with progression to longer sentences by age 5.
- By age 5 or 6, child has strong command of language use.

④ CONDITIONS AND CONCERNS COMMON TO DEVELOPMENTAL STAGE

Signs of Possible Developmental Delays: Potential Illness or Injury

- Accidents are the leading cause of death in children—falls, drowning, motor vehicle (pedestrian or passenger in car), and poisoning.
- Communicable diseases, intestinal parasite infections, conjunctivitis, and stomatitis are common conditions during this developmental stage.
- Accidental poison ingestion is a serious concern for this age group.
- Lead poisoning can be a concern for children in environments with lead-based paint.
- Physical or emotional abuse or neglect and sexual abuse can present a concern for some children.

⑤ NURSING IMPLICATIONS

- Unless contraindicated by physical condition, provide opportunities for child to climb and jump.
- Provide sedentary activities that allow the child to accomplish a task, such as building blocks, puzzles, and clay, when condition requires decreased activity.
- Nursing care and patient teaching addressing the detection, prevention of transmission, and eradication of communicable diseases, and prevention of complications is important.
- Evaluate environment for risk factors for lead paint ingestion and assess for signs of lead poisoning.
- Poison prevention education and practices, as well as instruction on emergency measure in the event of accidental poisoning, should be provided to parents.
- Assessment of parent–child interactions, family dynamics, and environmental factors should be performed and support data collected as evidence if suspicion of any form of abuse is present.

SCHOOL-AGED CHILD

Age range: 5 to 9 years (6 to 11 years)

Physical Milestones

- Growth is slower than during the preschool period.
- Growth is even and steady with weight gain approximately 5 pounds per year.
- Children are graceful and steady on their feet.

✔ ROUTINE CHECKUP

1. What activity would be appropriate for Andy, age 4, who is hospitalized for dehydration following a prolonged respiratory infection?
   a. A question game with his talking bear
   b. Solitary play with a colorful rattle
   c. A game of scrabble with a friend
   d. Group play with peers his age

Answer:

2. Dawn, age 2, is noted to have slight respiratory distress and continues to rub her nose. What might the nurse suspect is the problem, and what assessment should be made?

Answer:

- By the end of the period, boys and girls double their strength and physical abilities.
- Decreased head circumference relative to height; proportional appearance.
- Loss of baby teeth and appearance of larger adult teeth is noted.
- Body systems, including immune system, gastrointestinal system, bladder capacity, and heart, become mature.
- Bones are still developing and are subject to structural changes from stresses.
- Girls may begin to experience secondary sex characteristics at the end of this period as they progress toward adolescence.

Social Milestones

- Develop confidence in the security of the family and begin to explore relationships outside of family.
- Peer group becomes important, but parents are primary influence.
- Motivated by a sense of accomplishment; desires to complete task.
- Sense of success or failure has a strong impact on this age group.

Emotional Growth

- Greater understanding of complex emotions such as pride, shame, and personal responsibility; moral standards become more established.
- Understands ability to experience more than one emotion at a time.
- Considers events that contribute to emotional state.
- Greater ability to control emotions and responses; can conceal emotions.
- Uses strategies to redirect feelings.

Language Development

- Efficient language skills of preschool and early school age years are refined through grammar education.
- Ability to use words to express knowledge and concerns increases with education.
- Narrative skills improve with increased ability to provide directives and form grammatically correct sentences.
- Able to make inferences about what phrases mean including subtle/figurative statements.
- Able to think about own and the speech of others and to evaluate messages and correct if needed.

For developmental characteristics, see Table 2-2.

CONDITIONS AND CONCERNS COMMON TO DEVELOPMENTAL STAGE

Signs of Possible Developmental Delays

- Possible signs of developmental disorders such as increased motor activity, aggression, and **enuresis** (bedwetting) after the age of 5 years may be noted.
- Behavioral disorders such as attention deficit hyperactivity disorder may be noted.
- Learning disabilities such as **dyslexia** (letter reversal), dysgraphia (writing difficulty), or dyscalculia (calculation difficulty) may be noted.

Potential Illness or Injury

- Motor vehicle accidents as passenger or pedestrian are the leading cause of injury and death.
- Immunizations provide some protection against serious infections.
- Infection and reinfection with lice (pediculosis) can occur if due to child-to-child contact and sharing of clothing and hats.
- Thermal injury can occur secondary to accidental fire or exposure to sun.
- Common conditions in childhood include bacterial, viral, and fungal infections.
- Dental caries and malocclusion may occur in childhood and require treatment and preventive maintenance.
- Perform a full developmental assessment to determine possible contributors to enuresis and work with parents to manage enuresis and reduce the impact on child's self-esteem until condition resolves or successful treatment found.
- If developmental delays noted along with enuresis, refer for plan from pediatrician to promote developmental progression.

- Behavioral disorders such as attention deficit hyperactivity disorder, and tic disorder, as well as disorders such as school phobia, recurrent abdominal pain (RAP), conversion reaction (hysteria), depression, and schizophrenia may be noted.
- Risky behaviors may be noted due to peer pressure (i.e., drugs).

NURSING IMPLICATIONS

- Instruct client and family on importance of seat belt use and use of car seat until age or weight limit is reached.
- Educate and encourage parents to maintain health promotion activities: current immunizations and immunization records, regular checkup, and dental examinations.
- Instruct parents in proper treatment of home, siblings, and cautions to other child contacts to eradicate lice to prevent reinfection, and to monitor for signs of reinfestation.
- Monitor for signs of infection and instruct parents on importance of full cycle of antibiotics to fully cure infection.
- Minimize the stress of hospitalization and plan measures to detect and modify home or community stressors that may aggravate behavior disorders.
- Evaluate child's adjustment to school or other changes in home or environment and plan or refer child and family for treatment to disorder; monitor for medication side effects.
- Provide child and parent teaching on strategies to address peer pressure and avoid risky behavior.

PRETEEN (TWEENS)

Age range: 10 to 12 years

- Adolescence with changes related to puberty generally occur from age 10 to 12 (early) to 18 years.
- Girls may experience menstruation.
- Characteristics demonstrated in the preteen period are a blend of late childhood and early teen: The child is be**tween** stages and is moving into a phase of seeking increased autonomy and independence while still needing parental approval and support.
- Teen behaviors may be demonstrated at one moment with highly dependent childhood behaviors displayed in the next.
- High-risk behaviors may be demonstrated by a pediatric client in this stage in an attempt to show that he or she is "not a child."
- Preteens may act without full understanding of the consequences.

- ○ Gay, lesbian, or bisexual youth may experience barriers in developing self-identity.
- ○ Secondary characteristics in girls may develop in an expected pattern of five phases called the Tanner stages:
  - Stage 1 (prepubescence): Elevation of breast papilla, no pubic hair
  - Stage 2: Breast bud stage with areolar diameter enlargement; sparse growth of pubic hair along labia
  - Stage 3: Further enlargement of breast and areola; darker hair, coarse, sparse growth over entire pubis in triangle shape
  - Stage 4: Breast and areola project; coarse denser pubic hair restricted to pubic area
  - Stage 5: Mature breast configuration with blending of areolar into breast contour; adult growth of pubic hair spread to inner thigh

TEEN YEARS

Age range: 13 to 20 years (up to 22 years)

Physical Milestones

- ○ Experiences changes in body image due to rapid changes of puberty and secondary sex characteristics
  - Girls experience menstruation, if not started earlier.
  - Girls' peak growth spurt ends about age 18.
  - Boys develop body hair and experience voice changes.
  - Boys experience growth spurt (ends age 16) with high metabolic needs and large appetites.
- ○ Hormone changes can cause acne and increased perspiration.

Social Milestones

- ○ Greater focus on personal and interpersonal characteristics, beliefs, and emotional states while developing a sense of self and identity separate from parents.
- ○ Moral development with questioning of values is noted; spiritual development with questioning of family values and ideals noted.
- ○ Becomes less egocentric as age increases; better able to sympathize with others
- ○ Focus on mixed-gender friendships increases.

Emotional Growth

- ○ Demonstrates great rebellion against parents in attempt to gain increased autonomy and assert own identity.

TABLE 2–3 • Developmental Characteristics: Child to Teen ③				
Chronological Age Range	Developmental Theory	Stage or Phase	Defining Characteristics	Key Impact on Nursing Care
6 years to puberty	Freud Id, ego, superego Psychoanalytical	Latency stage	Sexual interest and social and intellectual skills developed	Encourage sibling and peer contact; assess for sex-related disease and pregnancy in older child and adolescents
Puberty onward		Genital stage	Sexual awakening interest in person outside family	
6 years old to puberty (10–11)	Erikson Life-span stages Psychoanalytical	Industry vs. inferiority	Developing sense of self-worth and talents	Provide activities based on interest, talents, and abilities Support self-esteem; be honest but maximize positive aspects of image and minimize defects
10 to 20 years (adolescence)		Identity vs. identity/role Confusion	Integrating multiple roles (sibling, student, worker), managing self image and peer pressure	
11 years to adulthood	Piaget: Social/cognitive	Formal operational stage	Reasons in more abstract, idealistic, and logical ways	Discuss condition openly with client and allow privacy to discuss concerns

- ◑ Emotional volatility (highs and lows) with moodiness, temper flares, and sulking during early adolescence that subside with aging toward adulthood.
- ◑ Great focus on physical appearance and concerns for "normal" development.
- ◑ Sexually active teens may have impaired self-image.
- ◑ Privacy and confidentiality are important to teens for trust building.
- ◑ Gay, lesbian, or bisexual youth may experience barriers in developing self-identity.

Language Development

- ◑ Able to communicate complex thoughts

Cognitive Development

- ◑ Thinks about one's own thoughts and emotions

CONDITIONS AND CONCERNS COMMON TO DEVELOPMENTAL STAGE

Signs of Possible Developmental Delays

- ◑ Depression may be noted with higher levels in girls than boys.
  - Poor peer relations, depressed or emotionally unavailable parents, parental marital conflict or financial problems, family disruption through divorce, poor self-image are contributing factors.
- ◑ Memory deficits and learning disorders may be a result of drug use or mental illness.
- ◑ Suicide ideation may manifest.
  - Preoccupation with themes of death
  - Talks of own death and desire to die
  - Loss of energy; exhaustion without cause
  - Flat affect; distant from others, social withdrawal
  - Antisocial or reckless behavior: alcohol, drugs, sexual promiscuity, fights
  - Change in appetite noted
  - Sleeping pattern changes noted: too little or too much
  - Decreased interest or decreased ability to concentrate
  - Gives away cherished items

❹ Potential Illness or Injury

- ◑ Risky behaviors, encouraged by peer pressure (i.e., violence/homicide, reckless driving, excessive and unprotected sexual intercourse, and adolescent pregnancy, smoking, substance abuse) are major causes of death and injury in adolescents.
- ◑ Mental health problems including depression, suicide, and eating disorders can lead to adolescent death and disability.
- ◑ Chronic illness requiring dietary intervention or a medication regimen can result in decreased self-esteem due to feeling of being different from and less "normal" than peers.
- ◑ Poor eating practices and decreased exercise contribute to obesity or malnutrition.
- ◑ Facial and body acne, aggravated by stress and hormones, is common in teens.

❺ NURSING IMPLICATIONS

- ◑ Effective interventions for teen clients must involve the teen in the planning and implementation.

- ◔ Teach adolescents and family strategies to reduce health-compromising behaviors and address peer pressure.
- ◔ Monitor for signs and plan interventions to address depression and suicidal ideation.
- ◔ Relate health-enhancing behaviors, such as nutritious eating, regular exercise, and driving safety with use of seat belts, to improved physical appearance and performance in school, athletics, or other activities of interest.
- ◔ Assist teen in planning care for chronic illness to minimize disruption of activities with peers.
- ◔ Provide opportunities for communication with adolescent in absence of parents to allow asking of personal questions.
- ◔ Daily hygiene and treatment with acne medication can reduce outbreak.

CONCLUSIONS

Knowledge and consideration of a child's developmental stage can contribute to planning of age-appropriate care. Recognition that the illness of a child can impact the child's growth and development allows the nurse to anticipate developmental delays or regressions and plan care accordingly. Additional key points:

- ◔ Age-appropriate care and teaching can reduce injury and illness children and adolescents may experience during the growth and development process.
- ◔ Developmental stage theories are not specific for an age, but include age ranges that may overlap.
- ◔ All levels of develop are important from physical to cognitive to psychosocial.
- ◔ Family interactions, or lack of, can impact growth and development.
- ◔ Illness can cause reversal to a younger developmental stage for a brief period.
- ◔ Nursing measures, including client and family teaching, must consider the developmental stage the child is demonstrating.

❓ FINAL CHECKUP

1. **Ellis, age 13, is admitted after experiencing diarrhea for the past 4 days. He is sullen and speaks only when his mother pushes him to answer questions. What should the nurse keep in mind when assessing Ellis?**
   a. Ellis likely has a communication deficit due to loss of electrolytes.
   b. Ellis would be more responsive to the nurse if his mother were absent.
   c. Ellis's behavior is not important because his chief complaint is diarrhea.
   d. Ellis is an adolescent and may also be quiet and sullen when he is well.

2. **A middle school nurse is teaching a class on sexual development to a group of 11-year-old girls. Which physical changes should be expected when the girls reach Tanner stage 3 of development? Select all that apply.**
   a. Height increases at a peak rate of 8 cm/year
   b. Breast buds palpable
   c. Pubic hair becomes dark, coarse, and spreads over mons pubis
   d. Adult breast contour
   e. Acne vulgaris develops

3. **Which factors should be considered when a nurse assesses a client's growth and development? Select all that apply.**
   a. Food preferences
   b. Language skills
   c. Religious preference
   d. Changes in personality and emotions

4. **An 8-year-old client is admitted to the emergency department with a broken arm. A nurse prepares the client for discharge and provides information to the child's parents regarding normal growth and development. Which information provided by the nurse is accurate regarding the development of an average 8-year-old client?**
   a. Requires continuous adult supervision
   b. Is interested in the opposite sex
   c. Has little control over small muscles
   d. Is accident prone, especially on the playground

5. **At what age do infants usually develop "object permanence"?**
   a. 1 to 3 months of age
   b. 4 to 7 months of age
   c. 8 to 10 months of age
   d. 10 to 12 months of age

6. **A nurse is assessing the development of a 2-year-old client in a wellness clinic. Which assessment finding is *least* typical for an average 2-year-old client?**
   a. Constantly in motion and tires easily
   b. May assert self by saying, "No!"
   c. Plays with other children
   d. May have an imaginary playmate

7. Jerry, age 15, is admitted through the emergency department after a car accident with minimal injury. The parents report that for the past months Jerry seems to have difficulty remembering and his grades have dropped. Which question might provide the most related information?

    a. Is Jerry a skilled driver based on his driving history?

    b. What classes are Jerry currently enrolled in?

    c. Does Jerry have a history of drug usage or mental illness?

    d. Is Jerry rebellious and less communicative than he was 6 years ago?

8. Adam, age 3, is admitted with anemia and is placed on bedrest. After several days of hospitalization and treatment his parents report that he has wet the bed several times, although he has been potty trained for over a year. Which is the most probable explanation for this situation?

    a. Children often revert to an earlier developmental stage when stressed.

    b. Three-year-olds are not fully potty trained and will have "accidents".

    c. Adam's anemia has progressed and is causing bladder irritation and voiding.

    d. Adam is being rebellious and letting his anger out by wetting the bed.

9. Johnny, a 15-year-old, has the physical development of a 7- to 8-year-old. Which of the following is referred to as his developmental age?

    a. Physiological

    b. Biological

    c. Sociological

    d. Chronological

ANSWERS

Routine checkup

1. a. Musical or talking toys are most appropriate at this age.
2. Nasal obstruction due to inhaled or inserted object is likely, so the nurse should examine the nose for an item that might have been inserted.

Final checkup

1. d	2. a, c, d	3. b, d	4. d
5. b	6. c	7. c	8. a
9. b			

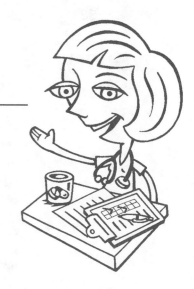

CHAPTER **3**

Pediatric Assessment

Learning Objectives

At the end of the chapter, the student will be able to

1 Discuss the role of communication skills in accurate assessment.

2 Determine assessment findings that deviate from the normal range for the pediatric client.

3 Discuss the steps in assessment of family and community.

4 Distinguish diagnostic findings that indicate pediatric health concerns.

5 Indicate appropriate nursing implications related to diagnostics and abnormal findings for pediatric clients.

 KEY WORDS

Biochemical tests	Edema	Petechiae
Blanching/capillary refill	Hypertelorism	Scoliosis
Body mass index (BMI)	Nuchal rigidity	Secondary sex characteristics
Chief complaint	Obesity	Skin turgor
Cyanosis	Overweight	Temperament
Ecchymosis	Pallor	

OVERVIEW

A comprehensive pediatric nursing history is one of the most crucial components of child care. Health assessment provides key information needed for diagnosis of a client condition and for planning of effective care to assist the client and family. You will move from assessing the client's and family's view of the problem through a client history and client support resources through a family/community assessment, to the physical examination and review of diagnostic test results. Understanding the expected findings (normal ranges) for the pediatric population will assist you in detecting abnormal findings. Assessment is used in initial contact with the client and throughout the course of the plan of care to evaluate degree of progress or lack of progress. Information found during the assessment is used to refine the plan of care to increase effectiveness and success in resolving or minimizing the client problem(s).

THE NURSING PROCESS

In providing care to the client and family, the nursing process provides a guide for comprehensive planning. After years of practice, the steps of the process might not be outlined distinctly as you proceed but will remain the foundation for care. The process includes assessment of the client and family relative to the problem and related concerns, as well as underlying family and dynamics that could impact support and resources needed by the client. Nursing diagnoses are statements that define the problems and potential problems indicated by the assessment findings. The North American Nurses Diagnosis Association (NANDA) has established a list of standard diagnoses for use by nurses for planning and communication about client care (see Appendix 1).

After determining a nursing diagnosis, the desired outcome of care and treatment is identified. Knowing the objective of the care, the desired result or outcome, helps guide the activities needed and gives a basis for evaluating the success of the care. The desired outcome is generally resolution, to the greatest degree possible, of the problem identified by the nursing diagnosis.

Nursing interventions are designed to help the client meet the desired outcome of resolving the problem(s) from their condition. Interventions include care to the client as well as client and family teaching. Continued monitoring and assessment is also an expected nursing intervention for comprehensive client care. Evaluation, and revision as indicated, is the final stage of the nursing process. Data gathered with continued monitoring are used to determine the degree to which outcomes were met and need to revise goals or interventions. New nursing diagnoses may be discovered and old nursing diagnoses may be deleted after reviewing data from continued monitoring and evaluation.

HEALTH ASSESSMENT: CLIENT HISTORY

COMMUNICATION

 Communication is important when performing a health assessment. To provide family-centered care:

- ① The child and family members must be included in the assessment process because each perspective is needed to gather complete data on the client's condition.
- ① Clear speech is necessary with use of regular terms instead of medical or nursing "jargon" that the child or family may not understand.

Culture alert **If English is a second language for the child or family, an interpreter may be needed to ensure that the questions asked and responses given are understood. Communication in the native tongue may be needed for full understanding of client concerns.**

Key considerations when communicating during a health assessment include the following:

- ① By encouraging parents to talk, nurses can identify information that affects all aspects of the child's life.
- ① Interviewing parents involves more than just fact gathering; this initial contact establishes the nature of future contacts and begins development of a trusting relationship with the nurse.
- ① Begin the interview with an introduction; explain the nurse's role and the purpose of the interview to establish a clear nurse to child/parent relationship.
- ① Treat the child/adolescent and parent as partners equal to the nurse in the care process.
- ① Use an interview process that is appropriate for the client's developmental stage:
  - • Use play with dolls or puppets with children; role playing may ease the anxiety of the interview process.
  - • Get on eye level with the child and actively engage children through play and verbal exchange.

Culture alert **Be aware of cultural variation in eye contact because direct eye contact might be considered disrespectful or evil.**

  - • Treat adolescents appropriately, neither as children nor adults. Find time without parents present to allow adolescents to ask questions or state concerns they may be embarrassed to discuss around parents.

◐ Touch is a powerful communication tool, especially for the infant who calms when cuddled or patted, or a parent who is distraught about a child's condition.

Culture alert **Be aware of cultural variation in physical contact, particularly across genders, which might be considered inappropriate or taboo.**

◐ Provide an interpreter or use technology to assist in translation of questions and of responses voiced in native tongue.
◐ Remember that nonverbal communication is as important as verbal. Smiling and maintaining a pleasant facial expression reduces client and parent anxiety.
◐ Attitude is also important in establishing a trust relationship with client and parents. Maintaining a nonjudgmental manner will help the child/parent feel comfortable and provide truthful information to the nurse.

NURSING HISTORY

Discuss or have parent complete a form containing the following information to provide contact data and clarify relationships to child:
◐ Demographic-biographical information (child name, age, address/phone number, caregiver name, relationship to child, etc.).
◐ Current state of health (i.e., fatigue, pain, weight gain or loss, activity tolerance, abilities or disability in communication, mobility, pain, etc.).
◐ Review of systems or head-to-toe approach should be used.
◐ **Chief complaint:** Current symptoms determine why the child was brought in for examination.
◐ Past history provides background for the problem and any additional problems that the child may have experienced. This assessment should include acute or chronic conditions as well as surgical procedures.

⚛ ASSESSMENT

Psychosocial Assessment
◐ Habits: Sleep pattern, that is, difficulty sleeping or excess sleep could indicate depression, drug reaction, or pain or discomfort from disease.
◐ Eating habits: Frequency and type of food intake; can reveal eating disorders, obesity, or malnutrition (failure to thrive in infant population) possibly due to poverty or could reveal abuse or neglect.
◐ Substance abuse: Drugs, tobacco, or alcohol (current or past); determine frequency and amount or usage.
◐ Sexual activity: Do not limit assessment to older adolescents because a child as young as age 8 or 9 may be sexually active.

NUTRITIONAL ASSESSMENT

An essential element in the assessment is evaluation of the child's nutritional status from a physical examination and a biochemical perspective, as well as the usual dietary intake. It is important to collect data from the child and family members regarding nutrition habits. Inquire about community access to variety of food types and factors impacting food choices, such as location of stores, fast-food choices due to time constraints, and economic barriers to purchase of sufficient quantities of fresh fruits and vegetables and low-fat cuts of meat, as well as fish and fowl choices. If the family practices vegetarianism, inquire about the specific foods allowed and assess adequacy of intake of nutrients from all food groups. Assess **overweight** (85–95% for body mass index [BMI]) or **obesity**, weight above 95th percentile for BMI in the child or family members because family eating habits will play a large part in childhood obesity moving into adulthood.

Culture alert **Assess dietary restrictions due to ethic cultural beliefs and taboos.**

Nutritional assessment should include
- ◑ Dietary intake
  - Dietary history by 24-hour recall, food diary, or record to note the nature and amount of foods and beverages consumed
- ◑ Clinical examination
  - Chart weight, height, and head circumference (for infants) on a growth chart; if child is <5th percentile or >95th, an insufficient or excess intake is likely present.
  - Calculate **body mass index (BMI):** Weight in kilograms divided by height in meters squared.
  - Delay of development of **secondary sex characteristics** (i.e., breasts in girls, pubic hair, testes) can indicate malnutrition or vitamin A and D deficit or excess.
  - Skin changes such as loss of **skin turgor,** elasticity of the skin, or **edema,** swelling or puffiness indicating dehydration or fluid overload.
  - Delayed wound healing (poor protein intake/malnutrition).
  - Flabby skin or stretch marks can indicate food/excesses.
  - Other physical changes noting malnourishment or excess dietary intake will be noted in the discussion of physical assessment.

Biochemical tests: Blood analysis of nutrients, electrolytes, and protein products
- ◑ Hemoglobin and hematocrit; low levels may reveal inadequate protein intake.
- ◑ Albumen, protein, creatinine, nitrogen; low levels could indicate low protein intake.

- Tissue from hair, nails, bone, and organs can reveal nutritional deficits or excess chemical elements.
- Urinalysis can reveal excess glucose or other electrolytes, as well as protein loss from renal damage that could indicate a risk for protein deficit.

An economic assessment could indicate a financial deficit that limits ability to buy food, indicating a need for assistance from social services.

FAMILY HISTORY AND REVIEW OF SYSTEMS

Questions about family history include items such as whether certain diseases/ conditions run in the family, the age and cause of death for blood relatives (to detect possible genetic conditions), and family members with communicable diseases (to detect possible infection or infestation).

Family Assessment

Family assessment is a most important aspect of the history because the emotional and physical health of the child or adolescent depends on the stability of the family structure and function. There are various definitions for the term *family,* which broadly means one or more adults living with one or more children in a parent–child relationship. Family also refers to those individuals who are important to the core or nuclear group. Family assessment involves exploration of family structure and composition as well as member relationships, characteristics, interactions, and dynamics. If the child is experiencing a major stressor, such as parental divorce, chronic illness, or death of a family member, or an issue such as behavioral or physical problems, or developmental delays that suggest family dysfunction, they are noted and an in-depth family assessment is indicated. In performing this assessment, consider the following:

Structure

- The number and composition of family members can determine the amount of support available to the child/adolescent during the health challenge.
- Questions should be open enough to encompass various family structures, such as "What are the names of the child's parent(s)?" instead of "Where is your husband or wife?"
- Inquire about all persons living in the household, or households in which the child resides at any time, and their relationships to the child and family to provide a full picture of the family structure or multiple family structure the child is exposed to.
- Ask about extended family and additional support such as from friends or church members, to determine the extent of resources available to the child and family.
- Inquire about family illness or deaths, previous separations, or divorces and the child's response to these events to determine use of previous coping skills.

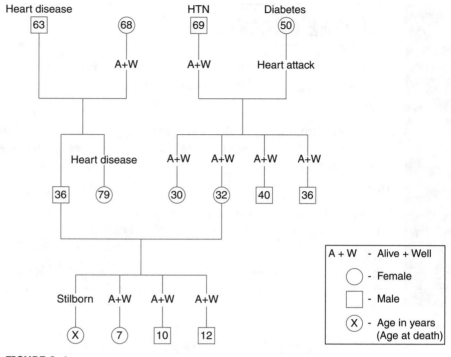

FIGURE 3-1

◑ A genogram, a diagram of the family composition and structure, can be helpful in viewing the family structure comprehensively if the core unit is circled and connections of other members of the family to this core are clearly indicated (Figure 3-1).

FAMILY FUNCTION

Family function assessment is focused on how members interact with one another. Several tests may be used to assess family function. A picture of the family from the child's perspective can be enlightening about the family relationships, as well as a way to observe family interactions. The important aspects of this assessment are the determination of the family's ability to

◑ Adapt to stressors.
◑ Grow and mature.
◑ Work in partnership in decision making.
◑ Demonstrate affection and caring among the family members.
◑ Demonstrate resolve or commitment to assist family members.
◑ Spend and value family time together.

✔ ROUTINE CHECKUP 1

1. When performing a family assessment, it is important to consider the _____ and the _____ of the child's family.

Answer:

2. When performing physical assessments on young children and infants, intrusive procedures must be completed first to ensure the accuracy of the assessment. True/False?

Answer:

3. Mark, age 4, has a hearing deficit. Why would the nurse need to speak with the social worker about services to support Mark and his family?

Answer:
_____
_____

PHYSICAL EXAMINATION

A systematic approach to the physical examination, proceeding from head to toe, is the best method of fully assessing a client. For infants and toddlers, however, intrusive procedures such as ear, eye, nose, and mouth examinations should be done last to keep the child calm for as long as possible during the physical examination. Use play as much as possible to encourage cooperation (e.g., "Where is your belly?" when palpating stomach). Allow child to handle equipment when appropriate (stethoscope). Normal findings for examination of most systems are similar across the age span, but some distinctions are noted at certain developmental stages.

General

- ◑ Overall appearance reveals cleanliness, well nourished, clothes well fitting, stature appropriate for age, posture straight, no signs of pain (frown/grimace).
- ◑ Behavior and personality, interactions with parents and nurse, **temperament** (behavioral style: calm or not). Note: If child is agitated, some assessments will need to be deferred until more cooperative and calm to minimize distress.

Skin Integrity (absence of lesions, drainage, etc.)

- ◑ Color: **Pallor** (pale appearance) or **cyanosis** (bluish tint) could indicate poor circulation or oxygenation; flushing could indicate increased blood flow to skin due to infection.

- ○ Texture, dryness or moisture, temperature, hair growth or lack of, could indicate fluid or nutritional deficits.
- ○ **Blanching/capillary refill** (pallor followed by return of flush after pressure; <3 seconds indicates circulatory adequacy).
- ○ Birthmarks or other skin color deviations (nonpathologic) may be noted.
- ○ **Ecchymosis** (blue/black areas or bruises often from trauma) or abrasions (indicating trauma, accidental or intentional), or **petechiae,** small pinpoint hemorrhages, could indicate a bleeding disorder due to lack of platelets.

Hair

- ○ Note color, distribution, quality, texture, elasticity, and cleanliness. Cultural variations in coarseness or curliness of hair may be noted, but hair and scalp should be clean without lesions.
- ○ Hair loss or dry, thin, and brittle hair can indicate nutritional deficits or a side effect from medication/cancer treatment.
- ○ Unusual hair distribution on face, arms, trunk, or legs could indicate pathology.
- ○ Presence or absence of hair in underarm or pubic regions could indicate premature or delayed pubertal changes or hormonal dysfunction. Balding in an infant could suggest need for more frequent position changes for sleep.
- ○ Inspect for scalp itching, which could indicate seborrhea, ringworm, or scalp infection or infestation, for example, lice (gray flakes from nits/ova adhering to hair, particularly in school-aged child who could be exposed from other children).

 Safety alert **Use gloves or a tongue blade during inspection for lice to avoid self-infestation. Also check scalp for ticks (smooth, oval, gray or brown bodies)**

Nails

- ○ Should be smooth and flexible.
- ○ If dry and brittle or ridges are noted, nutritional deficits may be present.
- ○ Clubbed (bulged and slightly cyanotic) fingertips may indicate respiratory or cardiac dysfunction.

Head and Neck

- ○ Head control should be noted by 4 months of age.
- ○ Shape and symmetry: Report extreme asymmetry for further evaluation.
- ○ Fontanels should be closed by 18 months of age.
- ○ Note reports of headaches, swollen neck glands, neck stiffness, or decreased range of motion.

Safety alert Nuchal rigidity, **pain with neck flexion or hyperextension of head, may indicate meningeal irritation and possible meningitis.**

- Report any shift in trachea (possible lung problem) or mass in the neck.

Eye and Vision

- Note size, symmetry, color, and movement of eye, as well as exterior structures and spacing between the eyes. Report deviations from expected straight palpebral fissures (upward slant normally noted in Asian clients). Down syndrome may be characterized by epicanthal folds, upward palpebral slant, and **hypertelorism** (large spacing between eyes).
- Eyelids should be smooth without drooping or malposition; note blink reflex.
- Examine pupil for roundness, equal size, reactivity to light, accommodation, and size, color, and clarity of iris (black and white speckling seen in Down syndrome).
- Lens of the eye normally not visible; white or gray spots could indicate cataracts.
- Report unusual eye movement, strabismus, excessively cross eyed.
- Prepare child for eye exam with ophthalmoscope, by showing instrument and explaining that light will be bright. Red reflex presence can rule out many conditions.
- Vision testing should be age appropriate; use Snellen chart for older children.

Ears and Hearing

- Inspect external ear structures for alignment, general hygiene, presence and amount of wax (can view partially without otoscope).
- Infant and children should respond to human voice.
- Use a game approach to encourage child's cooperation.

Safety alert **Gently restrain infant and young child during otoscope use to avoid injury.**

- Pull pinna of the ear down and back for infants and up and back for children >3 years of age to straighten the ear canal and visualize the inner ear structures.
- Auditory testing should be appropriate to age, ranging from loud noise to elicit startle reflex in infants to use of audiometry for detection of type and degree of hearing loss, if present.

Mouth, Throat, Nose, Sinuses, and Neck

- History can reveal high-risk circumstances: Frequent oral lesions, dental problems, or nose bleeds require in-depth examination.

○ Allow child to examine mouth of nurse, parent, or doll/puppet to decrease anxiety.
○ Report any flaring of the nostrils, which could indicate respiratory distress.
○ Note any bleeding, swelling, discharge, dryness, or blockage of nasal passages that could indicate trauma, irritation, or infection such as a cold.
○ Mouth and throat may reveal lesions of mouth or lips, redness, or drainage indicating infection.
○ Fissures, stomatitis, or glossitis may indicate fluid and nutritional deficits.
○ White patches in infants or children may indicate candidiasis; herpes simplex or a syphilitic chancre may be noted with adolescents.
○ Tonsil enlargement, redness, white patches, or drainage in throat could indicate tonsillitis or pharyngitis.
○ Inspect teeth for dental caries that could indicate poor hygiene and nutritional deficits, and also note malocclusion (poor biting relationship of teeth and poor teeth alignment) that could result in feeding problems and loss of teeth, self-image problems.
○ Palpate head and neck for lymph nodes and report swollen, tender, or warm nodes that may indicate the presence of infection.

Chest (heart, neck vessels, pulses, and blood pressure)

○ Note chest shape, symmetry, and movement. Report significant retraction of chest muscles, which could indicate respiratory distress.
○ Note nipples for symmetry; breast development usually occurs from 10 to 14 years of age.
○ Listen to heart with child in sitting and supine position; note heart murmurs and record the location and volume intensity.
○ Note history of congenital heart disease or hypertension.
○ Neck vein distention could indicate congestive heart failure.
○ Report if child reports experiencing chest pain, infant becomes fatigued or short of breath during feeding because these are signs of decreased circulation or cardiac function.
○ Resting pulse rates according to the age of the child are as follows:
  • Infants >3 months: pulse rate 100 to 200 beats/minute
  • 4 months to 2 years of age: 80 to 150 beats/minute
  • 2 years to 10 years: 70 to 110 beats/minute
  • 10 years to adulthood: 55 to 90 beats/minute
○ Blood pressure also varies according to age (systolic: age + 90; diastolic: 1 to 5 years, 56, and 6 to 18 years, age + 52). Average blood pressure
  • >2 years: 95/58 mm Hg
  • 2 to 5 years: 101/57 mm Hg
  • 6 to 10 years: 112/75 mm Hg
  • 11 to 18 years: 120/80 mm Hg

Lungs and Respiration

- ☾ Breath sounds should be clear; voice sounds heard through the lungs but syllables should be indistinct (vocal resonance). Syllables clearly heard when whispered (pectoriloquy), or sound increased in intensity or clarity (bronchophony), diminished or absent vocal resonance, or decreased or absent breath sounds could indicate lung congestion or consolidation.
- ☾ Abnormal breath sounds should be described instead of labeled to promote diagnosis and monitoring by various health-care providers.
- ☾ Respiratory rates vary with age:
  - <1 year: 30 to 35 breaths/minute
  - 2 to 3 years: 25 breaths/minute
  - 4 to 6 years: 21 to 23 breaths/minute
  - 8 to 12 years: 19 to 20 breaths/minute
  - 14 to 18 years: 16 to 18 breaths/minute

Abdomen

- ☾ Always auscultate before palpation or percussion of the abdomen to avoid altering current bowel sound pattern with artificial stimulation of bowel activity.
- ☾ Gently palpate abdomen; *do not* palpate abdomen if Wilms tumor is present.
- ☾ Examine all four quadrants of the abdomen.
- ☾ Report visible peristaltic waves, which may indicate pathologic state.
- ☾ Note absence or asymmetric abdominal reflex in infants and children >1 year of age.
- ☾ Have child cough, laugh, or blow up balloon to increase intraabdominal pressure while inspecting for hernia.
- ☾ Report hyperperistalsis indicated by hyperactive bowel sounds or an absence of bowel sounds, both of which may indicate a gastrointestinal disorder.
- ☾ Lack of tympany on percussion could indicate full stomach, or presence of fluid or solid tumor; avoid assessment of stomach immediately after meals.
- ☾ Note guarding and tenderness, particularly rebound tenderness, or pain that could indicate inflammation or infection.

Genitourinary

- ☾ Exam can be anxiety provoking for older child and adolescents, thus secure privacy (ask preference for parental presence), preserve modesty, and when possible offer same-sex examiner.
- ☾ If complaint of burning, frequency or difficulty voiding, obtain urine specimen for possible culture.
- ☾ Note urinary and genital structures, size, and appearance; explain anatomy for older child and caution that you will touch an area prior to doing so to prepare the child.

◐ Report undescended testes (cryptorchidism), urinary meatus that is not central at the tip of the shaft of the penis, large scrotal sac (possible hernia), or enlarged clitoris.

 Culture alert **Female circumcision will produce a different genital appearance. Note and report the appearance but try not to react and show disapproval.**

◐ If swelling, skin lesions, inflammation, drainage, or irregularities are noted, report for follow-up assessment for possible sexually transmitted disease (STD) or possible sexual abuse if STD noted in young child.
◐ Anal protrusions, hemorrhoids, lesions, irritation, or mucosal tags should be noted and may require follow-up.
◐ Diaper rash should be noted for treatment.
◐ Perianal itching might indicate the need for testing for pinworms.

Back and Extremities

◐ Note any lack or difficulty in mobility, uneven stance, or gait that might indicate uneven limbs or spinal curvature.
◐ With child standing erect and again with child bending forward, note if curvature of the spine (**scoliosis**) is present and report for further examination.
◐ Report rigidity in spinal column with movement from supine to sitting position that might indicate a neurologic problem (e.g., meningitis).
◐ Bowlegs (genu varum) or knock knee (genu valgum) that is asymmetric or extreme may indicate pathology and should be reported for further examination.

 # ROUTINE CHECKUP 2

1. Current symptoms that determine why the child was brought in for treatment are called the _____ _____.

Answer:

2. Obesity is defined as being overweight. True/False?

Answer:

3. A bulging of the veins in the neck could indicate congestive heart failure. True/False?

Answer:

◑ Muscle weakness or paresis (may indicate nutritional deficit) or extreme asymmetry of strength in extremities, hands, and fingers should be reported.

Developmental delays, detected through examination with tools such as the Denver II or other inventory, should be noted and reported along with any relevant historical data.

DIAGNOSTIC PROCEDURES

When preparing the client and family for diagnostic procedures, explain things as simply as possible and remain concrete and avoid abstractions. Be very clear about what the child needs to do (hold still, turn on side, etc.). Involve the older child when possible, in holding tape, counting while medicine is pushed, or other task. Give the adolescent choices and control whenever possible in assisting during the diagnostic procedure.

LABORATORY TESTS

4 Diagnostic findings, particularly biochemical tests, often vary based on the age of the client. The greatest age-related difference in test results is noted between those of the newborn or infant and test results of children >12 years of age to adulthood. Lab values should be interpreted with consideration for client age. The following are examples of tests that may be performed:

Biochemical tests involve blood analysis of nutrients, electrolytes, and protein products as described in the earlier discussion of nutrition assessment. These and other tests can indicate dysfunction in pediatric body systems:

◑ Complete blood count (CBC): Hematocrit, hemoglobin, red blood cell count, platelets. Decreased or increased levels may relate to respiratory, cardiovascular, renal, or bone marrow malfunction, or hydration problems (elevated hematocrit with hemoconcentration due to dehydration); decreased or elevated platelet levels can indicate risk for bleeding or clotting disorder.

◑ Prothrombin time (PT) or partial thromboplastin time (PTT): High levels mean blood is less likely to clot, indicating a risk for bleeding.

Blood chemistries

◑ Potassium, sodium, chloride, calcium, magnesium, phosphorus, and others indicate electrolyte imbalances due to deficits or excess in dietary intake, malabsorption, or medication side effects, or glucose elevation or decrease (diabetes or pancreatitis).

◑ Venous carbon dioxide, in addition to arterial blood gases, shows imbalances in respiratory system.

◑ Blood urea nitrogen and creatinine reveal renal damage.

◑ White blood cell (WBC) count and erythrocyte sedimentation rate (ESR) might be elevated in infection. WBC is decreased in bone marrow or immune system depression.

- Other serum/blood assessments specific to systems reveal adequacy or deficit in organ function. For example: AST, ALT (elevated in liver disease), HBeAg/HBsAg, IgM, IgG, anti-HBc (hepatitis B infection current or past), anti-HCV, HCV RNA (hepatitis C), amylase and lipase (gastrointestinal function), T3, T4, TRH, and TSH (elevated or depressed in thyroid disease), ACTH (pituitary function), or FSH, LH (gonad function).
- Peak or trough levels of medications may be drawn to guide treatments; elevations may result from renal malfunction or insufficient drug dosage.

Urine Testing

- Urinalysis may reveal decreased renal function or electrolyte imbalance such as excess glucose.
- Urine specific gravity may reveal low or high levels that may relate to fluid depletion or overload.
- Pulse oximetry might be decreased due to respiratory abnormalities.
- Scope procedures: Direct visualization of body cavity to detect tumor, ulceration or irritation, or foreign body and to obtain specimen (biopsy): bronchoscopy (lung blockage), gastroscopy (stomach irritation or blockage), colonoscopy (intestinal blockage or irritation), sigmoidoscopy (blockage).
- Scan or radioscope such as radiograph, magnetic resonance imaging (MRI), ultrasound, or sonogram allows for indirect view of deep body structures, detects tumors, foreign bodies, narrowing of body passages, or openings between chambers (such as between heart chambers).

 Nursing alert **Some procedures involve the use of contrast dyes to improve visualization of structures.**

- Assess client for allergy to shellfish or iodine because contrast can cause a severe allergic reaction (anaphylaxis) requiring lifesaving measures.
- Electromyography (EMG), nerve conduction studies, and/or electroencephalogram (EEG) may indicate problems in nerve conduction in the brain or neuromuscular system.

NURSING IMPLICATIONS

The nurse should exercise caution during diagnostic procedures and data interpretation with pediatric clients.

- A blood draw can be scary. Use careful language when speaking with young children, avoiding words with double meanings such as "shot" or "stick" that might cause a scary mental image.
- Explain that the smallest amount of blood possible is being taken to reassure the client and family.

- Warn the child that the needle injection will cause a brief pain that will pass quickly.
- Encourage the child to look away from the needle during the blood draw process.
- Store and label samples appropriately to avoid the need to repeat a test.
- Urine specimen collection may require attachment of a collection device to the perineum of a newborn or infant.
- Young children may need assistance in cleaning for a clean-catch urine specimen.
- Explain the procedure to the parent or family member who might assist the child if desired.

 Nursing alert **Be careful when interpreting lab values because the normal ranges of many lab values vary by age (newborn/infant, 2 to 12 years of age, and ≤12 years of age).**

ROUTINE CHECKUP 3

1. Platelet deficits would most likely occur with what condition?

   a. Cardiovascular problems
   b. Bone marrow malfunction
   c. Diabetes
   d. Respiratory disorders

Answer:

2. When interpreting lab vales it is important to remember that "normal ranges" may vary by age. True/false?

Answer:

CONCLUSION

Factors related to family and community can positively or negatively impact the care of the pediatric client. The nurse should deliver family-centered care to ensure that support systems are maximized and not disrupted so the client receives needed support throughout the illness and return to the home and community. Several key points should be noted from this overview chapter:

   1. Provision of family-centered care will require use of an organized nursing process to gather assessment data and plan age-appropriate interventions for the pediatric client.

2. Communication is critical to obtain information from and relay information to the child and family in the process of assessing and planning for client care; family members know more about the child and their information should be valued.

3. Cultural and ethnic differences and preferences should be considered and accommodated when possible during the nursing care process.

4. History assessment is important to determine exposures and chronic conditions, as well as habits that may influence a pediatric client's health status.

5. Nutritional assessment and support is important to maintain and to restore the health status of a child or adolescent.

6. Childhood obesity is a major concern and risk factor for obesity in adults.

7. Family assessment is important to determine support for the child during and after an illness.

8. A physical examination should be performed systematically to determine symptoms of conditions that require treatment and that may impact a child's growth and development.

9. Blood pressure, pulse, and respirations vary with age, consider normal based on average value for age.

10. Assessment procedures may need to be altered depending on pediatric condition—such as light palpation only for a child with a Wilms tumor—to avoid injury to client.

11. Involve the client and family in the assessment and diagnostic procedures with clear explanation of expected assistance.

12. Clearly explain what will be felt, seen, heard, or smelled by the child in preparation for a procedure.

13. Normal diagnostic findings and values should be interpreted based on the age of the child or adolescent to determine what is truly abnormal.

14. Assess for allergy to seafood, shellfish, or iodine because some procedures may require contrast dye that contains iodine.

? FINAL CHECKUP

1. **What type of community assessment should be done to determine if Dawn, a 5-year-old who is blind after a recent accident, should be discharged home?**
   a. Home
   b. Neighborhood
   c. School
   d. All of the above

2. **Iynuoma, age 11, has been admitted for observation. Which are the key considerations for communicating during her health assessment?**
   a. Recognizing cultural differences and getting an interpreter if needed
   b. Asking close-ended, direct questions to establish trust
   c. Teaching the child and the parents that the nurse is the expert in the care process
   d. All of the above

3. **Tommy, age 15, has several small sores, sparse pubic hair, and a BMI <65%. He is most likely suffering from which of the following?**
   a. Scoliosis
   b. Cyanosis
   c. Malnutrition
   d. None of the above

4. **July has low levels of hematocrit and albumen as well as high levels of glucose in her urine. The possible implication of these symptoms is which of the following?**
   a. A protein deficiency
   b. Renal damage
   c. A need for assistance from social services
   d. All of the above

5. **At 16 years of age, Susie is flat-chested, unusually pale, and she consistently suffers from swelling in her feet and legs. Susie's symptoms can be described as which of the following?**
   a. Edema, pallor, and delayed development
   b. Pallor, hypertelorism, and petechiae
   c. Edema, ecchymosis, and pallor
   d. None of the above

6. **The number and composition of family members, instances of family illness or death, and parental divorce are all aspects of which of the following?**
   a. Temperament
   b. A child's family data
   c. a and b
   d. None of the above

7. **Nuclear rigidity is:**
   a. A symptom of meningitis
   b. A symptom of cardiac dysfunction
   c. A headache symptom
   d. None of the above

8. **Hypertelorism is noted during the initial examination of a 3-year-old African American boy. He most likely suffers from which of the following?**
   a. Blindness
   b. Deafness
   c. Down syndrome
   d. None of the above

9. **White patches, redness, and excessive drainage are symptoms common to disorders of which of the following?**
   a. Ears and eyes
   b. Back and chest
   c. Skin and nails
   d. Mouth and throat

10. **Which of the following facts should the nurse involved in the health assessment of a pediatric client remember?**
    a. Family and community can positively or negatively impact patient care.
    b. Cultural and ethnic preferences should be accommodated when possible to maximize success of patient care.
    c. Deliverance of family-centered care assures support systems are maximized and not disrupted.
    d. All of the above.

ANSWERS

Routine checkup 1
1. Structure and function.
2. False.
3. An assessment of the family is needed to determine the need for resources and support of the community (such as signage to drivers in the community to be careful that a deaf child lives in the neighborhood).

Routine checkup 2
1. Chief complaints.
2. False.
3. True.

Routine checkup 3
1. b.
2. True

Final checkup

1. d	2. a	3. c	4. b
5. a	6. b	7. a	8. c
9. d	10. d		

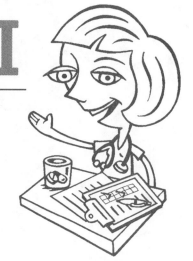

PART II

Systematic Exploration of Pediatric Conditions and Nursing Care

CHAPTER 4

Head and Neck: Eyes, Ears, Nose, and Throat

Learning Objectives

At the end of the chapter, the student will be able to

1. Discuss the pediatric risk factors for disruption of structures of the head and neck.

2. Discuss signs and symptoms related to pediatric head and neck conditions.

3. Evaluate diagnostic procedures associated with head and neck conditions.

4. Discuss treatment regimens associated with conditions of the head and neck.

5. Teach and support parents regarding prophylactic care and the treatment and care required for a child with conditions of the eye, ear, nose, and throat.

OVERVIEW

The head and neck regions of the body are the centers for most of the major senses of the body: vision, hearing, smell, and taste. In addition, conditions that affect the throat may impact eating and cause a decrease in the child's nutritional intake. The eyes, ears, nose, and throat present entry points for bacteria and foreign bodies. The airway of the young pediatric client is smaller in diameter than that of an adult; therefore obstruction from swelling or foreign bodies is a threat to oxygenation. Children exchange infectious organisms through play and sharing of food, drink, and clothing. Failure to treat a condition of the head and neck could lead to severe structural injury, such as possible loss of hearing or sight.

EYES

Conditions of the eye may involve the conjunctiva (infection), pupils (structural abnormality), cornea (opacity or scarring) or lens (spots/cataract), among other structural changes. Inflammations of the eyelids can be the result of invasion by organisms or foreign bodies or from blockage of the lacrimal (tear) duct. Examination of the external and internal eye can reveal many overt and covert problems. Refractive errors (disorders in which the shape of the eye causes light rays to bend before reaching the retina, result in the ability to clearly see close objects only (**myopia**) or distant objects only (**hyperopia**). Early identification of these conditions usually leads to corrective lenses (glasses or contact lens). Malalignment (such as strabismus) of the eyes may be noted in infants, but after 4 months of age **binocularity** (ability to focus on one visual field with both eyes) should be present; thus malalignment noted at the age of ≥5 months should be further explored.

STRABISMUS

1 What Went Wrong?

Malalignment of the eyes (cross-eye) with an inward deviation (**esotropia**) or an outward deviation (**exotropia**) of the eyes can result from muscle paralysis or congenital defect. Visual perspectives are not parallel so the brain receives two different images.

2 Signs and Symptoms

- Squinting of eyelids or frowning noted
- Difficulty judging distance when picking up objects
- Unable to see print or moving objects clearly
- Difficulty fixating on objects from one distance to another
- Closes one eye to see
- Tilts head to one side
- In combination with refractive error: headache, dizziness, **diplopia** (double vision), photophobia (light sensitivity)
- If untreated, may progress to blindness from disuse due to **amblyopia** (blindness in one eye because of the brain ignoring the extra signal coming from that eye)

3 Test Results

- Corneal light reflex test (Hirschberg test) shows the light falls off center in one eye and not symmetrically within each pupil.
- Cover test: When the strong eye is covered, the uncovered eye moves to attempt to adjust, revealing malalignment.
- Vision testing to determine accompanying refractive error.

4 Treatment

- Based on the cause of strabismus
  - Occlusion therapy (patching of stronger eye to exercise weak eye)
  - Surgery to increase visual stimulation to weaker eye

5 Nursing Intervention

- Monitor vision and eye movement to determine effectiveness of treatment.
- Instruct family to apply occlusion patching as ordered.
- Teach family to care for eye after surgery.

Nursing alert Early diagnosis and treatment is critical to prevent blindness in one eye secondary to amblyopia with brain suppressing image from that eye.

ACUTE CONJUNCTIVITIS

1 What Went Wrong?

- The cause of the inflammation of the conjunctiva often varies depending on the age of the child.
- Newborns may be infected during birth with Chlamydia or *Neisseria gonorrhoeae*, or herpes simplex virus with a resulting conjunctivitis.
- Infants may experience conjunctiva secondary to a nasolacrimal (tear) duct obstruction.
- Children may experience bacterial (most common), viral, allergic, or foreign body invasions resulting in conjunctivitis.

2 Signs and Symptoms

- Inflamed conjunctiva is noted with most forms of conjunctivitis in addition to
- Bacterial: Purulent drainage, early morning crusting of eyelids, and swollen lids.
- Viral: With general conjunctivitis, a report of upper respiratory tract infections may be reported, watery serous drainage, and swollen lids; with hemorrhagic conjunctivitis, the presence of enterovirus is noted, and severe inflammation, subconjunctival hemorrhage, and photophobia (sensitivity to light) may be noted.
- Allergic conjunctivitis may reveal itching, watery to viscous stringy discharge, and swollen lids.
- Conjunctivitis due to a foreign body may reveal tearing and pain in addition to inflammation.

3 Test Results

- Culture of the purulent drainage is often needed to identify the cause of the conjunctivitis.

4 Treatment

- Viral conjunctivitis is self-limiting and treatment is cleaning away of secretions.
- Bacterial conjunctivitis is treated with antibacterial agents:
  - Polymyxin (Polytrim) and bacitracin (Polysporin)
  - Sodium sulfacetamide (Sulamyd) or trimethoprim and polymyxin (Polytrim)
  - Supportive care of removal of dried secretions

5 Nursing Intervention

- Keep eye clean of secretions and crust, being careful not to contaminate.
  - Warm moist compress is effective for crust removal.
  - Older children can remove crust in warm flowing water from shower.

◐ Administer ophthalmic medication after cleansing of eye to reduce eye contamination.
◐ Client and parent teaching
  • Instruct parent and client to keep washcloth and towel separate to prevent use by other people.
  • Instruct the child and parents in good hand hygiene to minimize spread of infection.
  • Tissues should be discarded properly after use to avoid transfer of infection.
  • Never use the same tissue or area of washcloth on both eyes in order to avoid transfer of organisms to uninfected eye.

Nursing alert **Use separate tissue for each eye or different cloth to avoid contamination of uninfected eye with organisms from infected eye.**

EARS

❶ Conditions of the ear primarily occur in the middle and inner ear. The eustachian tube generally functions to protect the middle ear from nasopharyngeal secretions, to drain middle ear secretions into the nasopharynx, and to

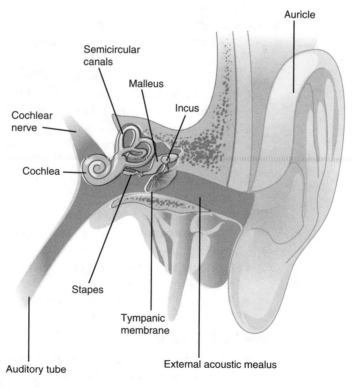

FIGURE 4-1

equalize pressure within the middle ear. Because the eustachian tube is shorter, straighter and wider, and more horizontal in the child than in the adult, organisms travel quickly from the pharynx to the middle ear. Persistent ear infection can result in partial or full hearing loss.

OTITIS MEDIA

Otitis media (OM), inflammation of the middle ear, is one of the most common diseases of early childhood.

What Went Wrong?

The primary cause of OM is a dysfunctioning eustachian tube:

- Secretions accumulate in the middle ear due to obstruction secondary to infection or allergy (intrinsic) or to enlarged adenoids or tumor (extrinsic).
- Ear infection is commonly caused by *Streptococcus pneumoniae*, *Haemophilus influenzae,* and *Moraxella catarrhalis.*
- Exposure to tobacco smoke (increases respiratory infection, decreases mucociliary function leading to eustachian tube blockage) and reflux of milk into the eustachian tube can contribute to development of OM.

Signs and Symptoms

- Symptoms commonly result from increased pressure in the ear or primary infection.
- Pain due to the pressure on surrounding structures
  - Infants may pull at ear or move head around.
  - Child may complain of earache.
  - Fever may spike as high as 40°C (104°F).
- Eardrum perforation due to excess pressure buildup is a common complication in OM, particularly in chronic disease.
- Cervical or preauricular lymph gland enlargement.
- **Rhinorrhea** (nasal drainage), vomiting, diarrhea if respiratory infection also present.
- Purulent drainage accumulation in the middle ear chamber; can drain to outer ear with rupture.
- Loss of appetite might be noted due to pain with chewing or sucking.
- **Tympanosclerosis** (eardrum scarring) is the deposition of hyaline material into the fibrous layer of the tympanic membrane.
- **Labyrinthitis** (infection of the inner ear) or **mastoiditis** (inflection of the mastoid sinus) could occur but are rare with the use of antibiotic therapy.
- Prolonged OM can result in complications including hearing loss.

Test Results

- Otoscopy reveals an intact membrane that appears bright red and bulging, with no visible landmarks or light reflex.

- Tympanometry may detect lack of movement of the tympanic membrane due to pressure buildup.
- Culture of drainage is used to determine involved organism.
- Acoustic reflectometry will reveal the presence of effusion in the middle ear.

Treatment

- Cautious use of antibiotics to treat infections to avoid penicillin resistance.
- Recurrent OM is treated with long-term antibiotic therapy and immunotherapy.
- Surgery such as a myringotomy with placement of tubes to facilitate drainage may be performed for severe pain.
- An adenoidectomy may be performed if blockage of the eustachian tube by adenoids is the cause of the OM.

Nursing Intervention

- Parent teaching about prophylactic care
  - Position infants as upright as possible during feeding to avoid reflux of formula into eustachian tube.
  - Avoid smoking around infants and children.
- Administer analgesics as ordered to provide pain relief.
- Heat pack application over the ear may relieve pain for some children.
- Position child on the affected side to promote drainage (if draining, or postoperatively after myringotomy).
- Assist in removal of drainage, when possible
  - Postoperative support may include wicks inserted loosely in the ear to promote drainage but prevent infection transfer to middle ear.
  - Frequent cleansing of outer ear and moisture barrier on ear to protect from purulent drainage.
- Family-centered care
- Educating the family in care of child
  - Analgesia for pain management
  - Postoperative care to prevent spread of infection and promote healing
- Providing emotional support to the child and family
  - Explain the process for management of drainage.
  - Encourage follow-up evaluation of hearing to detect any loss of hearing.

 Nursing alert **Instruct parents to position infant as upright as possible and not to lie an infant down and prop bottle in infant's mouth during feeding to avoid formula reflux into eustachian tube.**

✔ ROUTINE CHECKUP 1

1. The nurse notices an inward deviation of the eyes in a 3-month-old child. What actions would be appropriate for the nurse to take?
   a. Inform the doctor of the abnormality and assist the parents in planning for pending surgery.
   b. Document the finding and plan to follow up by observing the eyes at a future visit after the child is >4 months of age.
   c. Patch one eye and allow the other to strengthen, and then patch the opposite eye.
   d. Administer analgesics and instruct the parents to administer analgesics on a regular basis until the child is older and able to take the medication.

Answer:

2. Why should parents be taught to hold child upright during feedings to avoid otitis media?

Answer:

NOSE

Most pediatric conditions of the nose are discussed in Chapter 5 on respiratory conditions. Nose bleeds (**epistaxis**) can occur in many conditions and may require different treatment depending on the cause.

🔺 What Went Wrong?

Epistaxis can occur from trauma to the nasal mucosa or secondary to bleeding disorders involving a decrease in clotting factors, such as hemophilia.

🔺 Signs and Symptoms
- Bleeding from nasal passage (commonly the anterior septum)

🔺 Test Results
- Clotting factors: Prolonged values for prothrombin (PT), partial thromboplastin (PTT), and thrombin time (TT) may be noted in some conditions that cause epistaxis.
- Decreased platelets and fibrinogen levels may be noted, increasing risk for bleeding.

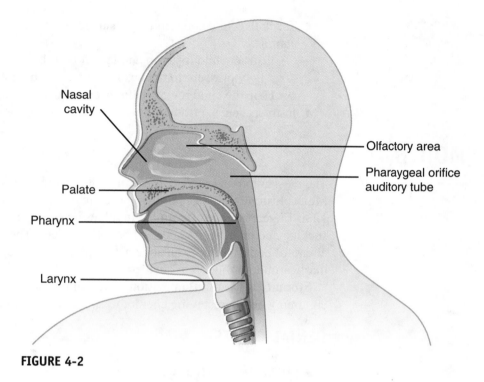

Nasal cavity

Olfactory area

Pharaygeal orifice auditory tube

Palate

Pharynx

Larynx

FIGURE 4-2

⚃ Treatment

- Apply pressure to the nose for a minimum of 10 minutes (thumb and forefinger to the bridge of the nose).
- Clotting factor, platelets, and fresh-frozen plasma may be administered.
- Nasal packing with cotton or wadded tissue may be applied to involved nostril(s).
- Ice or cold pack may be applied to the bridge of the nose for persistent bleeding.

⚄ Nursing Intervention

- Administer blood factors and monitor for adverse reactions:
  - Watch for signs of fluid volume overload because small children may experience congestive failure if fluid infusion is too large or rapid.
  - Monitor for infusion reaction including hemolysis if blood transfusion is given.

◑ Teach the child and family to manage nosebleeds through the following actions:
- Instruct child to sit up and lean forward.
- Apply pressure to the nose for a minimum of 10 minutes.
- Help the child remain calm because anxiety can aggravate bleeding.

◑ Instruct client to breathe through the mouth while nasal packing is in place.

MOUTH

The most common oral condition for children and adolescents is dental caries. Malocclusion is another problem noted in more than half of pediatric clients 12 to 17 years of age. Treatment involves discouraging habits such as thumb sucking and the placement of orthodontic devices. The nurse should refer the client for dental services and encourage proper brushing and flossing, particularly around orthodontic devices.

Stomatitis is an inflammation of the oral mucosa that can often impact children who are receiving chemotherapy and are immunocompromised.

DENTAL CARIES

① What Went Wrong?

◑ Dental caries are among the most common oral problems in children and adolescents. The most vulnerable victims are children 4 to 8 years of age with primary eruption of permanent teeth and 12 to 18 years of age with secondary eruption of permanent teeth.

◑ These are the major factors that contribute to the development of dental caries:
- The host: Improperly structured teeth with crowding prevents adequate cleaning and hereditary or health factors impacting the quality and quantity of saliva flow, and resistance or susceptibility to caries.
- Microorganisms: Microflora produces acids that digest and destroy teeth.
- Substrates: Particularly sucrose-containing substances consumed between meals and a protein matrix forming a dental plaque on the teeth demineralizes tooth enamel. Demineralization of enamel leads to tooth decay and development of dental caries.

② Signs and Symptoms

◑ Pain
◑ Visible decay
- Surface areas
- Fissures of the molars

3 Test Results

Radiograph: Caries between teeth and in fissures are typically noted by radiograph.

4 Treatment

- Prophylaxis/preventive treatment with fluoride applications, fluoride in the water, and sealants to tooth fissures and groves
- Removal of all decayed portions of a tooth and replacement of lost surfaces with durable material

5 Nursing Intervention

- Oral inspection
  - Refer for routine dental examination and for dental caries.
- Teach the client and parents
  - Prevention through oral hygiene: correct tooth brushing and flossing, and regular dental exams
  - Restriction of sugar treats, particularly chewy candies
  - Early treatment with fluoride in water and oral rinses
  - Brushing after intake of sugary liquids, including medications

STOMATITIS

1 What Went Wrong?

- Stomatitis, inflammation of the oral mucosa, including the cheek, lip, tongue, palate, and floor of the mouth, may be infectious or noninfectious. The most common form in children is aphthous stomatitis, or canker sore, which has an unknown origin or may be associated with trauma such as injury with toothbrush, biting of the cheek, or abrasion by braces.
- Herpetic gingivostomatitis (HGS) is caused by the herpes simplex virus (usually type 1) and is commonly referred to as a cold sore or fever blister.

Nursing alert **Use caution and wear gloves when touching areas near herpetic lesions to avoid spread of the infection through broken skin on the hand.**

2 Signs and Symptoms

- Aphthous stomatitis
  - Painful, small, whitish ulcerations surrounded by a red border.
  - Ulcers persist for 4 to 12 days and then heal.
  - Syndrome of periodic fever, aphthous stomatitis, pharyngitis, and cervical adenitis (PFAPA) may occur in some children (cause unknown).
- Herpetic gingivostomatitis
  - Fever.
  - Pharynx becomes edematous and erythematous.

- Severe, painful vesicles erupt on the mucosa.
- Cervical lymphadenitis.
- Foul breath odor.
- Recurrent form: Single or group vesicles on lips, precipitated by stress, trauma, exposure to sunlight, or immunosuppression.

Test Results
- Diagnosed by symptoms
- Culture may be performed

Treatment
- Symptom relief with acetaminophen in mild cases; codeine with severe pain
- Topical anesthetics: Orabase, Anbesol, Kank-a, Lidocaine (Xylocaine viscous), diphenhydramine (Benadryl) and Maalox mixed in equal parts for pain relief
- Antiviral agents for severe cases of HGS

Nursing Intervention
- Pain relief
  - Administer topical agents and analgesics for pain relief.
  - Provide medication before meals to promote adequate nutrition intake.
  - Provide straw for drinking to avoid painful lesions.
  - Perform mouth care with soft toothbrush, foam applicator, or cloth for comfort.
- Teach the client and parents:
  - Prevention of spread through careful handwashing and teaching to keep fingers out of mouth and avoid touching body with contaminated hands.
  - All objects placed in the mouth of the infected child should be washed thoroughly or discarded.
  - Use restraint as needed to prevent self-contamination by younger child.
  - Keep immunocompromised persons, infants, and other young children away from infected child to avoid exposure.
  - Inform parents and older children that type 1 HSV is not the herpes commonly associated with sexual activity, to avoid assumptions that the child is sexually active.

ROUTINE CHECKUP 2

1. How could dietary habits place a child at risk for dental caries?

Answer:

_____

_____

2. If the nurse observes aphthous stomatitis, what additional actions may be needed?
   a. Examine the area without wearing gloves to avoid irritation from the latex.
   b. Instruct the child or teen to avoid chewing ice until swelling subsides.
   c. Inform the parents that the child must be sexually active requiring treatment.
   d. Prepare to obtain a culture of the lesion to determine organism involved.

Answer:

THROAT

Most conditions affecting the throat present a risk for respiratory distress. Because the larynx and tracheal areas are smaller in children, obstruction from swelling is a true danger that requires immediate action by the nurse to prevent severe oxygen deficit. Actions must be taken to recognize airway obstruction early and restore an open airway as quickly as possible. Most of these conditions are addressed in the discussion of respiratory conditions in Chapter 5.

HEAD

PEDICULOSIS CAPITIS (HEAD LICE)

What Went Wrong?

○ Infestation of the scalp by lice (*Pediculus humanus capitis*) is a common parasite invasion among school-age children. The parasite lives by sucking blood from the host. The female lays **nits** (eggs) at the base of the hair shaft, and the nits hatch in a week to 10 days increasing the parasitic invasion.

 Nursing alert Lice infestation is often a source of embarrassment for the family due to association with lack of hygiene. Emphasize to the parents that anyone can be infected, and the usual cause is shared objects with an infected child and not lack of cleanliness.

🔑 Signs and Symptoms

- Gray-tan colored lice visible at the base of the hair
- Translucent empty nit cases on the scalp
- White specks (nits) close to the scalp
- Itching caused by the insects' movement and saliva on the scalp
- Scratch marks on scalp, particularly near ear, nape of neck, and back of head
- Inflammatory papules (elevated palpable lesion) due to infected lesions may be present.

🔑 Test Results

- Diagnosis is made with discovery of lice, nits, or nit cases on examination of scalp.

🔑 Treatment

- Shampoo with pediculicide preparation such as
  - Permethrin 1% cream rinse (Nix)
  - Pyrethrin with piperonyl butoxide (RID)
- Removal of nit cases
- Malathion 0.5% (children >2 years of age, 8- to 12-hour contact on scalp)
- Daily removal of nits with nit comb or other device to detect and remove lice

Nursing alert **If shampoo gets in the eye, flush well with water.**

🔑 Nursing Interventions

Prevention

- Provide client and family teaching regarding the spread of lice.
- Instruct parents, and provide education to community and schools, regarding the importance of not sharing clothing or personal items such as combs among children.
- Maintain the personal items of children in separate containers.
- Explain that children who were infected may return to school before nits are totally absent; remaining nits are often inactive or dead with no risk for further spread.

Assist with treatment

- Clean infested clothing and place in dryer for at least 20 minutes.
- Dry clean items that cannot be washed (or seal in a bag for 2 weeks to allow death of any parasites).
- Soak hair care items in lice-killing agent or boiling water.
- Systematically inspect the scalp of any child who scratches head, looking for lice, nits, or signs of infestation.

⑤ Family teaching and support
- ◐ Stress that cutting or shaving of hair is not needed to control spread of lice in order to avoid unnecessary distress for the child.
- ◐ Assist family to obtain financial support, as needed, for expensive pediculicides or insecticides.
- ◐ Support family by stressing that pediculosis is not a sign of poor sanitation.

 ## ✔ ROUTINE CHECKUP 3

1. Explain why manual removal of the nits may be needed if shampoo does not kill all lice.

Answer:

2. A 17-year-old young man complains of jaw pain and has swollen glands with tenderness along the jaw on palpation. What additional actions would be appropriate?
   a. Provide a burger and fries to encourage the adolescent to eat.
   b. Instruct the adolescent and parent regarding the need for limited activity until the swelling subsides.
   c. Inform the parents and the child that immediate surgery is needed to remove the infected tissue and prevent sterility.
   d. Provide loose pajamas for comfort if signs of orchitis are present.

Answer:

CONCLUSION

Conditions of the head and the neck present distinct challenges for the nurse to prevent disruption of a child's growth and development. Disruption in vision secondary to disorders in eye structures or function could result in loss of vision if treatment is delayed. These are the key points to remember:
- ◐ An ocular malalignment, such as strabismus, and associated refractive error can be detected with routine examination, and treatment by the nurse with family follow-up can prevent vision loss.
- ◐ Conjunctivitis can spread quickly among a group of children and to adults.
- ◐ Teaching the client and family about proper hygiene is important to control the spread of infection.
- ◐ Otitis media is related to dysfunction of the eustachian tube and can be aggravated by smoke and reflux of formula.

- Pain from otitis media is related to pressure from fluid buildup in the middle ear.
- Epistaxis (nosebleed) can occur in multiple conditions that affect clotting and is treated with external pressure to the nose or internal pressure from packing.
- Oral conditions such as dental caries and stomatitis require good hygiene to promote prevention and resolution.
- Mumps can occur if immunization has not been administered or condition has not previously been experienced. Caution must be taken to prevent spread of the condition due to exposure to saliva.
- Pediculosis capitis (head lice) can spread from a child through a group of children or a family if precautions are not taken.
- Treatment for head lice should be thorough and continue until the parasites are fully eradicated.

? FINAL CHECKUP

1. **When speaking to the child, the nurse notices that the child seems to hear well in the right ear but minimally in the left ear. What historical or physical finding might be significant in identifying a related problem?**
   a. A reported preference for fresh raw green vegetables.
   b. A history of untreated otitis media within the past month.
   c. The glands in the child's occipital region are flat and nontender.
   d. The child has experienced a recent increase in appetite.

2. **A nurse is conducting a vision screening during a physical exam of a 7-year-old child. The nurse realizes that the child cannot see *any* of the letters on the Snellen eye chart. What action by the nurse would be appropriate?**
   a. Notify the child's parents and refer the child to an optometrist.
   b. Inform the parents and child of the need to repeat the test using an age-appropriate tool.
   c. Move the child closer to the Snellen letter chart and repeat the test.
   d. Inform the parents and the child of the need for the pediatrician to prescribe eye drops to improve the child's vision.

3. **What teaching should the nurse provide for a child and family to reduce the risk of the child developing caries?**
   a. Teach the parents to serve steamed carrots at minimum twice weekly.
   b. Instruct the child and parents regarding the need to brush after meals.
   c. Encourage the child to eat soft candy rather than hard candy between meals.
   d. Provide water that is free of fluoride to prevent demineralization of teeth.

4. **While experiencing an upper respiratory infection, the parents report that their 1-year-old son has become irritable and constantly turns his head from side to side. He has a fever and drainage from the ear. What would you suspect is the problem?**
   a. Otitis media
   b. Mastoiditis
   c. Legg-Calvé-Perthes
   d. Osteomyelitis

5. **Treatment for epistaxis could include all *except* which intervention?**
   a. Packing the nose with cotton
   b. Rinsing the nares with warm fluid
   c. Applying cool compress to the nose
   d. Placing pressure on the exterior nose area

6. **A teen experiencing which of the following conditions would be able to continue work and regular activities immediately after treatment?**
   a. Pediculosis capitis
   b. Stomatitis
   c. Epistaxis
   d. All of the above

7. **A child with pediculosis capitis is most likely to exhibit what symptoms?**
   a. Itching at the bridge of the nose
   b. Inflammation of the nasal mucosa
   c. Bleeding from the scalp
   d. Redness of the tongue

8. **Nursing interventions in the treatment of a child with stomatitis could include what measures?**
   a. Administering aspirin to reduce fever
   b. Applying ice to the mucosa to reduce inflammation
   c. Monitoring for side effects from codeine administered for severe pain
   d. Avoiding medications like Maalox that could irritate the oral mucosa

9. **Which symptoms are appropriate for the form of conjunctivitis indicated?**
   a. Allergic conjunctivitis may reveal bloody drainage tearing.
   b. Foreign body-related conjunctivitis will reveal photophobia.
   c. Bacterial conjunctivitis may reveal sterile, clear watery drainage.
   d. Viral conjunctivitis will reveal swollen lids and serous drainage.

10. **What is the major reason a family might delay reporting a possible lice infestation?**
    a. Fear related to the surgery required for the treatment
    b. Shame associated with having a head lice infestation
    c. Concern that the nits might be destroyed during the treatment
    d. Ability to relieve itching with cool or cold compress application

ANSWERS

Routine checkup 1
1. b
2. When child is feeding while lying flat, reflux of formula into the eustachian tube is more likely to occur.

Routine checkup 2
1. Between-meal eating with high-sugar snacks contributes to plaque formation and demineralization of teeth.
2. d. A culture of the site will identify the organism and determine treatment.

Routine checkup 3
1. Removal of eggs (nits) reduces reinfestation of scalp with parasites.
2. b

Final checkup
1. b. Untreated otitis media can result in hearing loss.
2. a. The Snellen chart is the most accurate method for vision testing and inability to see should be evaluated by an optometrist.
3. b. Brushing to remove food from teeth will reduce the development of caries.
4. a. Otitis media in an infant may be manifested by tugging at ear or moving head from side to side.
5. b. Rinsing the nares with warm water will likely increase bleeding.
6. c. Once infection or infestation is resolved, activities can resume.
7. c. Itching may be noted due to saliva from the parasites.
8. c. Codeine may be administered for severe pain and side effects may occur.
9. d. Viral conjunctivitis can cause inflammation and drainage from the infection.
10. b. Infection with lice may carry a stigma that families may be ashamed to reveal.

CHAPTER 5

Respiratory Conditions

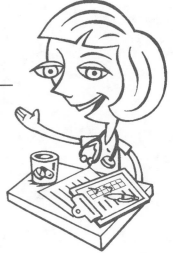

Learning Objectives

At the end of the chapter, the student will be able to

1 Describe the pathology for several illnesses of the respiratory system.

2 Describe the assessment signs and symptoms seen in children with respiratory difficulties.

3 Relate the assessment findings regarding respiratory difficulties specifically to the most common childhood illnesses in the upper and lower respiratory system.

4 Discuss the treatment recommended for viral and infectious disease processes of the upper and lower respiratory system.

5 Provide support to the child and family through education on measures that will encourage compliance and minimize physical and psychological morbidity of respiratory illnesses.

6 Recognize cardinal signs and symptoms of the respiratory system that suggest life-threatening emergencies.

KEY WORDS

Alveoli	Lymphadenopathy
Group A β-hemolytic streptococci (GABHS)	Palivizumab (Synagis)
	Respiratory syncytial virus (RSV)
Croup syndrome	Retractions
Enzyme-linked immunosorbent assay (ELISA)	Rhinorrhea
	Ribavirin (Virazole)
Epiglottitis	Steatorrhea
Epstein-Barr (EB) virus	Stridor
Influenza virus	Surfactant
Laryngitis	Tonsillectomy
Laryngotracheobronchitis (LTB)	Tracheostomy

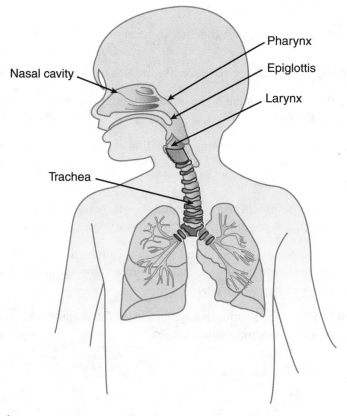

FIGURE 5-1

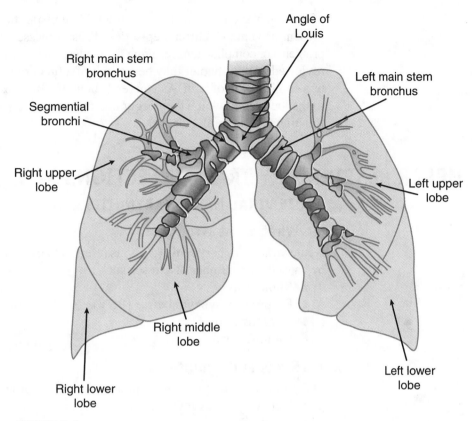

FIGURE 5-2

OVERVIEW

The respiratory tract consists of upper and lower airway structures. Upper airway structures begin with the oronasopharynx, the passageway connecting the nasal airway to the trachea. Because the oral area is a shared passageway to the esophagus as well as the pharynx and larynx, inflammation in the area can impact swallowing as well as breathing. The pharynx and upper trachea, which contains the glottis or vocal cords and epiglottis of the larynx, have an impact on speech as well as breathing. Lower airway structures include the lower trachea, bronchi, bronchioles, and **alveoli** of the lungs. The lungs are divided into a two-lobed lung on the left and a three-lobed lung on the right side of the chest. Infants and children have smaller airway structures than those of adults; thus obstruction of the airway can occur rapidly. In addition, the cartilage of the young pediatric airway and reactive bronchial smooth muscle places the pediatric client at risk for obstruction due to bronchial constriction.

This chapter examines the common respiratory illnesses that are seen in the childhood population. The text explores the illnesses as altered functions of the upper and lower respiratory tract. Most respiratory illnesses in children present as acute or chronic episodes. These illnesses may occur as primary problems or complications resulting from other illnesses. The respiratory illnesses reviewed in this chapter may be a result of a functional or structural problem or a combination of both. As you read about the illnesses, relate the alterations to the location in which they occur and the type of respiratory condition (i.e., functional, structural, or both).

UPPER RESPIRATORY TRACT INFECTIONS

ACUTE VIRAL NASOPHARYNGITIS

❶ What Went Wrong?

Acute viral nasopharyngitis (AVN) is referred to as the common cold and may be caused by a number of viruses such as

- Rhinovirus
- Respiratory syncytial virus (RSV)
- **Influenza virus**
- Parainfluenza virus

❷ Signs and Symptoms

Symptoms are more severe in infants than in children and adults. The most prevalent symptom is fever along with

- Irritability.
- Restlessness.
- Decreased appetite.
- Decreased activity.
- Nasal stuffiness and discharge.
- Muscular aches.
- Cough.
- Occasionally fever may recur or the child might experience otitis media.

❸ Test Results

The diagnosis for AVN is usually made on the client's history and physical exam. Affected children usually have a normal WBC count.

❹ Treatment

- There is no specific treatment for AVN.
- Effective vaccines are not available.
- Children are usually treated at home.
- Antipyretics are prescribed for mild fever and discomfort.
- Decongestants may be prescribed for children and infants >6 months of age.

5 Nursing Intervention
- A thorough nursing assessment is essential.
- Education and support to the caregiver
- Provide nursing care and teach family members to
  - Assess hydration.
  - Note color of nasal drainage, duration of fever.
  - 6 Monitor for the presence of respiratory distress or complications from a more severe condition:
    - Wheezing or shortness of breath
    - Respiratory rate >50 to 60 breaths/minute
    - Listlessness or irritability and crying
    - Persistent cough >2 days
    - Refusing food or drink
    - Poor sleeping pattern

TONSILLITIS AND PHARYNGITIS
What Went Wrong?
1 Tonsillitis and pharyngitis are common viral infections in children; however, 20% of acute tonsillitis and pharyngitis are caused by **group A β-hemolytic streptococci (GABHS)** and can lead to significant health problems.

2 Signs and Symptoms
- Sore throat.
- Difficulty swallowing.
- Fever.
- Most manifestations are by inflammation.
- As the palatine tonsils enlarge with edema, they may meet midline of the throat and cause the child to have difficulty swallowing and breathing.
- Mouth breathing leads to offensive mouth odor.
- Persistent cough.
- Children with GABHS may experience
  - Headache
  - Abdominal pain
  - Nausea
  - Vomiting
  - Diarrhea

3 Test Results
- Throat cultures positive for GABHS infection warrant antibiotic treatment.

Treatment
- Treatment of viral tonsillitis and pharyngitis is symptomatic.
- Warm saline gargles.

❍ Nonaspirin analgesics and antipyretics.
    ❍ If left untreated, GABHS infections can lead to
        • Scarlet fever
        • Otitis media
        • Suppurative infections of surrounding tissues
    ❍ **Tonsillectomy** is recommended for recurrent streptococcal infections and massive hypertrophy.
    ❍ ◢4◣ Tonsillectomies are reserved for children >3 years of age due to excessive blood loss and a potential for the tonsils to grow back.

◢5◣ Nursing Interventions

    ❍ Baseline assessment prior to the procedure.
    ❍ Postsurgical assessments include close monitoring with high alert for bleeding and infection.

Nursing alert ◢6◣ **Frequent swallowing following a tonsillectomy is a cardinal sign of bleeding at the surgical site.**

CROUP SYNDROME
◢1◣ What Went Wrong?

Croup syndrome is a very common viral syndrome applied to a symptom complex characterized by hoarseness and a cough described as "barking" that results from an inspiratory **stridor** sound produced when there is obstruction of the larynx and trachea. Croup syndrome affects the

    ❍ Larynx
    ❍ Trachea
    ❍ Bronchi to varying degrees, resulting in
        • Laryngotracheobronchitis (LTB)
        • Epiglottitis
        • Laryngitis

◢2◣ Signs and Symptoms

Manifestation of croup include a "barking" cough, nasal drainage, sore throat, and low-grade fever.

ACUTE LARYNGOTRACHEOBRONCHITIS
◢1◣ What Went Wrong?

Laryngotracheobronchitis (LTB) is the most common type of croup and primarily affects children <5 years of age. The disease process is an inflammation of the mucosa lining the larynx and trachea causing a narrowing of the airway. The typical patient with LTB is a toddler who develops the classic "barking" cough and acute stridor after several days of coryza.

Signs and Symptoms

- Brassy cough.
- Gradual onset of low-grade fever.
- The child struggles to inhale air past the obstruction and into the lungs producing an inspiratory stridor.
- The child may be in moderate respiratory distress with mild wheezing.
- Symptoms of hypoxia and airway obstruction may lead to respiratory acidosis and respiratory failure.

Test Results

These organisms are responsible for LTB:
- Parainfluenza virus types 1, 2, and 3
- RSV
- Influenza A and B
- *Mycoplasma pneumoniae*

Treatment

The major objective for treatment is medical management of the infectious process and maintaining an airway for adequate respiratory exchange. Children with mild croup without stridor are managed at home. High humidity with cool mist provides relief in most cases. Fluids are essentials for recovery. If the child is unable to take fluids, intravenous fluid therapy is initiated.

Nursing Interventions

- Vigilant observation and accurate of assessment of the respiratory status.
- Noninvasive cardiac, respiratory, and blood gas monitoring.
- Ensure intubation equipment is immediately accessible to the patient.
- Keep the child comfortable.
- Allow the parent or caregiver to lie next to the child in the mist tent to lessen anxiety.
- Modify treatment to cool moist mist blowing directly toward the patient from the hose when child will not tolerate mist tent.

ACUTE EPIGLOTTITIS

What Went Wrong?

Acute **epiglottitis** is a serious obstructive inflammatory process resulting from a bacterial infection that occurs principally in children between 2 and 5 years of age but can occur from infancy to adulthood. The obstruction is supraglottic as opposed to subglottic as in laryngitis. This disorder requires immediate attention.

✌ Signs and Symptoms

- ◑ Onset is abrupt without cough.
- ◑ Can rapidly progress to severe respiratory distress.
- ◑ Asymptomatic the night prior to onset.
- ◑ No spontaneous cough.
- ◑ The child is apprehensive.
- ◑ Voice is muffled with a froglike croaking sound on inspiration.
- ◑ Sore throat, reddened and inflamed.
- ◑ Drooling.
- ◑ Agitation.
- ◑ Fever.
- ◑ Dysphagia.
- ◑ Suprasternal.
- ◑ Substernal **retractions**.
- ◑ 🔟 Respiratory obstruction develops quickly and may lead to
  - Hypoxia
  - Acidosis
  - Reduced level of consciousness
  - Sudden death

The key difference between laryngotracheobronchitis (LTB) and epiglottitis is the presence of a cough in LTB.

➌ Test Results

- ◑ Positive for *Haemophilus influenzae*
- ◑ Chest films
- ◑ WBC with differential count

➍ Treatment

- ◑ Intensive observation by experience personnel.
- ◑ Endotracheal intubation.
- ◑ **Tracheostomy.**
- ◑ All invasive procedures should be performed in the operating room or areas equipped to initiate immediate intubation.
- ◑ Antibiotic therapy.

➎ Nursing Interventions

- ◑ Reassure the child and family to reduce anxiety.
- ◑ Avoid assessment of the oral cavity with a tongue blade.
- ◑ Allow the child to remain in the caregiver's lap and in the position that is most comfortable.

 🔟 *Nursing alert* **The onset of epiglottitis is abrupt and can rapidly progress to severe respiratory distress. The obstruction is supraglottic as opposed to sub-glottic as in laryngitis. This disorder requires immediate attention.**

ACUTE LARYNGITIS

1 What Went Wrong?

Acute **laryngitis** is most common in older children and adolescents. Viruses are usually the causative agents, and the disease is almost always self-limited without extended duration or sequelae.

2 Signs and Symptoms

- Hoarseness
- Coryza
- Sore throat
- Nasal congestion
- Fever
- Headache myalgia
- Malaise

3 Test Results

Virus are usually the causative agent.

4 Treatment

Treatment is supportive of the symptomatic presentation; fluids and humidified are highly encouraged.

5 Nursing Interventions

- Assist the patient to expectorate secretions adequately.
- Avoid the spread of infection.
- Maintain patent airway.

INFECTIOUS MONONUCLEOSIS

1 What Went Wrong?

Infectious mononucleosis is an acute common self-limiting infectious disease among young people <25 years of age. The disease course is usually mild but occasionally can be severe accompanied by serious complications.

2 Signs and Symptoms

Symptoms vary greatly in type, severity, and duration. The patient presents with
- Malaise
- Sore throat
- Fever with
  - Generalized **lymphadenopathy**
  - Splenomegaly
  - Skin rash over the trunk
  - Tonsils enlarged and reddened
  - Enlarged spleen
  - Possible jaundice

③ Test Results

- **Epstein-Barr (EB) virus** is the principal causing agent.
- The incubation period following exposure is 4 to 6 weeks.
- The diagnosis is established by atypical leukocytes and a positive heterophil agglutination test.
- Spot test to determine blood agglutination of significant agglutinins.

④ Treatment

- No specific treatment for this disease process
- Mild analgesics
- Force fluids and humidified air are usually sufficient.

⑤ Nursing Interventions

- When the spleen is enlarged, activities in which the child may receive a blow to the abdomen should be avoided.
- Diet counseling to meet growth and energy needs during the illness is recommended.
- Education should be directed to avoid secondary infections.
- Exposure to persons outside the family should be carefully considered, and adolescents should be supported and assured that the course of illness is temporary.
- Advise the patient and family that regular activities may resume when the acute phase of the illness has ended.

ROUTINE CHECKUP 1

1. The nurse teaches the caregiver of the infant diagnosed with nasopharyngitis to call the physician if which of the following occurs?
   a. Coughing.
   b. Infant becomes irritable.
   c. Shows signs and symptoms of an ear infection (correct answer).
   d. Low-grade fever.

Answer:

2. The nurse would expect which of the following to be appropriate for the infant diagnosed with staphylococcal pneumonia?
   a. Administer a course of antibiotics as prescribed.
   b. Monitor intake and output strictly to detect cardiac overload.
   c. Administer antitussives every 2 to 3 hours to relieve symptoms.
   d. Postural drainage every 2 hours.

Answer:

LOWER RESPIRATORY TRACT INFECTIONS

PNEUMONIA

What Went Wrong?

Pneumonia is an acute inflammation of the pulmonary parenchyma associated with alveolar consolidation. Viruses such as the following are primary causative agents:

- Cytomegalovirus
- Influenza
- Adenovirus
- RSV

Bacterial pneumonia most often caused by mycoplasma pneumonia occurs less frequently in children. Pneumonia can be classified as

- Lobar
- Interstitial or
- Bronchial

Lobar, as indicated, involves a significant portion of the lung; interstitial pneumonia includes the alveolar walls and peribronchial, and interlobular tissues. Bronchial pneumonia, as suggested by its name, involves the bronchi and lung fields.

Signs and Symptoms

Clinical manifestations include

- Cough
- Malaise
- Fever
- Prostration
- Anorexia
- Breath sounds
- Wheezes
- Fine crackles
- Headache
- Tachypnea
- Wheezing
- Gastrointestinal upset

Test Results

- Diagnosis is based on physical findings and a sputum culture.
- Chest films demonstrate the extent and location of the involvement.

Treatment

- The course of treatment is managed according to the etiology of the disease.
- Treatment for viral pneumonia is supportive to relieve symptoms.
- Bacterial pneumonia is treated with antibiotic therapy.
- The objective of treatment is effective ventilation and prevention of dehydration.

○ Oxygen therapy and chest physiotherapy may also be required.
○ Isolation is used as a precautionary measure when patients hospitalized until the causative agent is identified.

Nursing Intervention
○ Assess and monitor for manifestations that suggest increasing respiratory distress.
○ Provide symptomatic relief through supportive measures.
○ Encourage adequate fluid intake to remove secretions.
○ Administer pain medication to encourage deep breathing and respiratory therapy treatments.
○ Antibiotic therapy.

ASTHMA

What Went Wrong?
Asthma is a chronic inflammatory disorder of the airways. It is characterized by chronic inflammation, bronchoconstriction, and bronchial hyperresponsiveness. Asthma is the most common chronic respiratory illness in the childhood population.

Signs and Symptoms
○ Expiratory wheezing
○ Chronic cough
○ Dyspnea (shortness of breath or difficulty in breathing)
○ Nonproductive cough
○ Tachypnea
○ Chest pain
○ Irritability
○ Restlessness
○ Use of accessory muscles
○ Orthopnea (an increase in difficulty breathing when students are lying down)

Test Results
○ Physical assessment findings and client history
○ Peak expiratory flow (PEF) rates
○ Pulmonary function test (PFT)
○ Peak expiratory flow rate

Treatment
○ Prevent and minimize physical and psychologic morbidity.
○ Prevent and reduce exposure to airborne allergens and irritants.
○ Pharmacologic therapy to prevent and control asthma symptoms:
   • Reverse airflow obstruction
   • Long-term control medications
   • Quick-relief medications

- Corticosteroids
- Cromolyn sodium
- Metered-dose inhaler (MDI)
- Chlorofluorocarbons (CFCs)
- Corticosteroids
- β-adrenergic agents
- Salmeterol (Serevent)
- Methylxanthines
- Anticholinergics
- Leukotriene modifiers
- Exercise

NURSING INTERVENTIONS

- Assess how asthma impacts everyday life.
- Assess child and family's satisfaction with the effectiveness of the treatment program.
- Assist the child and family to avoid allergens.
- Teach child and family to modify the environment to relieve asthmatic episodes, (i.e., avoid excessive heat, cold, and other extremes of the weather or wind).
- Educate parents on reading food labels.
- Avoid foods known to provoke symptoms, foods such as monosodium glutamate (MSG), sulfites, bisulfites, and metabisulfites.
- Avoid aspirin with children who are sensitive and subject to aspirin-induced asthma.
- Monitor for and alert caregivers to signs of status asthmaticus, a life-threatening complication.

BRONCHIOLITIS
What Went Wrong?

Bronchiolitis is an acute viral infection of the bronchioles. The illness occurs most frequently in children <2 years of age during winter and spring. The **respiratory syncytial virus (RSV)** is responsible for 80% or most cases. The inflammatory process leads to airway edema and the accumulation of mucous and cellular debris. The obstruction in the airways leads to overinflation in some alveoli and atelectasis in others.

Signs and Symptoms

- Symptoms of upper respiratory infection (URI), such as sneezing, **rhinorrhea,** decreased appetite, low-grade fever, and coughing.
- Wheezing, retractions, crackles, nasal flaring, dyspnea, prolonged expiratory phase, and intermittent cyanosis.

Test Results

- ◑ The physical examination and medical history are the main diagnostic tools for bronchiolitis.
- ◑ It is difficult to identify the specific etiologic agent by clinical criteria alone.
- ◑ Nasal and nasopharyngeal secretions are tested by rapid immunofluorescent antibody (IFA) or **enzyme-linked immunosorbent assay (ELISA)**.

Treatment

- ◑ Most cases are treated at home with high humidity, adequate fluid intake, rest, and medications.
- ◑ Children with complicating conditions should be hospitalized.
- ◑ Mist therapy combined with oxygen by hood or tent are sufficient enough to alleviate dyspnea and hypoxia.
- ◑ **Ribavirin (Virazole)** is a specific aerosol antiviral medication for RSV bronchiolitis and reserved for severely ill infants and children with compromising illnesses.
- ◑ Two drugs are currently available for prevention of RSV bronchiolitis:
  - RSV immune globulin intravenous (RSV-GIV or RespiGam)
  - **Palivizumab (Synagis)**

Nursing Intervention

- ◑ Conduct continuous and thorough respiratory system assessments.
- ◑ Practice consistent handwashing and do not touch the mucous-secreting areas such as the nasal mucosa or conjunctiva.
- ◑ Assign isolation rooms to hospitalized patients.
- ◑ Nurses caring for patients with RSV bronchiolitis should not care for other patients who are considered high risk.

Nursing alert **Pregnant health-care providers should not care for a patient receiving ribavirin.**

CYSTIC FIBROSIS

What Went Wrong?

Cystic fibrosis (CF) is an inherited autosomal recessive trait disorder that affects the exocrine glands of the body. The condition is characterized by an alteration in sweat, electrolytes, and mucus production that leads to multisystem involvement. The white population experiences 95% of the occurrences.

Signs and Symptoms

The clinical symptoms vary widely and changes as the disease progresses. Chronic respiratory infections are persistently associated with CF. The majority of the patients also have some exocrine pancreatic insufficiency.

◑ Manifestations associated with respiratory infections:
- Cough
- Sputum production
- Hyperinflation of the alveoli
- Bronchiectasis
- Hemoptysis
- Pulmonary insufficiency

◑ Manifestations associated with gastrointestinal dysfunction:
- **Steatorrhea**
- Vitamin deficiencies A, D, E, and K
- Diabetes mellitus

➌ Test Results

◑ A quantitative sweat chloride test >60 mEq/L.
◑ Chest radiography
◑ Stool fat and enzyme analysis

➍ Treatment

◑ Chest physiotherapy (CPT)
◑ Postural drainage and percussion
◑ Exercise, deep breathing, and coughing
◑ Antimicrobial agents
- Inhaled antibiotics
- Intravenous antibiotics

◑ Oxygen therapy
◑ Replacement of pancreatic enzymes
◑ High-protein, high-caloric diet
◑ Salt supplementation during hot weather

➎ Nursing Interventions

◑ Pulmonary and gastrointestinal assessments
◑ Aerosol therapy
◑ Family education to prevent exacerbation of the disease
◑ Educating parents on chest physiotherapy and breathing exercises

RESPIRATORY DISTRESS SYNDROME

➊ What Went Wrong?

Premature infants born <36 weeks of gestation may develop respiratory distress syndrome or hyaline membrane disease (HMD) due to lack of **surfactant** to keep the alveoli open.

➋ Signs and Symptoms

◑ Breathing >60 breaths/minute
◑ Retractions (suprasternal and substernal)

- Grunting
- Nasal flaring
- Cyanosis
- Flaccidity

Test Results

- Diagnosis is based on infant's history, physical examination, lab results, and chest radiographs.
- Chest radiograph reveals fibrosis of the lungs.

Treatment

- Prenatal steroids
- Administration of exogenous surfactant
- Diuretics
- Bronchodilators
- Oxygen therapy

Nursing Interventions

- Ongoing physical examinations
- Observing and accessing the infant's response to respiratory therapy
- Monitoring pulse oximetry and arterial oxygen concentration
- Hyperventilation and suctioning when indicated

✔ ROUTINE CHECKUP 2

1. The nurse would know that which of the following would be appropriate for an infant diagnosed with staphylococcal pneumonia?
   a. Administer a course of antibiotics as prescribed.
   b. Intense intake and output measures to detect cardiac overload.
   c. Support the infant with intense antitussive therapy.
   d. Complete assessments hourly.

Answer:

2. An infant with bronchiolitis is hospitalized. The causative organism is respiratory syncytial virus (RSV). Which of the following would be an expected mode of treatment while hospitalized?
   a. Reverse isolation
   b. Airborne isolation
   c. Contact isolation
   d. Negative-pressure isolation

Answer:

SUDDEN INFANT DEATH SYNDROME

What Went Wrong?

No one cause has been identified for Sudden Infant Death Syndrome (SIDS) though several risk factors have been noted. The incidence of SIDS often peaks between 2-4 months of age with less than 5% of cases happening after 6 months of age. Breast fed infants have lower incidence of SIDS and the risk factors identified for SIDS occurence include:

- Sleeping on abdomen or with pillows or other soft materials around that could suffocate an infant
- Low birth weight infants
- Infants with low Apgar scores
- Exposure to tobacco smoke
- Respiratory disorders such as bronchopulmonary dysplasia
- Maternal habits such as smoking or drug use during pregnancy
- Central Nervous system abnormalities
- Male gender
- Possibly higher incidence in siblings of SIDS victims

Signs and Symptoms

- Unexplained death that occurs suddenly in an infant younger than one year of age
- Blood-tinged frothy fluid in mouth and nose
- Wet diaper that is full of stool indicating a devastating death experience
- Bedding may be greatly disturbed

Test Results

- Intrathoracic hemorrhage and pulmonary edema noted on autopsy

Treatment

- Avoid blaming or declaring that abuse, neglect, or wrong activity has occurred:
- Provide support to parents and family
- Autopsy will be ordered and performed

Nursing Interventions

- Parent and family discharge teaching after the birth of a child, particularly the birth of a sibling of a SIDS victim, related to methods of decreasing the risk factors for SIDS :
  - Stress "Back to Sleep" for infants to reinforce positioning of infant
  - Encourage removing pillows and loose linen from infant sleeping area
  - Encourage smoking cessation prior to pregnancy, during pregnancy, and after pregnancy in any area that would allow newborn exposure to smoke

- Promote good nutrition and prenatal care to promote health pregnancy and birth and decrease premature births
- ◐ Recognize the signs and symptoms of SIDS versus those of child abuse and

 Nursing alert **Avoid blaming or promoting guilt in the parents/guardians; avoid statements related to how the infant death could have been prevented**

- ◐ Reassure parents and family that the death could not have been predicted or prevented
- ◐ Reinforce the need for an autopsy to gain information about the death
- ◐ Arrange home followup for the family to help them with coping and handling guilt and greif
- ◐ Refer family to the national SIDS support group

CONCLUSION

The most common cause of illness in the infant and childhood population is an infection in the respiratory tract. Infections are described and treated according to areas of involvement. The upper respiratory tract involves the nose and pharynx. The lower respiratory tract consists of the epiglottis, larynx, and the trachea. These are the key points to remember:

- ◐ The common cold is referred to as acute viral nasopharyngitis and the prevalent symptom is fever.
- ◐ Illnesses of the upper respiratory tract frequently cause otitis media.
- ◐ Throat cultures positive for beta-hemolytic streptococci (GABHS) warrant antibiotic treatment.
- ◐ Untreated GABHS infections can lead to scarlet fever otitis media and suppurative infections of surrounding tissues.
- ◐ Constant swallowing after a tonsillectomy may indicate bleeding at the surgical site.
- ◐ Children with mild croup without stridor are managed at home with high cool humidity and increased fluids.
- ◐ If the airway is compromised due to epiglottitis, immediate attention is necessary and the nurse should prepare for intubation.
- ◐ The key difference between laryngotracheobronchitis (LTB) and epiglottitis is the presence of a cough in (LTB).
- ◐ When diagnosed with mononucleosis, patients should not participate in activities in which the patient may receive a blow to the abdomen.
- ◐ Viruses such as cytomegalovirus, influenza, adenovirus, and RSV are the most common causative agent for pneumonia in children.
- ◐ RSV is responsible for ≥80% cases of bronchiolitis in children.
- ◐ Pregnant health-care providers should not care for a patient receiving ribavirin.
- ◐ The quantitative sweat chloride test >60 mEq/L is used to diagnose cystic fibrosis.

? FINAL CHECKUP

1. **When caring for a child that has undergone a tonsillectomy, the nurse should do which of the following?**
   a. Observe for continuous swallowing.
   b. Encourage gargling with warm saline water.
   c. Apply warm compresses to the throat.
   d. Apply cold compresses to the throat.

2. **Which of the following statements best represents infectious mononucleosis?**
   a. Herpes simplex type 2.
   b. Leukopenia is often paired with the diagnosis.
   c. Amoxicillin is used to treat the pharyngitis.
   d. Physical assessment and blood test are used as test results to establish the diagnosis.

3. **A 3-year-old girl is seen in the emergency department. She has a croupy cough on inspiration, she is irritable, easily agitated, and drooling. She is most comfortable in the upright position. The nurse observes her and performs which of the following appropriate interventions?**
   a. Have her lie down in a more relaxed position.
   b. Use a tongue blade to examine her throat.
   c. Prepare the patient for a mist tent.
   d. Notify the physician and prepare for an emergency procedure.

4. **The nurse is assessing a child with croup and a sore throat in the ED. The child is drooling and agitated. The nurse should know that examining the child's throat using a tongue depressor might precipitate which of the following?**
   a. Profuse coughing
   b. Inspiratory stridor
   c. Complete obstruction
   d. Increased agitation

5. **The nurse allows the mother of a toddler with acute laryngotracheobronchitis to lie in the crib with the child. The nurse's rationale for this action is primarily which of the following?**
   a. Mothers of hospitalized toddlers often experience anxiety and extreme guilt.
   b. The mother's presence reduces anxiety and demands for oxygen thus reducing respiratory efforts.
   c. Separation anxiety is a major milestone to be accomplished in toddlerhood.
   d. The mother's assessment and report to the nurse is measurable in the respiratory assessment.

6. **An infant has been diagnosed with staphylococcal pneumonia. Nursing care of the child with pneumonia includes which of the following?**
   a. Administration of antibiotic
   b. Frequent complete assessment of the infant
   c. Round-the-clock administration of antitussive agents

7. A child has a chronic cough, no retractions but diffuse wheezing during the expiratory phase of respiration. This suggests which of the following?
   a. Asthma
   b. Pneumonia
   c. Croup
   d. Foreign body aspiration

8. Cystic fibrosis most often affects multiple systems of the body. The primary factor responsible for possible multiple clinical manifestations is which of the following?
   a. Hyperactivity of sweat glands
   b. Hypoactivity of parasympathetic nervous system
   c. Sweat chloride test >60 mEq/L
   d. Increased viscosity resulting in mucous gland secretions

9. Streptococcal pharyngitis should be treated with antibiotics to avoid which of the following?
   a. Otitis media
   b. Acute laryngitis
   c. Nephrotic syndrome
   d. Hemorrhagic fever

10. The causing agent for mononucleosis is which of the following?
   a. RSV
   b. Influenza
   c. Adenovirus
   d. Epstein-Barr

ANSWERS

Routine checkup 1
   1. c
   2. a

Routine checkup 2
   1. a
   2. b

Final checkup

1. a	2. d	3. d	4. c
5. b	6. a	7. a	8. d
9. a	10. d		

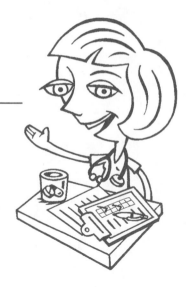

CHAPTER 6

Cardiovascular Conditions

Learning Objectives

At the end of the chapter, the student will be able to

1 Discuss the pediatric risk factors for disruption of cardiovascular function.

2 Discuss signs and symptoms related to cardiovascular conditions.

3 Evaluate diagnostic procedures associated with cardiovascular conditions.

4 Discuss treatment regimens associated with conditions of the cardiovascular system.

5 Teach and support parents regarding prophylactic care and the treatment and care required for a child with conditions of the heart and vasculature.

 KEY WORDS

β-Hemolytic streptococcus	Left-to-right shunt
Bradycardia	*Staphylococcus aureus*
Cardiac catheterization	Tachycardia
Digoxin	Tachypnea
Eisenmenger complex	

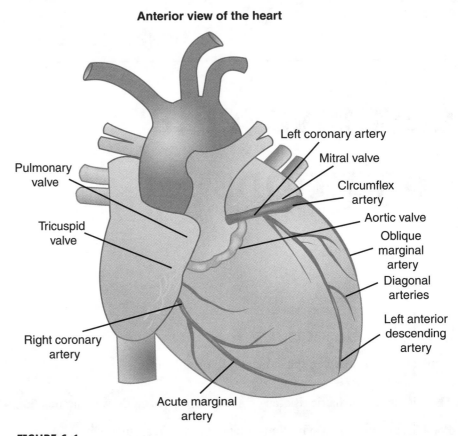

FIGURE 6-1

OVERVIEW

The heart is a hollow working muscle responsible for pumping blood through the body to provide oxygen and nutrients to the cells. A child's heart is about the size of his or her fist and beats faster than that of an adult. Heart rate slows from birth to adolescence when the rate is similar to the adult rate. The cardiovascular system includes the heart and blood vessels. The hematologic system involves the blood and organs that produce blood. Blood is needed to carry oxygen and nutrients to the cells and must be structurally sound and adequate in amount to ensure the health and proper functioning of the body.

The heart is a hollow muscle with four chambers: two atria and two ventricles. The right atria and ventricle receive blood from the body by way of the veins and the inferior and superior vena cava and move it to the lungs by way of the pulmonary arteries. The left atria and ventricle of the heart receive blood from the lungs and move blood out to the brain via the aorta and out to the arteries of the body. Valves, the aortic, pulmonary, mitral, and tricuspid, are

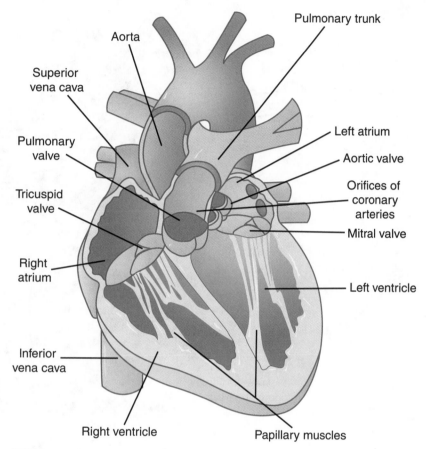

FIGURE 6-2A

in place between the chambers of the heart to prevent blood flow backward into the chamber after being pushed forward. The contraction of heart muscle is regulated by an electrical system that controls the speed at which the heart beats. If the tissues of the body require additional oxygen, the heart rate is increased.

CONGESTIVE HEART FAILURE

🔑 What Went Wrong?

Congestive heart failure (CHF) is the inability or failure of the cardiovascular system to provide adequate cardiac output to meet the metabolic demand of the body. CHF usually occurs secondary to congenital heart defects in which there are structural abnormalities leading to increased pressure or volume load to the ventricles.

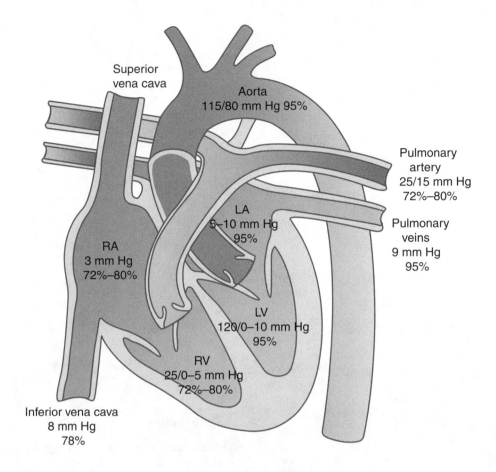

Superior
vena cava

Aorta
115/80 mm Hg 95%

Pulmonary
artery
25/15 mm Hg
72%–80%

Pulmonary
veins
9 mm Hg
95%

LA
5–10 mm Hg
95%

RA
3 mm Hg
72%–80%

LV
120/0–10 mm Hg
95%

RV
25/0–5 mm Hg
72%–80%

Inferior vena cava
8 mm Hg
78%

FIGURE 6-2B

The cause of congestive heart failure (CHF) can be classified as follows:

- Volume overload
- Pressure overload
- Decreased contractility
- High cardiac output demands

Signs and Symptoms

The signs and symptoms of CHF can be placed in three categories:

1. Impaired myocardial function
   Tachycardia
   Diaphoresis
   Poor perfusion
2. Pulmonary congestion
   Tachypnea

Mild cyanosis
Dyspnea
Costal retractions
Orthopnea
Wheezing
Cough
Hoarseness
Gasping and grunting respirations
3. Systemic venous congestion
Hepatomegaly
Edema
Weight gain
Ascites
Pleural effusions
Distended neck and peripheral veins

❸ Test Results

◐ Diagnosis is confirmed by child's clinical presentation:
- Dyspnea
- Retractions
- Tachypnea
- Activity intolerance

◐ The chest radiograph demonstrates cardiomegaly and increased pulmonary vascular markings.

◐ Electrocardiogram may reveal the etiology of CHF.

❹ Treatment

◐ Two groups of drugs are used to enhance myocardial integrity:
- Digitalis glycosides to improve contractility
- Angiotensin inhibitors to reduce the afterload on the heart

◐ Diuretic therapy is used to eliminate excess water and salt.

❺ Nursing Interventions

◐ Administer diuretic therapy.
◐ Assess heart rate, blood pressure, peripheral perfusion, excretion of urine.
◐ Assess for imbalanced nutrition.
◐ Evaluate for excessive fluid volume.
◐ Administer **digoxin.**
◐ Auscultate apical pulse.
◐ Administer digoxin when apical pulse is 90/70.
◐ Assess for vomiting that may be evidence of digoxin toxicity.
◐ Teach the caregiver the correct method to administer digoxin.

ATRIAL SEPTAL DEFECT

❶ What Went Wrong?

Atrial septal defect (ASD) is an abnormal opening between the atria that allows blood to flow from the left atrium into the right atrium. Left atrium pressure is slightly higher, which allows blood to flow from the left to right atrium. This abnormal blood flow causes

- Increase of oxygenated blood into the right atrium
- Right atrium and right ventricle enlargement

❷ Signs and Symptoms

- Patients are sometimes asymptomatic.
- ASD may precipitate CHF.
- A murmur characteristic of ASD is heard on auscultation.
- Increased pulmonary blood flow may lead to pulmonary vascular obstruction or emboli.

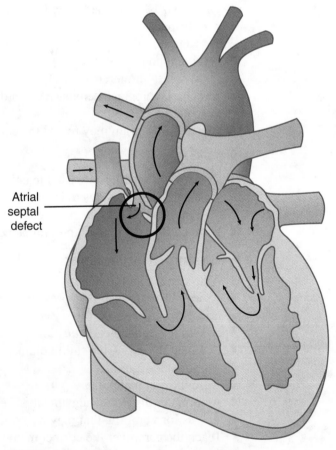

Atrial
septal
defect

FIGURE 6-3

③ Test Results

- **Cardiac catheterization:** Catheters are inserted into the heart via a large peripheral vein and advanced into the heart to measure pressures and oxygen levels in heart chambers and visualize heart structures and blood flow patterns. Reveals septal defect and any structural changes or defects.
- Pulse oximetry (SpO_2): Device used to evaluate the degree of oxygen saturation in the blood using a small infrared light probe. Oxygen level may be within normal range.
- Electrocardiogram: Detects normal electrical events and abnormal cardiac rhythms in the heart. Atrial septal defect is noted with right ventricular hypertrophy.
- Echocardiogram: Two-dimensional Doppler evaluation to detect evidence of valve leakage, cardiac anatomy, size, and function. Septal defect and ventricular hypertrophy are evident.

④ Treatment

- Treatment of choice is surgical patch closure.
- Open heart repair with cardiopulmonary bypass.
- ASD may require mitral valve replacement.

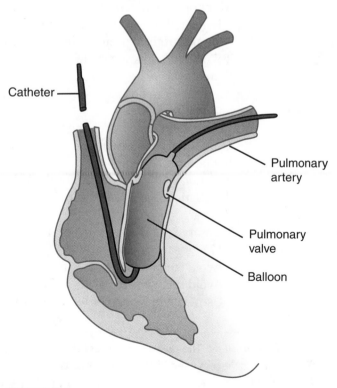

FIGURE 6-4

⑤ Nursing Interventions for Child Undergoing Cardiac Catheterization

◐ Prepare the patient for cardiac catheterization:
- Take complete nursing history.
- Patient must be NPO (*nil per os,* i.e., nothing by mouth) for 4 to 6 hours.
- Complete assessment including calculation of body surface area.
- Check for allergies; allergies to iodine, contrast dyes, and shellfish should be relayed to the physician prior to the procedure.
- Document baseline assessment of pedal pulses and pulse oximetry.
- Utilize child life specialists to alleviate anxiety for the child and family.
- Arrange a tour of the lab with the child if age appropriate.
- Explain specific aspects of the procedure such as the placement of the intravenous line and electrocardiogram (ECG) electrodes.
- Demonstrate how the skin will be washed with brown soap and how the skin will be numbed.
- Explain how the contrast affects the patient and how sedation will make the child feel.

◐ Care of the patient after cardiac catheterization:
- Monitor patient with cardiac monitor and pulse oximeter prior to discharge.
- Monitor the patient for
  ◦ Temperature and color distal to the catheter insertion site
  ◦ A pulse of the extremity distal to the catheter insertion site
- Take vital signs every 15 minutes for the first hour and hourly thereafter.
- Monitor for trends and assess for possible hypotension, tachycardia, and **bradycardia.**
- Check the pressure dressing for evidence of bleeding.
- Observe for bleeding at the insertion site or evidence of hematoma.
- Monitor intake and output for diuresis from contrast material.
- The patient and family should be provided with education upon discharge to
  ◦ Observe the site for signs of inflammation and infection.
  ◦ Monitor for fever.
  ◦ Avoid strenuous activities for a few days.
  ◦ Avoid tub baths for 48 to 72 hours.
  ◦ Use acetaminophen or ibuprofen for discomfort.

Nursing alert **The nurse should assess for latex allergies prior to catheterization. Some catheters used in the catheterization laboratory have latex balloons. If the child has a latex allergy, the balloon can precipitate a life-threatening reaction.**

Nursing alert **If bleeding occurs, apply direct continuous pressure 1 inch above the percutaneous skin site to localize pressure over the vessel puncture.**

Nursing Interventions for Child Undergoing Cardiac Surgery

◐ Provide preoperative care of the child undergoing cardiac surgery:
  - Make inquiries to parents and caregivers as to any questions they may have about the procedure.
  - Orient child and family to strange surrounding prior to surgery day.
  - Check chart for signed informed consent forms.
  - Check identification band with surgical personnel to ensure identity.
  - Ensure side rails are securely fastened.
  - Use restraints for transport.
  - Check laboratory values for signs of systemic alterations.
  - Bathe and groom the child.
  - Provide mouth care for comfort while NPO.
  - Cleanse operative site with prescribed method.
  - Administer antibiotics as ordered.
  - Remove jewelry, makeup, and prosthetics as needed.
  - Check for loose teeth.
  - Institute preoperative teaching to reduce anxiety.
  - Prepare child and family for postoperative procedures such as nasogastric tube, wound care, and monitoring apparatus.
  - Administer preoperative sedation.

◐ Provide postoperative care for the child undergoing cardiac surgery:
  - Make sure child is in safe position of comfort according to the physician's order.
  - Perform stat (from Latin *statim*, "immediately") orders.
  - Use proper handwashing.
  - Assess wound for bleeding and signs of infection.
  - Provide appropriate wound care.
  - Assess breath sounds.
  - Perform neurologic checks.
  - Take frequent vital signs.
  - Administer fluids to prevent hypotension.
  - Monitor fluids losses through chest tube.
  - Administer pharmacologic support as ordered.
  - Monitor electrolytes and supplement with infusion as ordered.
  - Administer sedatives and analgesics for comfort.
  - Allow caregivers to visit as soon as possible.

• Explain procedures and equipment to caregivers.
• Encourage caregivers to ask questions.
• Involve child life specialist and social services in the care to support the child and family.

ROUTINE CHECKUP 1

1. Beverly, age 5, is scheduled for a cardiac catheterization. What behavior would be appropriate for to do when teaching preoperatively?
   a. Direct teaching to her parents because she is too young to understand.
   b. Blend your approach to her level of development so that she can understand.
   c. Teach parent and Beverly several days before the procedure so they will be prepared.
   d. Give exact details of all the procedures so she will know what to expect.

Answer:

2. After cardiac catheterization, the nurse monitors the child's vital signs. The heart rate should be counted for how many seconds?
   a. 15
   b. 30
   c. 60
   d. 120

Answer:

VENTRICULAR SEPTAL DEFECT

What Went Wrong?

A ventricular septal defect (VSD) is an abnormal opening causing complications between the right and left ventricles. The defect may vary in size from a pinhole to the actual absence of the septum.

Signs and Symptoms

  ◑ Blood flows from the left ventricle into the pulmonary artery.
  ◑ Increased pulmonary blood flow and increased pulmonary resistance.
  ◑ CHF.
  ◑ In severe cases, patient may develop **Eisenmenger syndrome**.

Test Results

  ◑ Cardiac catheterization: Catheters are inserted into the heart via a large peripheral vein and advanced into the heart to measure pressures and

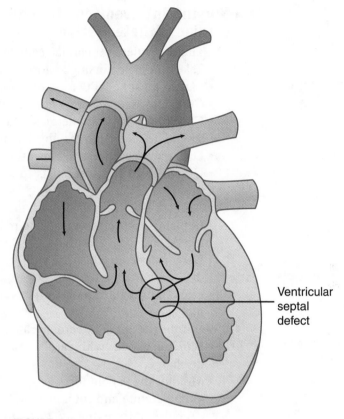

FIGURE 6-5

oxygen levels in the heart chambers and visualize heart structures and blood flow patterns. Ventricular defects and cardiomegaly will be evident.

- Pulse oximetry (Spo$_2$): Device used to evaluate the degree of oxygen saturation in the blood using a small infrared light probe. Oxygen saturation will be decreased.
- Electrocardiogram: Detects normal electrical events and abnormal cardiac rhythms in the heart. Signs of cardiomegaly noted.
- Echocardiogram: Two-dimensional Doppler evaluation to detect evidence of valve leakage, cardiac anatomy, size, and function. Septal defect, cardiomegaly and altered cardiac function noted.

4 Treatment

- Palliative approach includes pulmonary artery banding (band around the pulmonary artery).
- Complete surgical repair is the treatment of choice:
  - Pursestring technique for small defects
  - Dacron patch for larger openings

Nursing Interventions for Child Undergoing Cardiac Catheterization

◐ Prepare the patient for cardiac catheterization:
- Take complete nursing history.
- Patient must be NPO for 4 to 6 hours.
- Complete assessment including calculation of body surface area.
- Check for allergies; allergies to iodine, contrast dyes, and shellfish should be relayed to the physician prior to the procedure.
- Document baseline assessment of pedal pulses and pulse oximetry.
- Utilize child life specialists to alleviate anxiety for the child and family.
- Arrange a tour of the lab with the child if age appropriate.
- Explain specific aspects of the procedure such as the placement of the IV and ECG electrodes.
- Demonstrate how the skin will be washed with brown soap and how the skin will be numbed.
- Explain how the contrast affects the patient and how sedation will make the child feel.

◐ Care of the patient after cardiac catheterization:
- Monitor patient with cardiac monitor and pulse oximeter prior to discharge.
- Monitor the patient for
  ○ Temperature and color distal to the catheter insertion site
  ○ A pulse of the extremity distal to the catheter insertion site
- Take vital signs every 15 minutes for the first hour and hourly thereafter.
- Monitor for trends and assess for possible hypotension, tachycardia, and bradycardia.
- Check the pressure dressing for evidence of bleeding.
- Observe for bleeding at the insertion site or evidence of hematoma.
- Monitor intake and output for diuresis from contrast material.
- The patient and family should be provided with education upon discharge to
  ○ Observe the site for signs of inflammation and infection.
  ○ Monitor for fever.
  ○ Avoid strenuous activities for a few days.
  ○ Avoid tub baths for 48 to 72 hours.
  ○ Use acetaminophen or ibuprofen for discomfort.

Nursing Interventions for Child Undergoing Cardiac Surgery

◐ Provide preoperative care of the child undergoing cardiac surgery.
- Make inquiries to parents and caregivers as to any questions they may have about the procedure.
- Orient child and family to strange surrounding prior to surgery day.

- Check chart for signed informed consent forms.
- Check identification band with surgical personnel to ensure identity.
- Ensure side rails are securely fastened.
- Use restraints for transport.
- Check laboratory values for signs of systemic alterations.
- Bathe and groom the child.
- Provide mouth care for comfort while NPO.
- Cleanse operative site with prescribed method.
- Administer antibiotics as ordered.
- Remove jewelry, makeup, and prosthetics as needed.
- Check for loose teeth.
- Institute preoperative teaching to reduce anxiety.
- Prepare child and family for postoperative procedures such as nasogastric tube, wound care, and monitoring apparatus.
- Administer preoperative sedation.

◐ Provide postoperative care for the child undergoing cardiac surgery:

- Make sure child is in safe position of comfort according to the physician's order.
- Perform stat orders.
- Use proper handwashing.
- Assess wound for bleeding and signs of infection.
- Provide appropriate wound care.
- Assess breath sounds.
- Perform neurological checks.
- Take frequent vital signs.
- Administer fluids to prevent hypotension.
- Monitor fluids losses through chest tube.
- Administer pharmacologic support as ordered.
- Monitor electrolytes and supplement with infusion as ordered.
- Administer sedatives and analgesics for comfort.
- Allow caregivers to visit as soon as possible.
- Explain procedures and equipment to caregivers.
- Encourage caregivers to ask questions.
- Involve child life specialist and social services in the care to support the child and family.

PATENT DUCTUS ARTERIOSUS

⬤ What Went Wrong?

Patent ductus arteriosus (PDA) occurs when the artery connecting the aorta and the pulmonary artery in fetal circulation fails to close during the first few weeks of life. The continued patency allows blood from the aorta to flow back

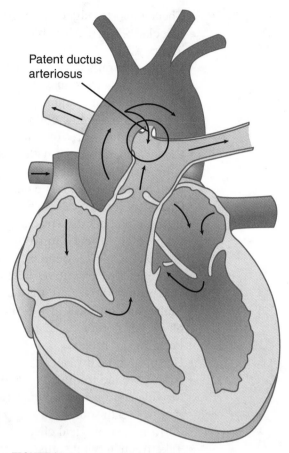

Patent ductus arteriosus

FIGURE 6-6

to the pulmonary artery resulting in a **left-to-right shunt.** This altered circulation causes

    ◑ Increased workload on the left side of the heart

    ◑ Pulmonary congestion and resistance

    ◑ Right ventricular hypertrophy

❷ Signs and Symptoms

    ◑ Patient may be asymptomatic.

    ◑ Characteristics of CHF.

❸ Test Results

    ◑ Cardiac catheterization: Catheters are inserted into the heart via a large peripheral vein and advanced into the heart to measure pressures and oxygen levels in the heart chambers and visualize heart structures and blood flow patterns. Patent ductus and right ventricular hypertrophy evident.

- Pulse oximetry (Spo$_2$): Device used to evaluate the degree of oxygen saturation in the blood using a small infrared light probe. Oxygen saturation decreased.
- Electrocardiogram: Detects electrical events normal and abnormal cardiac rhythms in the heart. Signs of ventricular hypertrophy noted.
- Echocardiogram: Two-dimensional Doppler evaluation to detect evidence of valve leakage, cardiac anatomy, size, and function. Septal defects and ventricular hypertrophy noted.

4 Treatment

The palliative approach includes
- Administration of indomethacin (prostaglandin inhibitor)
- Application of coils to occlude the PDA

Surgical treatment includes ligation and clipping of the patent vessel.

5 Nursing Interventions for Child Undergoing Cardiac Catheterization

- Prepare the patient for cardiac catheterization:
  - Take complete nursing history.
  - Patient must be NPO for 4 to 6 hours.
  - Complete assessment including calculation of body surface area.
  - Check for allergies; allergies to iodine, contrast dyes, and shellfish should be relayed to the physician prior to the procedure.
  - Document baseline assessment of pedal pulses and pulse oximetry.
  - Utilize child life specialists to alleviate anxiety for the child and family.
  - Arrange a tour of the lab with the child if age appropriate.
  - Explain specific aspects of the procedure such as the placement of the IV and ECG electrodes.
  - Demonstrate how the skin will be washed with brown soap and how the skin will be numbed.
  - Explain how the contrast affects the patient and how sedation will make the child feel.
- Care of the patient after cardiac catheterization:
  - Monitor patient with cardiac monitor and pulse oximeter prior to discharge.
  - Monitor the patient for
    - Temperature and color distal to the catheter insertion site
    - A pulse of the extremity distal to the catheter insertion site
  - Take vital signs every 15 minutes for the first hour and hourly thereafter.
  - Monitor for trends and assess for possible hypotension, tachycardia, and bradycardia.
  - Check the pressure dressing for evidence of bleeding.
  - Observe for bleeding at the insertion site or evidence of hematoma.

• Monitor intake and output for diuresis from contrast material.
      • The patient and family should be provided with education upon discharge to
        ○ Observe the site for signs of inflammation and infection.
        ○ Monitor for fever.
        ○ Avoid strenuous activities for a few days.
        ○ Avoid tub baths for 48 to 72 hours.
        ○ Use acetaminophen or ibuprofen for discomfort.

🔑 Nursing Interventions for Child Undergoing Cardiac Surgery

◑ Provide preoperative care of the child undergoing cardiac surgery:
      • Make inquiries to parents and caregivers as to any questions they may have about the procedure.
      • Orient child and family to strange surrounding prior to surgery day.
      • Check chart for signed informed consent forms.
      • Check identification band with surgical personnel to ensure identity.
      • Ensure side rails are securely fastened.
      • Use restraints for transport.
      • Check laboratory values for signs of systemic alterations.
      • Bathe and groom the child.
      • Provide mouth care for comfort while NPO.
      • Cleanse operative site with prescribed method.
      • Administer antibiotics as ordered.
      • Remove jewelry, makeup, and prosthetics as needed.
      • Check for loose teeth.
      • Institute preoperative teaching to reduce anxiety.
      • Prepare child and family for postoperative procedures such as nasogastric tube, wound care, and monitoring apparatus.
      • Administer preoperative sedation.
◑ Provide postoperative care for the child undergoing cardiac surgery:
      • Safe position of comfort.
      • Perform stat orders.
      • Use proper handwashing.
      • Assess wound for bleeding and signs of infection.
      • Provide appropriate wound care.
      • Assess breath sounds.
      • Perform neurologic checks.
      • Take frequent vital signs.
      • Administer fluids to prevent hypotension.
      • Monitor fluids losses through chest tube.
      • Administer pharmacologic support as ordered.
      • Monitor electrolytes and supplement with infusion as ordered.
      • Administer sedatives and analgesics for comfort.

• Allow caregivers to visit as soon as possible.
• Explain procedures and equipment to caregivers.
• Encourage caregivers to ask questions.
• Involve child life specialist and social services in the care to support the child and family.

 ROUTINE CHECKUP 2

1. A chest radiograph will be ordered for which of the following purposes?
   a. Display the bones of chest and vessels of the heart.
   b. Evaluate the vascular anatomy outside of the heart.
   c. Show a graph of the electrical activity of the heart.
   d. Determine heart size and pulmonary blood flow patterns.

Answer:

2. Surgery for patent ductus arteriosus (PDA) prevents which of the following complications?
   a. Cyanosis
   b. Pulmonary vascular congestion
   c. Decreased workload on left side of heart
   d. Left-to-right shunt of blood

Answer:

COARCTATION OF THE AORTA

① What Went Wrong?

Coarctation of the aorta (COA) is a narrowing located near the insertion of the ductus arteriosus. This alteration results in

◐ Increased pressure in the head and neck area
◐ Decreased pressure distal to the obstruction in the body and lower extremities

② Sign and Symptoms

◐ High blood pressure and bounding pulses in the upper extremities.
◐ Lower extremities cool with decreased pulses and blood pressure.
◐ Symptoms of CHF.

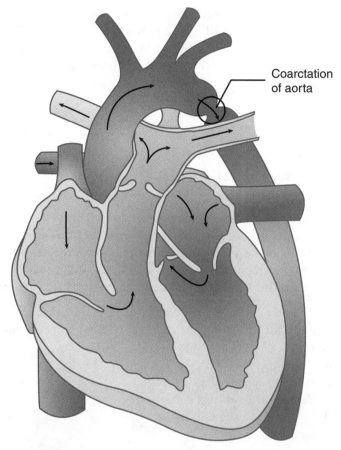

Coarctation
of aorta

FIGURE 6-7

○ Hypertension.
○ Older children experience headaches, fainting, and epistaxis.

❸ Test Results

○ Cardiac catheterization: Catheters are inserted into the heart via a large peripheral vein and advanced into the heart to measure pressures and oxygen levels in heart chambers and visualize heart structures and blood flow patterns. Reveals location of aortic narrowing and VSD or PDA if present.
○ Pulse oximetry (Spo_2): Device used to evaluate the degree of oxygen saturation in the blood using a small infrared light probe. May be normal or decreased if CHF is present.
○ Electrocardiogram: Detects electrical events normal and abnormal cardiac rhythm in the heart. Signs of right and left ventricular hypertrophy noted.
○ Echocardiogram: Two-dimensional Doppler evaluation to detect evidence of valve leakage, cardiac anatomy, size, and function.

④ Treatment
- Balloon angioplasty
- Resection of the coarcted portion with end-to-end anastomosis of the aorta
- Enlargement of the constricted section by a graft prosthetic

⑤ Nursing Interventions for Child Undergoing Cardiac Catheterization
- Prepare the patient for cardiac catheterization:
  - Take complete nursing history.
  - Patient must be NPO for 4 to 6 hours.
  - Complete assessment including calculation of body surface area.
  - Check for allergies; allergies to iodine, contrast dyes, and shellfish should be relayed to the physician prior to the procedure.
  - Document baseline assessment of pedal pulses and pulse oximetry.
  - Utilize child life specialists to alleviate anxiety for the child and family.
  - Arrange a tour of the lab with the child if age appropriate.
  - Explain specific aspects of the procedure such as the placement of the IV and ECG electrodes.
  - Demonstrate how the skin will be washed with brown soap and how the skin will be numbed.
  - Explain how the contrast affects the patient and how sedation will make the child feel.
- Care of the patient after cardiac catheterization:
  - Monitor patient with cardiac monitor and pulse oximeter prior to discharge.
  - Monitor the patient for
    - Temperature and color distal to the catheter insertion site
    - A pulse of the extremity distal to the catheter insertion site
  - Take vital signs every 15 minutes for the first hour and hourly thereafter.
  - Monitor for trends and assess for possible hypotension, tachycardia, and bradycardia.
  - Check the pressure dressing for evidence of bleeding.
  - Observe for bleeding at the insertion site or evidence of hematoma.
  - Monitor intake and output for diuresis from contrast material.
  - The patient and family should be provided with education upon discharge to
    - Observe the site for signs of inflammation and infection
    - Monitor for fever
    - Avoid strenuous activities for a few days
    - Avoid tub baths for 48 to 72 hours
    - Use acetaminophen or ibuprofen for discomfort

❺ Nursing Interventions for Child Undergoing Cardiac Surgery

◑ Provide preoperative care of the child undergoing cardiac surgery:
  - Make inquiries to parents and caregivers as to any questions they may have about the procedure.
  - Orient child and family to strange surrounding prior to surgery day.
  - Check chart for signed informed consent forms.
  - Check identification band with surgical personnel to ensure identity.
  - Ensure side rails are securely fastened.
  - Use restraints for transport.
  - Check laboratory values for signs of systemic alterations.
  - Bathe and groom the child.
  - Provide mouth care for comfort while NPO.
  - Cleanse operative site with prescribed method.
  - Administer antibiotics as ordered.
  - Remove jewelry, makeup, and prosthetics as needed.
  - Check for loose teeth.
  - Institute preoperative teaching to reduce anxiety.
  - Prepare child and family for postoperative procedures such as nasogastric tube, wound care, and monitoring apparatus.
  - Administer preoperative sedation.

◑ Provide postoperative care for the child undergoing cardiac surgery:
  - Make sure child is in safe position of comfort according to the physician's order.
  - Perform stat orders.
  - Use proper handwashing.
  - Assess wound for bleeding and signs of infection.
  - Provide appropriate wound care.
  - Assess breath sounds.
  - Perform neurologic checks.
  - Take frequent vital signs.
  - Administer fluids to prevent hypotension.
  - Monitor fluids losses through chest tube.
  - Administer pharmacologic support as ordered.
  - Monitor electrolytes and supplement with infusion as ordered.
  - Administer sedatives and analgesics for comfort.
  - Allow caregivers to visit as soon as possible.
  - Explain procedures and equipment to caregivers.
  - Encourage caregivers to ask questions.
  - Involve child life specialist and social services in the care to support the child and family.

AORTIC STENOSIS

❶ What Went Wrong?

Aortic stenosis (AS) is a narrowing or a stricture of the aortic valve that results in

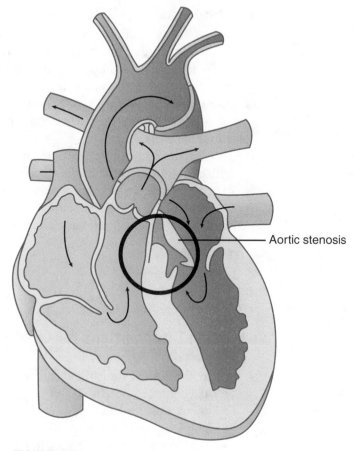
Aortic stenosis

FIGURE 6-8

- Resistance to blood flow in the left ventricle
- Decreased cardiac output
- Left ventricular hypertrophy
- Pulmonary venous and pulmonary arterial hypertension

The hallmark result of AS is hypertrophy of the left ventricular wall, which leads to increased end-diastolic pressure and pulmonary hypertension.

Signs and Symptoms

- Faint pulses
- Hypotension
- Tachycardia
- Poor feeding
- Exercise intolerance
- Chest pain
- Dizziness
- Characteristic murmur

3 Test Results

- Cardiac catheterization: Catheters are inserted into the heart via a large peripheral vein and advanced into the heart to measure pressures and oxygen levels in heart chambers and visualize heart structures and blood flow patterns. Reveals septal defect and left ventricular hypertrophy.
- Pulse oximetry (Spo_2): Device used to evaluate the degree of oxygen saturation in the blood using a small infrared light probe. Decreased oxygen saturation levels.
- Electrocardiogram: Detects electrical events normal and abnormal cardiac rhythm in the heart. Evidence of ventricular hypertrophy.
- Echocardiogram: Two-dimensional Doppler evaluation to detect evidence of valve leakage, cardiac anatomy, size, and function. Reveals Aortic stenosis and any other cardiac defects.

4 Treatment

- Balloon angioplasty
- Excision of a membrane
- Cutting of the fibromuscular ring

5 Nursing Interventions for Child Undergoing Cardiac Catheterization

- Prepare the patient for cardiac catheterization:
  - Take complete nursing history.
  - Patient must be NPO for 4 to 6 hours.
  - Complete assessment including calculation of body surface area.
  - Check for allergies; allergies to iodine, contrast dyes, and shellfish should be relayed to the physician prior to the procedure.
  - Document baseline assessment of pedal pulses and pulse oximetry.
  - Utilize child life specialists to alleviate anxiety for the child and family.
  - Arrange a tour of the lab with the child if age appropriate.
  - Explain specific aspects of the procedure such as the placement of the IV and ECG electrodes.
  - Demonstrate how the skin will be washed with brown soap and how the skin will be numbed.
  - Explain how the contrast affects the patient and how sedation will make the child feel.
- Care of the patient after cardiac catheterization:
  - Monitor patient with cardiac monitor and pulse oximeter prior to discharge.
  - Monitor the patient for
    - Temperature and color distal to the catheter insertion site
    - A pulse of the extremity distal to the catheter insertion site
  - Take vital signs every 15 minutes for the first hour and hourly thereafter.

- Monitor for trends and assess for possible hypotension, tachycardia, and bradycardia.
- Check the pressure dressing for evidence of bleeding.
- Observe for bleeding at the insertion site or evidence of hematoma.
- Monitor intake and output for diuresis from contrast material.
- The patient and family should be provided with education upon discharge to
  - Observe the site for signs of inflammation and infection.
  - Monitor for fever.
  - Avoid strenuous activities for a few days.
  - Avoid tub baths for 48 to 72 hours.
  - Use acetaminophen or ibuprofen for discomfort.

5 Nursing Interventions for Child Undergoing Cardiac Surgery

○ Provide preoperative care of the child undergoing cardiac surgery:
  - Make inquiries to parents and caregivers as to any questions they may have about the procedure.
  - Orient child and family to strange surrounding prior to surgery day.
  - Check chart for signed informed consent forms.
  - Check identification band with surgical personnel to ensure identity.
  - Ensure side rails are securely fastened.
  - Use restraints for transport.
  - Check laboratory values for signs of systemic alterations.
  - Bathe and groom the child.
  - Provide mouth care for comfort while NPO.
  - Cleanse operative site with prescribed method.
  - Administer antibiotics as ordered.
  - Remove jewelry, makeup, and prosthetics as needed.
  - Check for loose teeth.
  - Institute preoperative teaching to reduce anxiety.
  - Prepare child and family for postoperative procedures such as nasogastric tube, wound care, and monitoring apparatus.
  - Administer preoperative sedation.
○ Provide postoperative care for the child undergoing cardiac surgery:
  - Make sure child is in safe position of comfort according to the physician's order.
  - Perform stat orders.
  - Use proper handwashing.
  - Assess wound for bleeding and signs of infection.
  - Provide appropriate wound care.
  - Assess breath sounds.
  - Perform neurologic checks.

- Take frequent vital signs.
- Administer fluids to prevent hypotension.
- Monitor fluids losses through chest tube.
- Administer pharmacologic support as ordered.
- Monitor electrolytes and supplement with infusion as ordered.
- Administer sedatives and analgesics for comfort.
- Allow caregivers to visit as soon as possible.
- Explain procedures and equipment to caregivers.
- Encourage caregivers to ask questions.
- Involve child life specialist and social services in the care to support the child and family.

TETRALOGY OF FALLOT

What Went Wrong?

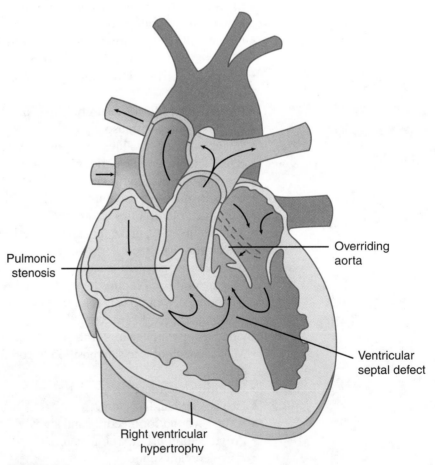

FIGURE 6-9

The classic form of tetralogy of Fallot (TOF) has four defects:
- Ventricular septal defect
- Pulmonic stenosis
- Overriding aorta
- Right ventricular hypertrophy

❷ Signs and Symptoms
- Cyanosis
- Hypoxia
- Anoxic spells when infant's oxygen supply exceeds blood supply

❸ Test Results
- Cardiac catheterization: Catheters are inserted into the heart via a large peripheral vein and advanced into the heart to measure pressures and oxygen levels in heart chambers and visualize heart structures and blood flow patterns. Reveals the four defects.
- Pulse oximetry (Spo_2): Device used to evaluate the degree of oxygen saturation in the blood using a small infrared light probe. Decreased according to degree of deoxygenation.
- Electrocardiogram: Detects electrical events normal and abnormal cardiac rhythm in the heart. Signs of right ventricular hypertrophy noted.
- Echocardiogram: Two-dimensional Doppler evaluation to detect evidence of valve leakage, cardiac anatomy, size, and function. The four defects are revealed.

❹ Treatment
- Blalock-Taussig procedure to increase pulmonary blood flow
- Complete repair by
  - Closing the VSD
  - Resectioning the infundibular stenosis
  - Enlarging the right ventricular outflow tract

❺ Nursing Interventions for Child Undergoing Cardiac Catheterization
- Prepare the patient for cardiac catheterization:
  - Take complete nursing history.
  - Patient must be NPO for 4 to 6 hours.
  - Complete assessment including calculation of body surface area.
  - Check for allergies; allergies to iodine, contrast dyes, and shellfish should be relayed to the physician prior to the procedure.
  - Document baseline assessment of pedal pulses and pulse oximetry.
  - Utilize child life specialists to alleviate anxiety for the child and family.
  - Arrange a tour of the lab with the child if age appropriate.

- Explain specific aspects of the procedure such as the placement of the IV and ECG electrodes.
- Demonstrate how the skin will be washed with brown soap and how the skin will be numbed.
- Explain how the contrast affects the patient and how sedation will make the child feel.

○ Care of the patient after cardiac catheterization:

- Monitor patient with cardiac monitor and pulse oximeter prior to discharge.
- Monitor the patient for
  ○ Temperature and color distal to the catheter insertion site
  ○ A pulse of the extremity distal to the catheter insertion site
- Take vital signs every 15 minutes for the first hour and hourly thereafter.
- Monitor for trends and assess for possible hypotension, tachycardia, and bradycardia.
- Check the pressure dressing for evidence of bleeding.
- Observe for bleeding at the insertion site or evidence of hematoma.
- Monitor intake and output for diuresis from contrast material.
- The patient and family should be provided with education upon discharge to
  ○ Observe the site for signs of inflammation and infection.
  ○ Monitor for fever.
  ○ Avoid strenuous activities for a few days.
  ○ Avoid tub baths for 48 to 72 hours.
  ○ Use acetaminophen or ibuprofen for discomfort.

⑤ Nursing Interventions for Child Undergoing Cardiac Surgery

○ Provide preoperative care of the child undergoing cardiac surgery:

- Make inquiries to parents and caregivers as to any questions they may have about the procedure.
- Orient child and family to strange surrounding prior to surgery day.
- Check chart for signed informed consent forms.
- Check identification band with surgical personnel to ensure identity.
- Ensure side rails are securely fastened.
- Use restraints for transport.
- Check laboratory values for signs of systemic alterations.
- Bathe and groom the child.
- Provide mouth care for comfort while NPO.
- Cleanse operative site with prescribed method.
- Administer antibiotics as ordered.
- Remove jewelry, makeup, and prosthetics as needed.
- Check for loose teeth.

- Institute preoperative teaching to reduce anxiety.
- Prepare child and family for postoperative procedures such as naso-gastric tube, wound care, and monitoring apparatus.
- Administer preoperative sedation.

◑ Provide postoperative care for the child undergoing cardiac surgery:

- Make sure child is in safe position of comfort according to the physician's order.
- Perform stat orders.
- Use proper handwashing.
- Assess wound for bleeding and signs of infection.
- Provide appropriate wound care.
- Assess breath sounds.
- Perform neurologic checks.
- Take frequent vital signs.
- Administer fluids to prevent hypotension.
- Monitor fluids losses through chest tube.
- Administer pharmacologic support as ordered.
- Monitor electrolytes and supplement with infusion as ordered.
- Administer sedatives and analgesics for comfort.
- Allow caregivers to visit as soon as possible.
- Explain procedures and equipment to caregivers.
- Encourage caregivers to ask questions.
- Involve child life specialist and social services in the care to support the child and family.

TRANSPOSITION OF GREAT ARTERIES

➊ What Went Wrong?

◑ In transposition of great arteries (TGA), the pulmonary artery rises from the left ventricle and the aorta exists from the right ventricle.

◑ There is no communication between the systemic and pulmonary circulation.

◑ Life is sustained due to defects associated with the TGA.

◑ The common defects are patent ductus arterious and ventricular septal defects.

➋ Signs and Symptoms

◑ Severely cyanotic

◑ Characteristics of CHF

➌ Test Results

◑ Cardiac catheterization: Catheters are inserted into the heart via a large peripheral vein and advanced into the heart to measure pressures and oxygen levels in heart chambers and visualize heart structures and blood

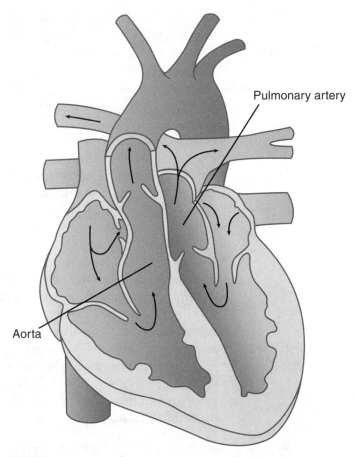

Pulmonary artery

Aorta

FIGURE 6-10

flow patterns. Reveals vessel transposition and septal defects and cardiomegaly.

- Pulse oximetry (Spo$_2$): Device used to evaluate the degree of oxygen saturation in the blood using a small infrared light probe. Oxygen saturation levels are low
- Electrocardiogram: Detects electrical events normal and abnormal cardiac rhythm in the heart. May be normal for newborn and later show signs of ventricular hypertrophy
- Echocardiogram: Two-dimensional Doppler evaluation to detect evidence of valve leakage, cardiac anatomy, size, and function. Will reveal vessel transposition and septal defects.

Treatment

- Intravenous prostaglandin E to increase blood mixing so that oxygen saturation if $\geq 75\%$.

◐ Atrial septostomy (Rashkind procedure) performed during catheterization to increase mixing and maintain cardiac output.
◐ Arterial switch procedure to connect the main artery to the proximal aorta and the ascending aorta to the proximal pulmonary artery.
◐ Coronary arteries are switched from the proximal aorta to the proximal pulmonary artery, which creates a new aorta.

5 Nursing Interventions for Child Undergoing Cardiac Catheterization

◐ Prepare the patient for cardiac catheterization:
  • Take complete nursing history.
  • Patient must be NPO for 4 to 6 hours.
  • Complete assessment including calculation of body surface area.
  • Check for allergies; allergies to iodine, contrast dyes, and shellfish should be relayed to the physician prior to the procedure.
  • Document baseline assessment of pedal pulses and pulse oximetry.
  • Utilize child life specialists to alleviate anxiety for the child and family.
  • Arrange a tour of the lab with the child if age appropriate.
  • Explain specific aspects of the procedure such as the placement of the IV and ECG electrodes.
  • Demonstrate how the skin will be washed with brown soap and how the skin will be numbed.
  • Explain how the contrast affects the patient and how sedation will make the child feel.

◐ Care of the patient after cardiac catheterization:
  • Monitor patient with cardiac monitor and pulse oximeter prior to discharge.
  • Monitor the patient for
    ○ Temperature and color distal to the catheter insertion site
    ○ A pulse of the extremity distal to the catheter insertion site
  • Take vital signs every 15 minutes for the first hour and hourly thereafter.
  • Monitor for trends and assess for possible hypotension, tachycardia, and bradycardia.
  • Check the pressure dressing for evidence of bleeding.
  • Observe for bleeding at the insertion site or evidence of hematoma.
  • Monitor intake and output for diuresis from contrast material.
  • The patient and family should be provided with education upon discharge to:
    ○ Observe the site for signs of inflammation and infection.
    ○ Monitor for fever.
    ○ Avoid strenuous activities for a few days.

○ Avoid tub baths for 48 to 72 hours.

○ Use acetaminophen or ibuprofen for discomfort.

Nursing Interventions for Child Undergoing Cardiac Surgery

◑ Provide preoperative care of the child undergoing cardiac surgery:

- Make inquiries to parents and caregivers as to any questions they may have about the procedure.
- Orient child and family to strange surrounding prior to surgery day.
- Check chart for signed informed consent forms.
- Check identification band with surgical personnel to ensure identity.
- Ensure side rails are securely fastened.
- Use restraints for transport.
- Check laboratory values for signs of systemic alterations.
- Bathe and groom the child.
- Provide mouth care for comfort while NPO.
- Cleanse operative site with prescribed method.
- Administer antibiotics as ordered.
- Remove jewelry, makeup, and prosthetics as needed.
- Check for loose teeth.
- Institute preoperative teaching to reduce anxiety.
- Prepare child and family for postoperative procedures such as nasogastric tube, wound care, and monitoring apparatus.
- Administer preoperative sedation.

◑ Provide postoperative care for the child undergoing cardiac surgery:

- Make sure child is in safe position of comfort according to the physician's order.
- Perform stat orders.
- Use proper handwashing.
- Assess wound for bleeding and signs of infection.
- Provide appropriate wound care.
- Assess breath sounds.
- Perform neurologic checks.
- Take frequent vital signs.
- Administer fluids to prevent hypotension.
- Monitor fluids losses through chest tube.
- Administer pharmacologic support as ordered.
- Monitor electrolytes and supplement with infusion as ordered.
- Administer sedatives and analgesics for comfort.
- Allow caregivers to visit as soon as possible.
- Explain procedures and equipment to caregivers.
- Encourage caregivers to ask questions.
- Involve child life specialist and social services in the care to support the child and family.

BACTERIAL ENDOCARDITIS

1 What Went Wrong?

Bacterial endocarditis (BE) is an infection of the valves and inner lining of the heart. It mostly affects children with

- Valvular abnormalities
- Prosthetic valves
- Ventricular septal defects
- Patent ductus arteriosus
- Tetralogy of Fallot
- Rheumatic heart disease

The most common causing agent is

- *Streptococcus viridans*
- *Staphylococcus aureus*
- Gram-negative bacteria

2 Signs and Symptoms

- Slow-onset low-grade intermittent fever
- Malaise
- Myalgias
- Arthralgias
- Headache
- Diaphoresis
- Weight loss

3 Test Results

- Growth of organism and identification of causative agent

4 Treatment

- High-dose antibiotics such as ampicillin, methicillin, cloxacillin, streptomycin, or gentamicin
- Blood cultures often used to identify organism

5 Nursing Intervention

- Counsel parents for the need of prophylactic antibiotic therapy before procedures and dental work.
- Counsel children to maintain good oral health to avoid infections from oral cavities.
- Teach patient and family to notify physician of any in behavior such as
  - Lethargy
  - Malaise
  - Anorexia
  - Extensive hospitalization for parenteral therapy.

RHEUMATIC FEVER

1 What Went Wrong?

Rheumatic fever (RF) is an inflammatory disease that occurs after an infection with group A **β-hemolytic streptococcal** pharyngitis. The illness is self-limited and involves

- Joints, skin, brain, serous surfaces, and heart.
- Cardiac valve damage is the most significant complication.

2 Signs and Symptoms

- Lesions called Aschoff bodies
- Carditis involving the endocardium , pericardium, and myocardium
- Apical systolic murmur
- Polyarthritis
- Erythema marginatum, a clear rash often over trunk and proximal portion of extremities
- Subcutaneous nodules
- Chorea

3 Test Results

- There is no single definitive laboratory test to diagnose RF.
- Clinical and laboratory findings are considered along with evidence of a recent streptococcal infection.

4 Treatment

- Ten-day course of antibiotic therapy
- Salicylates to control the inflammatory process

5 Nursing Interventions

- Promote compliance with the medication regimen.
- Support child and family and return to recovery.
- Prevent reoccurrence of the illness.

? FINAL CHECKUP

1. **Which of the following is a common sign of digoxin toxicity?**
   a. Seizures
   b. Vomiting
   c. Bradypnea
   d. Tachycardia

2. **When a uncorrected cardiac defect allows blood to shunt from the (high pressure) left side of the heart to the (lower pressure) right side, which of the following can occur?**
   a. Cyanosis
   b. Congestive heart failure
   c. Decreased pulmonary blood flow
   d. Bounding pulses in upper extremities

3. **Ventricular septal defect may result in which of the following blood flow patterns?**
   a. Obstructive blood flow to pulmonary artery
   b. Increased pulmonary blood flow
   c. Decreased pulmonary blood flow
   d. Mixed blood flow

4. **Which of the following describes congestive heart failure (CHF)?**
   a. Poor valve function
   b. Consequence of existing congenital cardiac defect
   c. Inherited disorder associated with a variety of defects
   d. Decreased workload on an abnormal myocardium

5. **Which of the following defects causes blood flow to be obstructed?**
   a. Aortic stenosis
   b. Patent ductus arteriosus
   c. Atrial septal defect
   d. Transposition of the great arteries

6. **Which of the following structural defects constitutes tetralogy of Fallot?**
   a. Ventricular septal defect, overriding aorta, right ventricular hypertrophy, pulmonary stenosis
   b. Foramen ovale patency, ventricular septal defect, overriding aorta, right ventricular hypertrophy
   c. Aortic stenosis, ventricular septal defect, overriding aorta, left ventricular hypertrophy
   d. Pulmonary stenosis, ventricular septal defect, aortic hypertrophy, left ventricular hypertrophy

7. **Alice should not be given her digoxin (Lanoxin) after her heart surgery if her apical pulse is less than which of the following?**
   a. 60 beats/min
   b. 90 beats/min
   c. 100 beats/min
   d. 120 beats/min

8. **After cardiac catheterization, the heart rate should be counted for how many seconds?**
   a. 15
   b. 30
   c. 60
   d. 120

9. **Which of the following actions by the practitioner would be important in the prevention of rheumatic fever?**
   a. Encourage routine hypertensive screenings.
   b. Conduct routine occult blood screenings.
   c. Refer children with sore throats for throat cultures.
   d. Recommend salicylates instead for minor discomforts.

10. **Surgery for patent ductus arteriosus (PDA) prevents which of the following complications?**
    a. Cyanosis
    b. Left-to-right shunt of blood
    c. Decreased workload on left side of heart
    d. Pulmonary vascular congestion

ANSWERS

Routine checkup 1
    1. b
    2. c

Routine checkup 2
    1. d
    2. b

Final checkup

1. b	2. b	3. b	4. b	5. a	6. a
7. b	8. c	9. c	10. d		

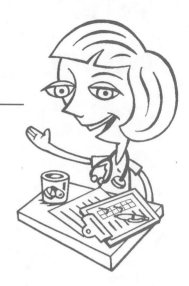

CHAPTER 7

The Hematologic System

Learning Objectives

At the end of the chapter, the student will be able to

1 Discuss the pediatric risk factors for disruption of hematologic function.

2 Discuss signs and symptoms related to hematologic conditions.

3 Evaluate diagnostic procedures associated with hematologic conditions.

4 Discuss treatment regimens associated with conditions of the hematologic system.

5 Teach and support parents regarding the treatment and care required for a child with conditions of the bone marrow and blood.

6 Relate the impact of heredity on genetic hematologic conditions.

 KEY WORDS

Anemia	Hemopoiesis
Ecchymosis	Leukocytopenia
Epistaxis	Megalokaryocyte
Hemarthrosis	Thrombocytopenia

OVERVIEW

◐ Blood cells are produced in the bone marrow beginning with the stem cell, which then become a lymphoid cell that then becomes a lymphocyte (B or T) myeloid cell, which changes to either an erythrocyte (red blood cell) or a granulocyte or monocyte (white blood cells) or **megalokaryocyte** (platelets precursor). Intrinsic factor stimulates the formation of blood cells (**hemopoiesis**) cell growth.

◐ The spleen, which is located in the left upper quadrant of the abdomen, is responsible for filtration of the blood, break down of hemoglobin, removal of old white blood cells, and storage of red blood cells and platelets.

◐ The liver is the primary site for the production of clotting factors. The liver uses vitamin K to produce prothrombin and factors VII, IX, and X.

◐ Normal coagulation/clotting involves a local response of vasoconstriction and release of a factor to stimulate platelet adhesion (sticking together) to form a plug and stop bleeding. Clotting factors act to stimulate formation of a fibrin clot by way of an

- Intrinsic pathway with factor XII, factor XI, I, II, V, VIII, IX, X, high molecular weight kininogen (HMK), and prekallikrein (KAL). Partial thromboplastin time (PTT) is used to measure function of factors.

- Extrinsic pathway with factor VII, I, II, V, VII, and X. Prothrombin time (PT) measures the function of factors in this pathway.

ANEMIA

A low red blood cell count, including a low hematocrit or hemoglobin level, results in a state referred to as **anemia.** With decreased blood cells the delivery of oxygen and nutrients is decreased, resulting in poorly nourished or poorly oxygenated body cells and malfunction of body organs and systems. Anemia results when the bone marrow that produces blood, or the kidney that stimulates blood production, is damaged or suppressed. Anemia can also result when a nutritional component needed to form blood, iron, is insufficient, or when blood cells that are produced are poorly structured, sickled, and malfunction.

APLASTIC OR HYPOPLASTIC ANEMIA

⚑ What Went Wrong?

The bone marrow can be damaged due to exposure to radiation, infections (human parvovirus, hepatitis), toxic substances, including radiation or medications administered to suppress cancer cells or eradicate microorganisms, or can result from unknown causes. The condition can be primary (congenital) or secondary (acquired) possibly due to autoimmune disease. The damage to the bone marrow results in the decreased production of white blood cells, red blood cells, and platelets. Hypoplastic anemia results in low red blood cells

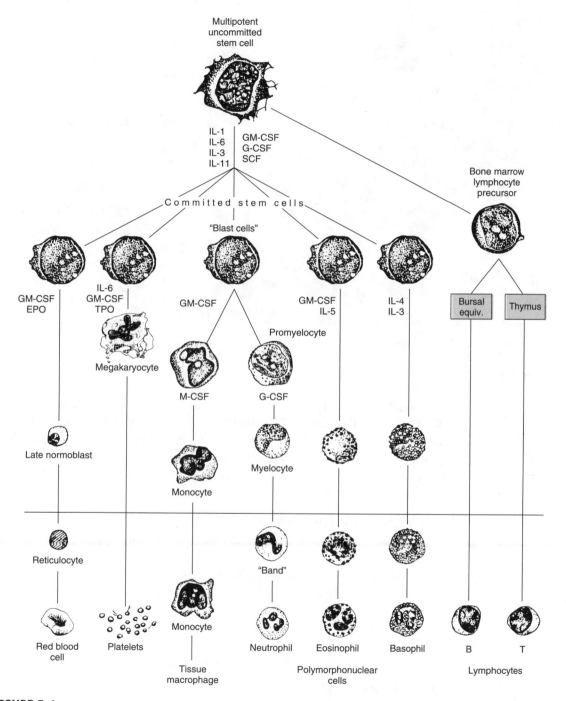

FIGURE 7-1

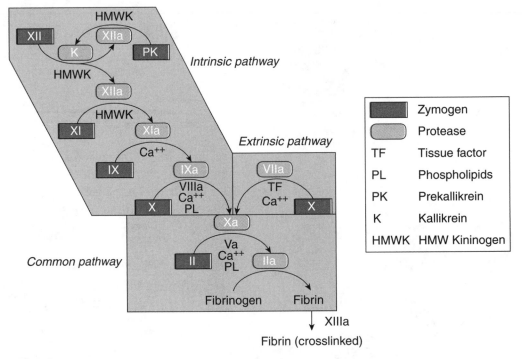

FIGURE 7-2

with either normal or decreased white blood cell count or platelets. Decreased white blood cells (**leukocytopenia**) place the client at risk for infection, low red blood cells results in decreased cell oxygenation and nutrition, and low platelets can predispose a client to bleeding. Prognosis depends on the extent and duration of decreased blood cell production and client vulnerability due to chronic disease or debility.

Signs and Symptoms

- Weakness and fatigue due to deoxygenated, malnourished body tissues
- Pallor due to decreased red blood cells
- Infections due to low white blood cells
- Bruising (ecchymosis) secondary to low platelet count (**thrombocytopenia**)
- Hemorrhage
  - Small superficial bleed (petechiae)
  - Nosebleed (epistaxis)
  - Other mucosal bleeding (oral, gastrointestinal, vaginal)

Test Results

- Bone marrow aspiration may reveal fatty yellow bone marrow.
- Complete blood count values reveal low red blood cell count, low white blood cell count, low hemoglobin, low hematocrit, and low platelet counts.

◐ Pulse oximetry and blood gases may reveal hypoxia in severe anemia.
◐ Acidosis may result in a decreased serum pH level.
◐ Electrolyte imbalance may be noted due to acidosis.

④ Treatment

◐ Bone marrow replacement/transplant to replace stem cells
◐ Immunosuppressive therapy to suppress autoimmune response
  • Antilymphocyte globulin (ALG)
  • Antithymocyte globulin (ATG)
  • Cyclosporine A (CSA)
  • Granulocyte macrophage colony-stimulating factor (GM-CSF)
  • Cyclophosphamide for immunosuppression

Nursing alert **Chemotherapeutic drugs can result in nausea and vomiting, alopecia, and mucosal ulceration and thus support measures should be taken.**

◐ Androgens may be added to ATG to stimulate erythropoiesis.
◐ Red blood cell transfusion with severe anemia.
◐ Platelet transfusion if decreased platelet level is severe.

Nursing Intervention

◐ Similar to care of a client with leukemia:
  • Reinforce physician's explanation of diagnosis and treatment plan.
  • Explain procedure at child's level of understanding including what will be seen, felt, heard, and smelled; use drawings when appropriate.
  • Provide antiemetic and appetite stimulant to increase nutritional intake.
  • Offer foods after antiemetic takes effect to reduce nausea and maximize caloric intake.
  • Allow to eat any food that is tolerated; avoid forcing food during nausea episode.
  • Rinse mouth to remove unpleasant taste sensation.
  • Maintain contact after discharge and between remissions to encourage follow-up care and respond to questions or provide emotional support.
  • During intravenous administration of ATG, monitor site closely to prevent infiltration or extravasation.
  • Maintain careful asepsis to prevent infection.
  • Meticulous mouth care with soft toothbrush to prevent infection, irritation, and bleeding from oral ulceration.
  • Liquid, bland, or soft diet as tolerated.

IRON DEFICIENCY ANEMIA

What Went Wrong?

Inadequate intake or excessive loss of iron causes this widespread nutritional disorder. Causes of this disorder could include

- Decreased supply due to poor eating habits, excessive milk or extended breastfeeding, and delayed solid food intake or rapid growth rate
- Inadequate stores of iron at birth, found in low birthweight babies, maternal iron deficiency, or fetal blood loss
- Impaired absorption due to presence of inhibitors such as gastric alkalinity or malabsorption disorders such as lactose intolerance or inflammatory bowel disease or chronic diarrhea
- Increased body need for iron due to prematurity, adolescence, or pregnancy
- Loss of iron due to parasites or blood loss

One molecule of the heme in hemoglobin contains an atom of iron; thus insufficient iron results in deficient hemoglobin production.

❷ Signs and Symptoms

- Infant may appear underweight due to malnourishment or overweight due to intake of excessive milk with minimal solid food ingestion.
- Characteristic symptoms: irritability, glossitis, stomatitis, koilonychias (concave/spoon fingernails).
- Plasma protein leakage noted with edema, growth retardation.
- Poor muscle development.
- Weakness and fatigue due to deoxygenated, malnourished body tissues.
- Pallor due to decreased red blood cells.
- Infections due to low white blood cells.
- Hemorrhage due to decreased platelets:
  - Small superficial bleed (petechiae)
  - Nosebleed (**epistaxis**)
  - Bruising (**ecchymosis**)
  - Other mucosal bleeding (oral, gastrointestinal, vaginal)
- Tachycardia and tachypnea may be present due low blood levels and need to circulate blood more frequently to oxygenate body cells.

❸ Test Results

- Complete blood count values reveal low red blood cell count, low white blood cell count, low hemoglobin, low hematocrit, and low platelet counts.
- Decreased serum proteins, albumen, transferrin, and gamma globulin.
- Reticulocyte count normal or slightly reduced.
- Serum iron concentration (SIC) about 70 mg/dL; total iron-binding capacity to detect transferrin iron binding globulin (TIBG) usually elevated >350 mg/dL for children 6 months to 2 years of age or >450 mg/dL for persons >2 years of age.

◐ Transferrin saturation—SIC divided by TIBC multiplied by 100—if below 10% = anemia.
◐ Guaiac stool to detect chronic bleeding.
◐ Pulse oximetry and blood gases may reveal hypoxia in severe anemia.
◐ Acidosis may result in a decreased serum pH level.
◐ Electrolyte imbalance may be noted due to acidosis.

④ Treatment

Prevention with nutrition:

◐ Breast milk or iron-fortified milk during first year.
◐ Iron supplement with milk or iron-fortified cereal by age 4 to 6 months (2 months of age in premature infants).
◐ Iron drops to breast-fed premature infants after 2 months of age.
◐ Limit formula to 1 L/day and encourage iron-rich solid foods.
◐ Avoid fresh cow's milk to avoid allergy and gastrointestinal blood loss.
◐ Supplemental iron (intramuscular [IM] or intravenous [IV] if unable to absorb gastrointestinally).
◐ Iron-fortified cereal.
◐ Vitamin B_{12} IM to treat deficiency due to failure of gastric mucosa to secrete intrinsic factor needed to absorb vitamin B_{12} (pernicious anemia more common in adults).
◐ Packed red blood cells if anemia severe.
◐ Oxygen supplement if severe hypoxia noted.

Nursing Intervention

◐ Monitor vital signs for signs of circulatory or respiratory distress due to low blood levels and poor oxygenation.
◐ If tolerated, administer oral iron compound between meals because high stomach acid enhances absorption:
  • Ferrous sulfate
  • Ferrous gluconate
  • Ferrous fumarate

Nursing alert **Liquid iron agents should be taken with a straw to avoid contact with teeth and resulting staining.**

◐ Administer iron with meals to reduce nausea and diarrhea (if necessary).
◐ Parenteral (IM or IV) iron if unable to absorb oral dose:
  • Iron dextran IM or IV
  • Iron sodium gluconate IV
  • Iron sucrose complex IV

Nursing alert **Use Z-track injection to prevent staining of the skin.**

◐ Request stool softener as indicated to treat constipation from iron.

⑤ Client and Family Teaching

◐ Teach proper nutrition as per treatment plan.
◐ Inform family of dietary sources high in iron such as green leafy vegetables.
◐ Administer with juices because vitamin C enhance absorption.
◐ Stress the importance of follow-up blood testing to determine if hemoglobin and hematocrit are adequate and iron administration is effective.
◐ Teach family to administer iron properly:
  • Oral medication with straw if liquid form is administered; avoid substances that impair absorption (tea, antacid, milk).
  • Teach the Z-track method for IM injections.
◐ Caution family and client that stool will be dark green to black due to iron content.

Nursing alert **Avoid administering iron with tea, antacid, or milk to maximize absorption.**

SICKLE CELL ANEMIA

① What Went Wrong?

In sickle cell anemia (SCA)/Hgb SS cell disease, an abnormal gene results in production of an irregular red blood cell called hemoglobin (Hgb) S that replaces some of the normal hemoglobin A. The red blood cells collapse into a crescent shape (sickling) when stressed such as during dehydration, hypoxemia, or acidosis. When cells sickle, clumping is noted that obstructs small blood vessels and blocks blood flow. These cells also have a short lifespan, resulting in early destruction due to damaged cell membrane and low blood count: anemia. This condition is an autosomal recessive condition requiring the gene from both parents. Some clients inherit one gene and may exhibit the sickle cell trait, which may or may not be symptomatic under severe conditions such as hypoxia during exertion in low-oxygen settings (high altitude). Clients of African descent have a high incidence of sickle cell anemia. Sickle cell anemia is a chronic illness with distress resulting from blocked and inadequate circulation and tissue/organ damage that cause pain and over time organ failure and death.

❷ Signs and Symptoms

- ◐ Acute pain due to blocked blood vessels and tissue ischemia, found in
  - Extremities: swelling of hands, feet, and joints—dactylitis (hand-foot syndrome)
  - Abdomen
  - Chest: pain and pulmonary disease
  - Liver: jaundice and hepatic coma
  - Kidney: hematuria and impaired function
  - Brain: stroke
  - Genitalia: painful erection (priapism)
- ◐ Crisis episodes due to
  - Vasoocclusion: most common crisis due to blocked blood flow from sickling
  - Sequestration
  - Aplastic crisis due to extreme drop in red blood cells (RBC) (often viral trigger)
  - Megaloblastic anemia with excess need for folic acid or vitamin B_{12} resulting in deficiency
  - Hyperhemolytic crisis—rapid RBC destruction—anemia, jaundice, and reticulocytosis
- ◐ Sickling episodes have exacerbation with remissions after effective treatment.
- ◐ Fatigue secondary to the anemia.
- ◐ Fever during a sickling episode possibly due to infection that provoked distress.
- ◐ Pooling of blood (sequestration) in organs resulting in enlargement:
  - Splenomegaly
  - Hepatomegaly
- ◐ Organ damage due to vessel blockage:
  - Heart (cardiomegaly) with weakened heart valves and heart murmur
  - Lungs, kidneys, liver, and spleen malfunction and failure
  - Extremities: avascular necrosis due to vascular blockage resulting in skeletal deformities (hip, shoulder, lordosis, and kyphosis) and possible osteomyelitis
  - Central nervous system (seizures, paresis)
  - Eyes: visual disturbance, possible progressive retinal detachment and blindness
- ◐ Growth retardation may also be noted.

❸ Test Results

- ◐ Low RBCs.
- ◐ Sickled cells noted per stained blood smear.
- ◐ Sickle-turbidity test (Sickledex).

- Hemoglobin, hematocrit, and platelets.
- Hemoglobin electrophoresis: separation of blood into different hemoglobins to determine the form of hemoglobinopathies (hemoglobin defects).
- Newborn screening for SCA: detects hemoglobin defects early.
- Pulse oximetry and blood gases may reveal hypoxia in severe anemia.
- Acidosis may result in a decreased serum pH level.
- Electrolyte imbalance may be noted due to acidosis.

Treatment

- Hydration to thin blood and decrease sickling and vascular blockage.
- Minimize infection; antibiotics may be ordered, vaccines recommended to avoid meningitis, pneumonia, and other infections.
- Oxygen supplement to decrease tissue ischemia.
- Pain medication: oral or intravenous analgesics such as opioids.
- Electrolyte replacements may be ordered to correct imbalances.
- Blood replacement with packed cells if anemia is severe.
- Bed rest with mild range of motion during episodes.

Nursing Intervention

- Pain control; fear of addiction is not the issue during a crisis.
- Fluid intake: Monitor intravenous fluids closely to avoid fluid overload.
- Intake and output to regulate volume and monitor kidney function.
- Rest periods during the day to avoid fatigue.
- Mild range of motion to retain mobility.

Nursing alert **Avoid cold and cold compresses with increased vasoconstriction and pain.**

Family Teaching

- Teach proactive care to prevent episodes/crisis:
  - Adequate fluid intake to prevent dehydration
  - Avoiding infection or early treatment
  - Moderate activity and adequate rest to avoid fatigue and hypoxia
- Early signs of impending crisis: splenic palpation to detect sequestration
- Stress need for immediate care if there are signs of crisis.
- Genetic testing and counseling:
  - Explain that SCA is an autosomal recessive condition requiring the gene from both parents.
  - Encourage testing of siblings to allow for childbearing planning.

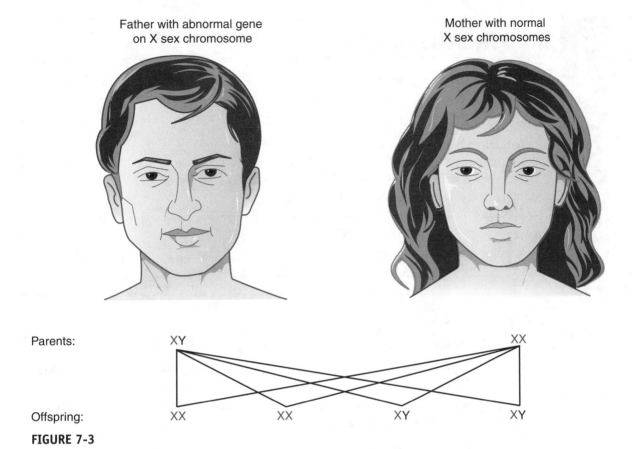

Father with abnormal gene
on X sex chromosome

Mother with normal
X sex chromosomes

Parents: XY   XX

Offspring: XX   XX   XY   XY

FIGURE 7-3

- Explain that each pregnancy when both parents are carriers presents a 25% chance a child will be born with the disease and a 50% chance the child will have the sickle cell trait.
- Refer for counseling and family planning if additional childbearing is desired.
- Discuss alternative parenting options (insemination, adoption, etc.).

◑ Support child and family with emotional responses, grieving, and coping:
- Allow ventilation of anger, concerns, fears, and questions.
- Support during depression over chronic illness.
- Provide honest responses regarding care during episodes.
- Use positive terms and avoid words like "crisis" when discussing vasoocclusive or other problem episodes with the child and family.
- Encourage child in control of condition and lifestyle needed to avoid episodes and promote maximum development.

ROUTINE CHECKUP 1

1. Why should a client with sickle cell anemia be concerned if he or she marries a person with the sickle cell trait?

Answer:

2. What defect is most commonly caused by anemia?
   a. Increased red blood cell count and blood viscosity
   b. Depressed hematopoietic system and hyperactivity
   c. Increased presence of abnormal hemoglobin
   d. Decreased capacity of blood to carry oxygen

Answer:

_____

_____

HEMOPHILIA

Hemophilia is a group of congenital bleeding disorders due to a deficiency of specific coagulation proteins. This condition occurs most commonly in persons of African descent, possibly as a genetic adaptation in trait carriers as protection from malaria.

What Went Wrong?

Hemophilia results most often from a genetic defect and most commonly a deficiency of factor VIII (hemophilia A) or factor IX (hemophilia B, or Christmas disease). However, a third of hemophilia cases occur from gene mutation. The X-linked form of the condition is passed when an affected male (XhY) mates with a female carrier (XhX) producing a 1 in 4 chance of the offspring having a girl or having a boy with the disease, having a female carrier, or having a child without the disease or trait. The female carrier can also be symptomatic.

❷ Signs and Symptoms

- ◗ Bleeding of varied degrees depending on severity of deficiency:
    - • Spontaneous bleeding
    - • Bleeding with trauma
    - • Bleeding with major trauma or surgery
- ◗ **Hemarthrosis** (bleeding into the joints) in the knees, elbows, and ankles begins with stiffness, tingling, or ache as early sign of bleeding, progressive damage.
- ◗ Warmth, redness, swelling, and severe pain and loss of movement.

- ◑ Epistaxis (not most frequent bleed).
- ◑ Hematomas may cause pain at the site due to pressure.
- ◑ Intracranial bleeding can cause changes in neurostatus and progress to death.

Nursing alert **Bleeding from the mouth, throat, or neck could result in airway obstruction and warrants immediate attention.**

❸ Test Results

- ◑ History of bleeding with X-linked inheritance evidenced is diagnostic.
- ◑ Clotting factor function testing will reveal an abnormality in ability to form fibrinogen or generate thromboplastin:
  - • Whole blood clotting time
  - • PT
  - • PTT
  - • Thromboplastin generation test (TGT)
  - • Prothrombin consumption test
  - • Fibrinogen level
- ◑ Pulse oximetry and blood gases may reveal hypoxia in severe anemia.
- ◑ Acidosis may result in a decreased serum pH level.
- ◑ Electrolyte imbalance may be noted due to acidosis.

❹ Treatment

- ◑ Factor VIII concentrate to replace the missing clotting factor.
- ◑ DDAVP (1-deamino-8-D-arginine vasopressin) for mild hemophilia (type 1 or IIA) to increase production of factor VIII.
- ◑ Corticosteroids for chronic hemarthrosis, hematuria, acute hemarthrosis.
- ◑ Ibuprofen or other nonsteroidal antiinflammatory drug (NSAID) for pain relief.

Nursing alert **NSAIDs should be used cautiously because they inhibit platelet function.**

- ◑ Epsilon aminocaproic acid (EACA, Amicar) blocks clot destruction.
- ◑ Exercise and physical therapy with active range of motion as client tolerates to strengthen muscles around joints.

Nursing alert **After acute episode, avoid passive range of motion due to possible joint capsule stretching with bleeding. Client should control active range of motion according to pain tolerance.**

Nursing Intervention

- Maintain protective environment to prevent injury to client.
- Monitor closely for signs of bleeding.
- Treat bleeding episodes promptly.
- Apply pressure to nares if nosebleed is noted.
- Minimize crippling due to contractures and joint damage from bleeding:
  - Promote complete absorption of blood from joints.
  - Mild exercise of limbs during confinement to prevent disuse.
  - Encourage regular exercise regimen at home.

⑤ Client and Family Teaching

- Protective care to prevent injury: Child-proof rooms with rounded corners, padding, and so on, to minimize injury to mobile infant or toddler.
- Noncontact sports and activities with minimum injury potential such as golf, swimming.
- Safety equipment to minimize injury.
- Soft toothbrush with water irrigation for mouth care to prevent oral bleeding.
- Electric razor instead of blades for shaving.
- Teach to recognize bleeding episode in early stages and early treatment:
  - RICE (rest, ice, compression, and elevation) to control bleeding
- Medical identification bracelet and notification of school nurse regarding condition.
- Teach child to control condition and lifestyle needed to avoid episodes and promote maximum development.
- Refer as needed for financial support if insurance ceases to cover client when older than age 21 and is removed from parental insurance.
- Provide support for emotional stress to patient and family related to chronic condition.
- Genetic counseling:
  - Encourage testing of siblings to allow for childbearing planning.
  - Explain that each pregnancy when both parents are carriers presents a 25% chance a child will be born with the disease and a 50% chance the child will have the sickle cell trait.
  - Refer for counseling and family planning if additional childbearing is desired.
  - Discuss alternative parenting options (insemination, adoption, etc.).

Nursing alert **Avoid aspirin compounds and substitute acetaminophen because aspirin impairs platelet function.**

IDIOPATHIC THROMBOCYTOPENIC PURPURA

Idiopathic thrombocytopenic purpura (ITP), a hemorrhagic condition, is an acquired disorder with an unknown cause that is possibly autoimmune in origin. It occurs between 2 and 10 years of age with recovery within 6 months.

What Went Wrong?

Excessive destruction of platelets results in deficiency (thrombocytopenia) leading to bleeding disorders. Bone marrow may be normal with large young platelets noted. The disorder may be acute or chronic.

Signs and Symptoms

- Petechiae, or bruising, due to bleeding in superficial skin surfaces.
- Bleeding from mucous membranes.
- Prolonged bleeding from wounds.
- Fatal hemorrhage is rare.

Test Results

- Platelet count <20.000 mm³
- White cell count to rule out leukemia
- Testing to rule out lupus or lymphoma

Treatment

- Supportive treatment
- Prednisone
- Anti-D antibody (if client is >1 year of age or <19 years of age)
- Intravenous immune globulin (IVIG)
- Splenectomy (after 5 years of age) for clients with severe chronic ITP to remove risk of hemorrhage followed by prophylactic penicillin and vaccines to prevent influenza, meningitis, or pneumonia

Nursing Intervention

- Supportive care:
  - Protective environment with padding to prevent injury.
  - Limit activity until platelets 50,000 to 100,000/mm³.
- Client and family teaching:
  - Teach to avoid all contact sports.
  - Medical examination with any abdominal or head trauma to rule out internal bleeding.
- Premedicate with acetaminophen 5 to 10 minutes before anti-D antibody infusion and monitor for reaction of fever, chills, or headache. Treat with Benadryl and Solu-Cortef and observe client closely.

Nursing alert **Teach client and family to avoid using aspirin or NSAIDs for pain management due to effect on platelets.**

ROUTINE CHECKUP 2

1. Common symptoms of hemophilia in children include (a) —————,
   (b) —————, (c) —————, (d) —————.
   Answers:

2. What data in a 6-year-old client's history would alert the nurse most to watch the client closely for signs of thrombocytopenia?
   a. The client has reported frequent backache and weight loss.
   b. The client reports urinating three times a day.
   c. The mother mentioned blood on the pillow some mornings.
   d. The school history indicates hyperactivity when doing class work.
   Answer:

3. Idiopathic thrombocytopenic purpura (ITP) commonly results in what finding?
   a. Blood clots
   b. Pallor
   c. Dry membranes
   d. Bruising
   Answer:

BETA-THALASSEMIA

Thalassemia is an inherited disorder involving deficiency in production of globin chains in hemoglobin. The beta form of the disorder is the most common and is found most often in persons of Greek, Italian, and Syrian descent. An alpha form of thalassemia is found in people of Chinese, Thai, African, and Mediterranean descent possibly due to genetic mutation because of intermarriages or spontaneous mutation.

What Went Wrong?

Thalassemia is an autosomal-recessive disorder in which the alpha or beta polypeptide chains in hemoglobin A are impacted. In beta-thalassemia there is a decreased synthesis of the beta chains with an increased synthesis of alpha chains resulting in defective hemoglobin and damaged red blood cells (hemolysis) and resulting anemia.

An overproduction of RBCs (immature cells) may result in compensation for the hemolysis. Folic acid deficiency may result from increased demand on bone marrow.

❷ Signs and Symptoms

- ◐ Anemia with accompanying:
  - • Pallor.
  - • Fatigue.
  - • Poor feeding.
  - • Progressive chronic anemia: Hypoxia, headache, irritability, precordial and bone pain, and anorexia may be noted.
- ◐ Thalassemia minor occurs with trait carrier condition and is nonsymptomatic.
- ◐ Thalassemia intermedia manifests with splenomegaly and moderate to severe anemia.
- ◐ Thalassemia major (Cooley anemia) is severe anemia.
- ◐ Excessive iron storage in organs without organ damage (hemosiderosis) or with cellular damage (hemochromatosis) may be noted.
- ◐ Retarded growth; particularly delayed sexual maturation is commonly noted.
- ◐ Bronzed complexion: iron-containing pigment may be noted due to breakdown of RBCs and excess iron.
- ◐ If untreated, bone changes such as enlarged head and other facial changes may be noted.

❸ Test Results

- ◐ RBC count is low.
- ◐ Hemoglobin and hematocrit levels are decreased.
- ◐ Hemoglobin electrophoresis analyzes the hemoglobin variants and helps distinguish the type and severity of thalassemia.

❹ Treatment

- ◐ Maintain adequate hemoglobin levels to reduce bony deformities and expansion of the bone marrow.
- ◐ Provide blood cells to promote growth and maintain activity tolerance:
  - • Transfusions of RBCs as needed to keep Hgb >9.5 g/dL
- ◐ Deferoxamine (Desferal), an iron chelating agent, with oral vitamin C may be administered to promote iron excretion (may help growth if given early at 2 to 4 years of age).
- ◐ Bone marrow transplantation may be done in some children.
- ◐ Splenectomy may be done to decrease destruction of blood cells, if severe splenomegaly is noted.

Nursing alert **After splenectomy, client is at risk for infection and should receive vaccines to prevent influenza, meningitis, and pneumonia in addition to regular immunizations.**

Nursing Intervention

- Promote adherence to treatment regimen.
- Support child during illness and distressing treatments.
- **5** Promote child and family coping:
  - Anticipate adolescent concerns related to appearance.
- Monitor closely for complications of the condition and treatment:
  - Multiple transfusions and iron buildup
  - Infection postsplenectomy
- **6** Genetic counseling:
  - Encourage testing of siblings to allow for childbearing planning.
  - Explain that each pregnancy when both parents are carriers presents a 25% chance a child will be born with the disease and a 50% chance the child will have the thalassemia trait.
  - Refer for counseling and family planning if additional childbearing is desired.
  - Discuss alternative parenting options—insemination, adoption . . . etc.

CONCLUSION

The hematology system is responsible for red blood cells that provide oxygen and nutrients to the cells of the body and white blood cells that protect the body from infections as well as the platelets and other clotting mechanisms that control bleeding. Conditions that impact the production of blood cells can cause a deficiency and result in poor tissue oxygenation and nourishment, and conditions that result in decreased clotting factors or platelets contribute to bleeding problems. Key information discussed in this chapter includes the following:

- Aplastic anemia results when the bone marrow is damaged and production of red and white blood cells and platelets is noted.
- Pallor is a common sign of anemia due to vasoconstriction and low red blood cells.
- Decreased red blood cells result in decreased cell oxygenation leading to fatigue.
- Low blood oxygen levels leads to tachycardia and tachypnea in an attempt to increase blood and oxygen supply to tissues.
- Emotional support is needed to encourage the child to continue to function to the maximum within limitations.
- A thorough history and physical can provide critical data for diagnosis and treatment planning.
- Possible causes of anemia include genetically transmitted traits for defective or absent blood elements or clotting factors.

❍ Physical assessment of a child with anemia may reveal cardinal symptoms:
- Pallor
- Fatigue
- Hypoxia

❍ Absence of adequate white blood cells increases susceptibility to infection.

❍ Insufficient platelets (thrombocytopenia, aplastic anemia) increase client susceptibility for bleeding.

❍ 6 Genetic conditions should involve client and family support including genetic counseling so family planning can be done and risks known.

❍ Test results for the anemias will often include low red blood cell count (anemia) and low platelet count.

❍ Bone marrow support is needed to maintain adequate production of red blood cells.

❍ Hemophilia results in bleeding due to a disruption in clotting factor synthesis.

❍ ITP results in bleeding due to the reduction in platelet function.

❍ Bleeding may be noted if platelets are reduced:
- Diagnostic tests in coagulation-related conditions may include clotting factors and
  - Whole blood clotting time
  - PT
  - PTT
  - TGT
  - Prothrombin consumption test
  - Fibrinogen level

❍ Rest and support treatment such as oxygen and adequate nutrition are beneficial to client success.

? FINAL CHECKUP

1. **A mother states that her 3-year-old girl was tired all the time and did not run with her siblings. The nurse assesses that the child has pale skin and mucous membranes and has muscle weakness. The child's hemoglobin on admission is 6.4 g/dL. After notifying the physician of the assessment findings, which of the following is the nurse's next intervention?**
   a. Push oral and intravenous fluids to correct the dehydration.
   b Decrease environmental stimulation to prevent seizures.
   c. Have the laboratory repeat the analysis with a new specimen.
   d. Decrease energy expenditure to decrease cardiac workload.

2. **Vasopressin would be a major treatment for which condition?**
   a. Beta-thalassemia
   b. Iron deficiency anemia
   c. Hemophilia
   d. Idiopathic thrombocytopenic purpura

3. **What is the most common reason a nurse could provide to a young girl in vasoocclusive sickle cell crisis regarding the need for the infusion of large volumes of fluid? The fluid is necessary to do which of the following?**
   a. Provide the iron to replace depleted stores.
   b. Infuse nutrients that will help her to fight the infection in her body.
   c. Increase her energy so she will not be as tired.
   d. Help her blood flow better to reduce blockages that cause pain.

4. **What is a primary reason why iron deficiency anemia is common during infancy?**
   a. Unfortified cow's milk is a poor iron source.
   b. Iron is not stored during fetal development.
   c. Fetal iron stores are exhausted by 1 month of age.
   d. Dietary iron cannot be started until 12 months of age.

5. **Which statement best describes iron deficiency anemia in infants?**
   a. Destruction of bone marrow and hematopoietic system depression is involved.
   b. It is easily diagnosed because of infant's frail, emaciated appearance.
   c. It results from an inadequate intake of milk and the premature addition of solid foods.
   d. Decreased red blood cells lead to reduction in the amount of oxygen available to tissues.

6. **The nurse should include what information when teaching the mother of a 8-month-old infant about administering liquid iron preparations?**
   a. Stop immediately if nausea and vomiting occur.
   b. Administer iron with meals to help absorption.
   c. Adequate dosage will turn the stools a tarry green color.
   d. Allow preparation to mix with saliva and bathe the teeth before swallowing.

7. **In what condition is the normal adult hemoglobin partly or completely replaced by abnormal hemoglobin?**
   a. Aplastic anemia
   b. Sickle cell anemia
   c. Iron deficiency anemia
   d. Thalassemia major

8. The parents of a child with hemophilia are concerned about subsequent children having the disease. The mother is a carrier and the father does not have the disease. Which statement best addresses their concern?
   a. Hemophilia is not an inherited condition.
   b. All subsequent siblings will have hemophilia.
   c. Each sibling has a 25% chance of having hemophilia.
   d. There is a 50% chance of siblings having hemophilia.

9. The symptoms noted in sickle cell anemia result primarily from which of the following?
   a. Decreased blood viscosity
   b. Deficiency in coagulation factor
   c. Increased blood cell destruction
   d. Decreased cell affinity for oxygen

10. What should be included in the plan of care for a preschool-age child who is admitted in a vasoocclusive sickle cell crisis (pain episode)?
    a. Pain management
    b. Administration of heparin
    c. Factor VIII replacement
    d. Electrolyte replacement

ANSWERS

Routine checkup 1
   1. If they have children, there is a 50% chance they will have a child with sickle cell disease.
   2. d

Routine checkup 2
   1. Bleeding, hemarthrosis, pain, neurostatus changes.
   2. c
   3. d

Final checkup
1. d	2. c	3. d	4. a	5. d
6. c	7. b	8. c	9. c	10. a

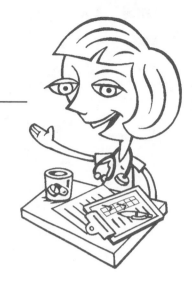

CHAPTER 8

Oncology Conditions

Learning Objectives

At the end of the chapter, the student will be able to:

1 Using appropriate terms, describe theories related to cell mutation resulting in cancers in children.

2 Assess a child with a cancerous process, such as leukemia or rhabdomyosarcoma.

3 Discuss the common treatment plan for a child with cancer.

4 Discuss the nursing implications when caring for a child receiving cancer therapy.

5 Determine the care needs of families of children with cancer.

 KEY WORDS

Benign	Malignant	Osteogenic sarcoma
Cachexia	Metastasis	Retinoblastoma
Ewing sarcoma	Neoplasm	Rhabdomyosarcoma
Leukemia	Neuroblastoma	Sarcoma
Lymphoma	Oncogenic virus	Tumor staging

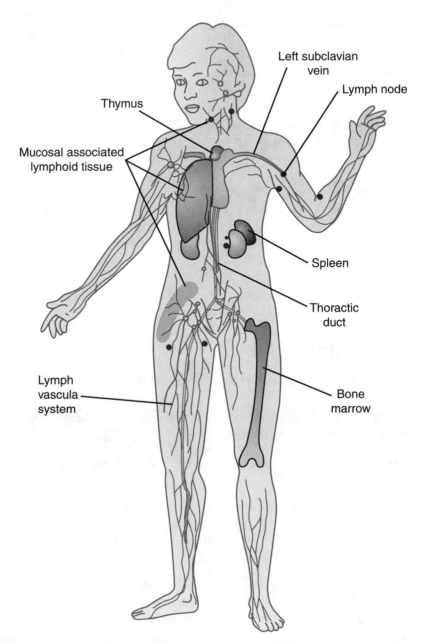

FIGURE 8-1

OVERVIEW

The physical changes and psychological stressors resulting when children develop cancer can create many challenges for the child and family. Nursing care is aimed at promoting continued growth and development of the child with the best quality of life possible. Family-centered care is provided to maximize support for the child and family members.

Family and friends may view a diagnosis of cancer as meaning the child's life will end in a short period of time, and they might withdraw from the child. Family may also become overbearing and restrict the child's continued growth. Teaching and support by the nurse is needed to correct misconceptions and keep the parents updated on the child's progress.

Knowledge of the impact of cancer conditions and the associated treatments helps the nurse anticipate problems and plan the assistance needed to reduce discomforts and maximize the strengths of the child and family during the process of the illness and treatments. Because cancer conditions involve multiple systems, the nurse must consider that multiple imbalances can and often do occur simultaneously in one client.

Symptoms and history can be invaluable when determining what imbalances may be present in the client. The nurse must explore historical data, along with monitoring of lab results and physical assessment data, to become and remain aware of client needs and advocate for the client in order to minimize complications that could worsen the client's condition.

Understanding the normal ranges of laboratory test values is critical to determining what are important and essential data to report and act on. Close monitoring of laboratory values by the nurse in concert with the medication or treatment is critical. The nurse should review this sampling of cancer conditions and consider how other cancer conditions may impact similar organs of the body or similar functions in the body and place the client at risk for complications and imbalances.

CANCER DEFINED

Cancer refers to the presence of **malignant** cells, cells that grow and proliferate in a disorderly, uncontrolled, and chaotic fashion. The term **neoplasm** usually refers to a new *abnormal* growth in the body. The growth can be **benign** (limited growth) or malignant (cancerous). Cancer in children is not common but is still the second leading cause of death in children <14 years of age. The most frequent type of cancer in children is immature blood cell overgrowth, or **leukemia** (acute lymphocytic or acute nonlymphocytic). Other childhood cancers include:

- **Lymphomas** (cancers of the lymph system): Non-Hodgkin or Hodgkin
- Central nervous system (CNS) tumors: Gliomas, medulloblastomas, ependymoma
- Solid tumors: Neuroblastoma, Wilms tumor, retinoblastoma, rhabdomyosarcoma, Ewing sarcoma, osteosarcoma, hepatoblastoma, germ cell tumor

Understanding the processes of abnormal cell growth will help the nurse explain to parents what is happening to their child and why certain treatment measures are needed at various stages of cell growth. These are the key points:

- New cells do not respond to normal communication instructing cells to stop growing when touching another cell; thus overgrowth occurs.
- Theories on what went wrong—childhood neoplasm development:
  - Gene theory, familial predisposition for cell mutation.
  - In utero exposure to carcinogen.
  - Exposure to carcinogen such as secondary smoke or asbestos.
  - Previous cancer produces high risk for additional cancer.
  - **Oncogenic virus** theory: A virus such as Epstein-Barr causes cancer.
  - Tumor suppressor cell deficit: Lack of suppression results in overgrowth, such as with retinoblastoma

SIGNS AND SYMPTOMS

CLIENT HISTORY

- Present illness: Active disease or in remission state
- Previous illness: Immunization history, surgeries, previous cancer events
- Developmental stage: Milestones achieved

FAMILY ASSESSMENT

- Family history of cancer: Note type, treatment, and outcome; note pediatric cancers.
- Family type and concerns related to child's condition and treatment.
- Presence of other family crises—family member illness, divorce, financial burdens—could decrease emotional and financial support for the child with cancer.
- Stress from the cancer diagnosis and subsequent long-term treatment of the child with cancer can destabilize a family and exacerbate existing problems.
- Sibling responses to the cancer diagnosis can range from fear for self to grief and fear about loss of a sibling.

SYMPTOMS

- Vague symptoms such as headache, fatigue, or general skeletal aches may be reported.
- May report nosebleeds (low platelet count).
- Weight loss in an apparently healthy child, particularly **cachexia** (weight loss along with muscle loss and poor appetite), is a common symptom of cancer.

PHYSICAL ASSESSMENT

- Review of symptoms may indicate level of cancer progression.
- Physical assessment may reveal cardinal symptoms of cancer:
  - Unusual lump or swelling (i.e., abdominal mass or swollen lymph glands)
  - Unexplained fatigue or pallor (due to anemia)
  - Easy bruising (ecchymosis and petechiae)
  - Persistent pain or limping gait
  - Prolonged unexplained fever or illness
  - Sudden changes in eye or vision
  - Rapid or excessive weight loss
- Children experiencing relapse of cancer condition may have residual symptoms from previous treatments.
- Visual assessment may reveal squinting, swelling, or strabismus, indicating eye tumor; presence of a white reflex instead of a red reflex indicates retinoblastoma.

TEST RESULTS

Laboratory Tests

- Complete blood count: May reveal leukemia or anemia from bone cancer.
- Chemistries (i.e., sodium, potassium, glucose, blood urea nitrogen [BUN], creatinine): May reveal liver or renal involvement and damage.
- Urinalysis: May reveal renal involvement.

Other Tests

- Lumbar puncture: May reveal leukemia, brain tumors, or spread to spinal cord.
- Imaging studies: Radiologic studies of the chest, abdomen, bone or skull; intravenous pyelogram (kidney conditions); computed tomography (CT), ultrasound, nuclear scan, and magnetic resonance imaging (MRI)
- Biopsy: Specimen of tumor is surgically removed for classification and staging of cancer. Bone marrow aspiration or biopsy may reveal cancer presence.
- Tumor staging: The malignant tumor's extent and progress is determined:
  - Stage I tumor is contained and can be completely removed.
  - Stage II tumor cannot be completely removed.
  - Stages III and IV tumors reveal **metastasis** (tumor spread beyond the original site or spread systemically):
    - Stage III tumor in regional lymph nodes.

- ◦ Stage IV tumor has spread to distant lymph nodes, bone, bone marrow, liver, and other organs.
    - ◦ Stage IV-S presents as localized tumor with spread to liver, skin, and bone marrow but without metastasis to bone.
  - • TNM system designation: Describes the tumor's size (T), its presence in the lymph nodes (N), and its metastasis (M) spread to other organs, if any. It is not helpful for those childhood tumors that are **sarcomas** (tumors derived from connective tissue, that is, bone, muscle, cartilage, blood vessels, or lymphoid tissue).

❸ TREATMENTS

- ◗ Surgical removal of tumor from involved body part(s)
- ◗ Thoracotomy for removal of cancer in the lungs
- ◗ Radiotherapy to destroy tumor
- ◗ Chemotherapy to assist in tumor destruction:
  - • Vincristine
  - • Cisplatin
  - • Actinomycin D
  - • Cyclophosphamide
  - • VP-16
  - • Doxorubicin
  - • Ifosfamide
  - • Etoposide

Nursing alert **While children are receiving chemotherapy, parents should not give them aspirin due to increased risk of bleeding and possible development of Reye syndrome.**

❹ NURSING INTERVENTIONS

- ◗ Provide nutritional support:
  - • Increased metabolism associated with cancer growth greatly increases nutritional needs and with cancer treatment, nutritional intake may be disturbed due to nausea or discomfort with eating.
  - • Assess for adequate nutritional intake: No further weight loss, lab values indicating adequate protein levels.
  - • Minimize exposure to germs because immune system compromise also results from treatment and places child at risk for infection.
  - • Provide emotional support because great emotional stress is also experienced by the child and family.
  - • Provide pain relief to address acute pain related to pressure of cancer tumor inside the bone.

- Address potential for disturbed body image related to hair loss due to radiation treatment by helping family plan in advance for hair coverings.
- Provide initial and continued assessment:
  - Analyze child's height and weight and note weight loss or growth delays.
  - Refer child with major joint swelling or pain for further orthopedic evaluation.

FAMILY AND CHILD SUPPORT

- Support the child and parents from the time of diagnosis through chemotherapy and other procedures such as surgery or radiation therapy.
- Explain treatment protocol to parents and include the child with cancer in planning care, as age permits.
- Promote the growth and development of the child and family coping.
- Prepare child and family for tests and knowledge of chemotherapy treatment side effects and complications to monitor for; involve child in decision making as much as possible.

Nursing alert **Parents should be cautioned to maintain regular health maintenance regimen during cancer therapy but *not* to continue immunizations that involve live-virus exposure due to child's compromised immune status.**

- Explain measures parents need to take to make their child more comfortable during therapy (i.e., not forcing food if the child is nauseated, playing games or reading stories while treatment is administered).
- When planning with parents and child, take into account their current stage of grief: Denial, anger, bargaining, depression, and acceptance.
- Consider the family's financial capabilities, and help them make any necessary financial arrangements for care.
- Encourage family and child to keep all follow-up examinations, despite fear of reports of cancer return; early detection leads to more effective treatment.
- Refer family for counseling and provide referral to community agencies to address resource needs for information or emotional or financial problems.
  - American Cancer Society (www.cancer.org)
  - National Cancer Institute (www.cancer.gov)
  - Children's Oncology Group (www.childrensoncologygroup.org)
  - Candlelighters Childhood Cancer Foundation (www.candlelighters.org)
  - The Leukemia & Lymphoma Society (www.leukemia-lymphoma.org)

Symptom Alleviation

- Evaluate for signs of infection and report for early treatment and eradication.

◑ Monitor for signs of septic shock.

◑ Monitor for complications of cancer treatment:

 Nursing alert **It is critical to monitor for signs of complications and report immediately so that the drug may be discontinued or reduced.**

- Fever.
- Bleeding: Administer platelets, move body parts gently, avoid punctures.
- Anemia: Regular, not strenuous, supervised activity with rest periods.
- Nausea and vomiting: Administer antiemetic and appetite stimulant.

 Nursing alert **Children may develop a hatred of foods offered during periods of nausea so avoid offering favorite foods during chemotherapy administration.**

◑ Mucosal ulceration can occur with chemotherapy. Offer bland soft diet, clean mouth with soft applicator, rinse mouth with salt water, and provide local anesthetics to relieve oral pain.

◑ Hemorrhagic cystitis: Fluid intake, frequent voiding, early-day drug administration, and drug to inhibit the condition.

◑ 🔔 Neurologic problems may result from the neurotoxic effects of chemotherapy. Nursing care addresses:

- Constipation: Physical activity, provide stool softeners and laxatives.
- Foot drop, extremity weakness or numbness: Apply footboard, inform parents and teachers so expectations of physical ability can be adjusted.
- Alopecia: Patchy baldness may be noted; hair returns in 3 to 6 months.
  ○ Prepare for head cover or wig prior to onset of alopecia to maintain self-esteem.
  ○ Reduce shock of hair loss with advance notice and suggest loose cap to collect hair that falls out during the night.

◑ Steroid effects: Alert child and family of possible body changes such as moon face, mood changes.

◑ Watch for oncologic emergencies. Report and initiate treatments as ordered:

- Acute tumor lysis syndrome.
- Hyperleukocytosis.
- Overwhelming infection.
- Obstruction (compression of mediastinal structures could result in vena cava syndrome—monitor for and treat respiratory distress.

✔ ROUTINE CHECKUP 1

1. Common symptoms of cancer in children include (a)_____,
   (b)_____, (c)_____, and
   (d)_____.
   Answer:
   _____

2. What data in a 12-year-old client's history would alert the nurse most to watch the client closely for signs of cancer?
   a. The client has reported frequent headache and weight loss.
   b. The client reports urinating three times a day.
   c. The dietary history reveals a high intake of fruit and vegetables.
   d. The school history indicates hyperactivity when doing class work.
   Answer:

3. (a)_____, (b)_____, (c)_____, and
   (d) _____ are four existing theories of the causes of childhood neoplasm development.
   Answer:
   _____

PEDIATRIC ONCOLOGY CONDITIONS

LEUKEMIA

What Went Wrong?

Leukemia, the most common cancer in childhood, is a group of cancer diseases of blood-forming tissues such as the bone marrow and lymphatic system. The problem in leukemia is the production of an excessive number of immature (still in the stem, or "blast," stage) white blood cells (WBCs). Crowding from these excessive immature cells compromises the production of other cells in the bone marrow. The leukemias are categorized by subtype into two major classifications: acute lymphoid leukemia (ALL)/blast stem leukemia, the most common type in children, and acute myelogenous leukemia (AML), most frequent in adults and the most common form of leukemia overall. The primary difference is the type of leukocyte (WBC) involved. In ALL, the immature WBCs are lymphocytes, and in AML the WBCs involved are cells from the myeloid line, primarily granulocytes or monocytes.

Signs and Symptoms

- Common assessment findings:
  - Diagnosis suspected by history and physical data.

TABLE 8–1 • Impact of Leukemia on Blood Cells			
Cell Type	Compromise	Resulting Impact	Residual Effects
Red blood cells (RBCs)	Low production (anemia)	Decreased oxygen transport	Shortness of breath with exertion Activity intolerance
			Pallor
Platelets	Decreased production	Decreased clotting	Bleeding tendency
White blood cells (WBCs)	Decreased functional WBCs	Decreased immune function.	Susceptibility to infection
Immature leukocytes	Excessive production of nonfunctional cells	Crowding within bone and pressure	Pain in bone and joints
		Thinning of bone shaft and weakening	Pathologic fractures

- History: Describe onset as acute to vague (insidious) with few symptoms.
- Cold that does not resolve completely.
- Pallor, fatigue, listlessness, irritability, fever, and anorexia may be noted.
- May mimic symptoms of rheumatoid arthritis symptoms or mononucleosis.
- Regular physical can reveal lab values indicating disease.

The result of this crowding depends on the cells that are compromised, as shown in Table 8-1.

Test Results

- Peripheral blood smear used for initial diagnosis—immature leukocytes noted (See Table 8-2).
- Bone marrow aspiration or biopsy used for definitive diagnosis—hypercellular with blast cells dominating.
- Lumbar puncture done after diagnosis to determine CNS involvement (rarely noted).
- Chest CT scan and bone scans to detect metastasis to lung.

Treatments

- Chemotherapy is performed with or without cranial irradiation in four phases:

TABLE 8–2 • Staging: Cell Subtype Classification by Morphology for Treatment and Prognosis			
Leukemia Type	**Staging System**	**Factors Examined**	**Findings**
Acute lymphoid leukemia (ALL) (most common form); Acute myelogenous leukemia (AML)	French-American-British (FAB) system Eight subgroups (not as related to prognosis)	Morphology (structure) and cytochemical reactivity of leukemia cells	L1 (85% of cases and best prognosis), L2, and L3

Note: Cytochemical markers are also used for staging leukemia because leukemic cell reactions to different chemicals differentiate between ALL and AML

Chromosome studies may be performed because some children with chromosome abnormalities (trisomy 20, 21, and others) are higher risk for types of leukemia.

Cell-surface immunologic markers can be used to identify type of cell involved. The common ALL antigen (CALLA)-positive children have best survival rate.

- Induction: Complete remission of leukemic cells (<5% blast cells)
  - Steroids and vincristine, L-asparaginase, and possibly doxorubicin
  - 4- to 6-week session
- Intensification or consolidation therapy: Decrease tumor burden
  - L-asparaginase, high-dose methotrexate, leucovorin rescue, vincristine, doxorubicin, steroids, cytarabine, and mercaptopurine
  - 6 months of treatment: Combinations dependent on cell type
- CNS prophylactic therapy: Decrease CNS invasion
  - Intrathecal chemotherapy: Methotrexate, cytarabine, and hydrocortisone
  - Possible cranial irradiation
- Maintenance: Maintain remission with irradiation as cell type indicates:
  - Combined drug regimen: Varied drugs (discontinue if toxic side effects [myelosuppression with low neutrophil count <1000/mm^3])
- Reinduction with relapse: Use of prednisone and vincristine and other chemotherapy
- Bone marrow transplantation (BMT) used to treat children with ALL and AML:
  - Reserved for second remission with ALL
  - May be used with first AML remission to improve prognosis
- Radiotherapy to destroy tumor

Nursing Interventions

- Reinforce physician's explanation of diagnosis and treatment plan.
- Explain procedure at child's level of understanding including what will be seen, felt, heard, and smelled; use drawings when appropriate.

◐ Maintain contact after discharge and between remissions to encourage follow-up care and respond to questions or provide emotional support.

◐ Provide antiemetic and appetite stimulant to increase nutritional intake.

◐ Offer foods after antiemetic takes effect to reduce nausea and maximize caloric intake.

◐ Allow to eat any food that is tolerated; avoid forcing food during nausea episode.

◐ Rinse mouth to remove unpleasant taste sensation.

LYMPHOMAS

What Went Wrong?

Lymphomas are lymph or reticuloendothelial system malignancies; they account for about 15% of all malignancies. Lymphomas are categorized as Hodgkin (most common in adults) or non-Hodgkin (most frequently occurring in childhood). They both occur more frequently in boys than in girls and most frequently in adolescents (Hodgkin, ages 15 to 19 years; non-Hodgkin <15 years of age). Metastasis occurs through lymphatic channels and spreads late in the disease, to the lung, liver, and bone marrow.

Signs and Symptoms

◐ Common assessment findings:
- History: May report anorexia, malaise, night sweats, and loss of weight.
- Cold that does not resolve completely.
- Pallor, fatigue, listlessness, irritability, and anorexia; fever may be noted.
- May mimic symptoms of rheumatoid arthritis symptoms or mononucleosis.
- Physical can reveal a painless, enlarged, rubbery-feeling lymph node (cervical).

Test Results

◐ Sedimentation rate elevated.

◐ RBCs decreased.

◐ Lymph node biopsy confirms diagnosis: Reed-Sternberg cells (large multinucleated cells—nonfunctioning monocyte-macrophage cells).

◐ Lymphangiogram for visualization of the lymphatic system with dye to mark disease (dye can stain skin for up to 12 months).

◐ Chest radiograph (large mediastinal nodes), CT scan (enlarged abdominal lymph nodes), and bone scans to stage the disease.

Staging

◐ Four subcategories: Lymphocyte predominant, nodular sclerosing (most common in children), mixed cellularity, and lymphocyte depletion.

◐ Staged by regional involvement: CT and multiple lymph node and bone marrow biopsies:

◐ **Non-Hodgkin Lymphoma or Hodgkin Lymphoma**

- Stage 1: One lymph node area or maximum of one extralymphatic site (IE)
- Stage II: Two or more lymph node regions, or one added extralymphatic site or organ involved, on same side of diaphragm or abdomen (IIE)
- Stage III: Lymph node regions on both sides of diaphragm, or one extralymphatic site (IIIE), spleen (IIIS), or both (IIISE)
- Stage IV: Cancer has spread throughout body with one or more extra-lymphatic sites with or without lymph node involvement

3 Treatments

◐ **Non-Hodgkin lymphoma:** Similar to leukemia treatment with induction, consolidation, and maintenance phases based on lymphoblastic or nonlymphoblastic cells:

- Lymphoblastic lymphoma: Multiple chemotherapy regimens—commonly cyclophosphamide or ifosfamide, vincristine, intrathecal chemotherapy such as L-asparaginase, prednisone, daunomycin, 6-thioguanine, cytosine arabinoside, and BCNU.
- Nonlymphoblastic cells: Cyclic drug combinations with cyclophosphamide and methotrexate plus anthracycline

◐ **Hodgkin treatment** also involves irradiation and chemotherapy:

- Treatment:
  - Aggressive irradiation: Involved field (IF), extended field (EF) including involved area and adjacent nodes, or total nodal irradiation (TNI).
  - Mechlorethamine (nitrogen mustard), vincristine (Oncovin), procarbazine, and prednisone, a protocol commonly called MOPP therapy.
  - Cyclophosphamide and cytarabine and other chemotherapy may be used.
  - Five-year survival for stage I or II is 90%; stage III or IV is 60 to 90%.

  Relapse in adulthood is possible.

4 Nursing Interventions

◐ Reinforce physician's explanation of diagnosis and treatment plan.

◐ Explain procedure at child's level of understanding including what will be seen.

◐ Address fear related to diagnostic tests, procedures, and treatments.

- Reinforce physician's explanation of diagnosis and treatment plan.
- Explain procedure at child's level of understanding including what will be seen, felt, heard, and smelled; use drawings when appropriate.

- Maintain contact after discharge and between remissions to encourage follow-up care and respond to questions, or provide emotional support.
◐ Provide antiemetic and appetite stimulant.
◐ Offer foods after antiemetic takes effect.
◐ Allow to eat any food that is tolerated; avoid forcing food during nausea episode.
◐ Rinse mouth to remove unpleasant taste sensation.
◐ Address activity intolerance secondary to thyroid damage from treatment and resulting hypothyroidism.
- Maintain child's activity within level of tolerance.
◐ Provide age-appropriate diversion toys, books, or other activities for child or adolescent.

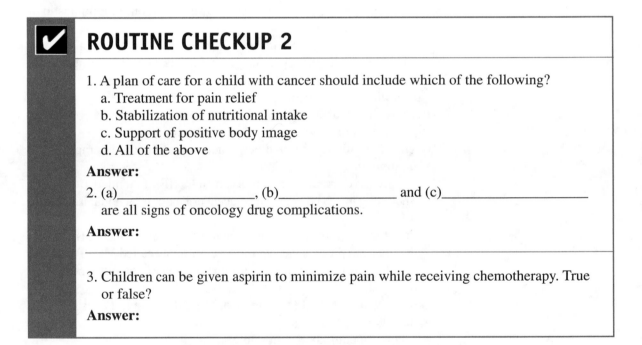

✔ ROUTINE CHECKUP 2

1. A plan of care for a child with cancer should include which of the following?
   a. Treatment for pain relief
   b. Stabilization of nutritional intake
   c. Support of positive body image
   d. All of the above

Answer:

2. (a)_____, (b)_____ and (c)_____ are all signs of oncology drug complications.

Answer:
_____

3. Children can be given aspirin to minimize pain while receiving chemotherapy. True or false?

Answer:

SARCOMAS (BONE TUMORS)

What Went Wrong?

An **osteogenic sarcoma,** the most common bone tumor, is a malignant tumor of long bone involving rapidly growing bone tissue. It occurs more often between ages 10 and 25 years and more in boys than girls. The most common tumor location is the distal femur (40 to 50% frequency), followed by the tibia (20%), and then the proximal humerus (10 to 15%). Metastasis, commonly to the lungs, occurs early because bones are highly vascular. Other sites of metastasis are the brain and other bone tissue.

Ewing sarcoma is a malignant tumor in the bone marrow of the midshaft of the long and trunk bone, most commonly the femur, pelvic bone, tibia, fibula, scapula, ribs and skull. It occurs most commonly between the ages of 4 and 25 years. Metastasis to the lungs and bones is often present at time of diagnosis, with eventual spread to the CNS and lymph nodes.

Signs and Symptoms

- Common assessment findings:
  - History of trauma to leg (client related pain to trauma and delayed trip to doctor)
  - Taller than average height due to rapid bone growth
  - Pain, warmth, and swelling at the tumor site
  - Pathologic fracture of the bone as tumor invades and weakens bone

Test Results

- Diagnosis by biopsy of suspicious area
- Elevated serum alkaline phosphatase due to rapidly growing bone cells
- Blood count, urinalysis
- Radiograph (will reveal an unusual "onion skin" reaction—fine lines on the film)
- Chest CT scan and bone scans to detect metastasis to lung
- Intravenous pyelogram or kidney MRI to detect metastasis to kidney.
- Bone marrow aspiration for Ewing sarcoma

Treatments

- Surgical removal of involved bone part replaced with an internally placed bone or metal prosthesis.
- Amputation of bone above the joint (commonly total hip amputation); not routine for Ewing sarcoma unless tumor is respectable or radiotherapy results in useless or deformed leg
- Thoracotomy for removal of cancer in the lungs
- Osteogenic sarcoma:
  - Chemotherapy to shrink tumor before surgery:
    - Methotrexate
    - Cisplatin
    - Doxorubicin
    - Ifosfamide
  - 60% or more adolescents cured with vigorous treatment
- Ewing sarcoma:
  - Radiotherapy to destroy tumor
  - Chemotherapy to assist in tumor destruction:

○ Vincristine
        ○ Cisplatin
        ○ Actinomycin D
        ○ Cyclophosphamide
        ○ VP-16
        ○ Doxorubicin
        ○ Ifosfamide
        ○ Etoposide
     • Three-year survival increased to 80% with vigorous treatment

Nursing Interventions

    ◐ Address fear related to diagnostic tests, procedures, and treatments to promote cooperation from the child and parents—responses to verbal directives with minimal resistance.

    ◐ Reinforce physician's explanation of diagnosis and treatment plan.

    ◐ Explain procedure at child's level of understanding including what will be seen, felt, heard, and smelled.

 Nursing alert **Instruct the child not to put weight on the affected limb due to danger of a pathologic fracture.**

    ◐ Explain what child is expected to do during test and care activities.

    ◐ Use distraction techniques to reduce focus on procedure and fear:
        • Involve client in procedure if possible—holding tape, repeat steps.

    ◐ Position leg gently to avoid disruption of neurologic or circulatory function.

    ◐ Address potential injury related to surgery and bone prosthesis:
        • Elevate limb to reduce swelling.

    ◐ Assess neurologic and circulatory system for absence of disruption:
        • Dry or moist desquamation followed by hyperpigmentation expected.
        • Minimal skin irritation and absence of ulceration.
        • Extremity distal to incision warm to touch.
        • Capillary refill <5 seconds.
        • No report of tingling or numbness in distal extremity.

 Nursing alert **Instruct adolescents to avoid excessive stress on leg that has received extensive radiation (no football, no weight lifting with pressure on that leg) because leg may not be as strong as normal afterward.**

    ◐ Assess pain level on a pain scale prior to and after treatment.

    ◐ Administer analgesic to control pain.

- Reduce risk for injury, decreased skin integrity, related to radiotherapy.
- Position leg gently to avoid disruption of neurologic or circulatory function.
- Dress child in loose-fitting clothing over treated site to reduce pressure and pain at site.
- Protect affected skin area from direct sunlight and temperature extremes from heat pads or ice packs.
- Elevate limb to reduce swelling.
- Encourage activity and use of extremity as tolerated when therapy is complete.
- Assess client for adequate nutritional intake:
    - No weight loss
    - Lab work reveals protein levels within normal range
- Provide antiemetic and appetite stimulant.
- Offer foods after antiemetic takes effect to minimize nausea and increase intake.
- Allow to eat any food that is tolerated; avoid forcing food during nausea episode.
- Rinse mouth to remove unpleasant taste sensation.

What Went Wrong?

Other Solid Tumors: Nephroblastoma (Wilms tumor), a malignant tumor composed of metanephric mesoderm cells of the upper pole of the kidney, accounts for 20% of the solid tumors found in children. Most cases (approximately 80%) are discovered in children <5 years of age with most cases occurring between the ages of 3 and 4 years. Increased incidence is seen among siblings, and Wilms tumor is associated with several congenital anomalies, most commonly including hemangioma, aniridia (lack of color in the iris), cryptorchidism, hypospadias, pseudohermaphroditism, cystic kidneys, and talipes disorders. The tumor is primarily located in the intraabdominal and kidney area. The metastatic spread is most often to the lungs, regional lymph nodes, liver, bone, and eventually spreads to the brain by the bloodstream.

Signs and Symptoms

- Presents most commonly as firm, nontender, mass deep within the flank and confined to one side of the body (may be confused with liver on palpation but does not move with respiration).
- Other symptoms may result from organ compression from tumor, metabolic alterations from the tumor, or metastasis.
- Hematuria may be noted in less than half of cases.
- Tumor may seem to appear suddenly if it hemorrhages into itself doubling in size in a short time.
- Anemia with accompanying pallor, anorexia, and lethargy may be noted.

- Hypertension due to tumor excretion of renin may occur on occasion.
- Metastasis may reveal symptoms dependent on location.
  - Dyspnea, cough, shortness of breath, and chest pain with chest involvement

Test Results

- History (familial history of cancer) and physical examination are important.
- Diagnosis by biopsy of fully excised tumor to prevent seeding by rupture of encapsulated tumor mass.
- Hematologic studies (may reveal polycythemia due to excess erythropoietin secretion or anemia from deficient erythropoietin secretion or from hemorrhage).
- Blood chemistry (including creatinine and BUN), urinalysis, and glomerular filtration rate may be used to assess renal function.
- Abdominal ultrasound and other radiographic studies.
- CT scan, MRI, and bone scans to detect metastasis to lung.
- Inferior venacavogram may reveal involvement with vena cava.

Treatments

- Multimodal treatment with surgical removal of tumor and chemotherapy
- Irradiation added based on stage of tumor and to shrink tumor before surgery
- Chemotherapy to shrink tumor before surgery and as follow-up:
  - Chemotherapy agents of choice:
    - Vincristine
    - Actinomycin D
    - Cyclophosphamide
    - Doxorubicin
- Partial or total nephrectomy (removal of kidney) may be necessary.
- If both kidneys involved, bilateral nephrectomy (last resort if sibling transplant is possible)

Nursing Interventions

- Interventions are similar to those with other solid tumors.
- Preoperative care:
  - Monitor closely for signs of renin release: Hypertension.

Nursing alert **Protect abdomen from trauma; tumor must *not* be palpated unless absolutely necessary and only with gentle pressure to avoid possible rupture and spread of cancer cells. Post sign above bed as reminder to reduce risk of deep palpation.**

◐ Postoperative care:
- Recovery period is rapid.
- Support is needed if renal function is severely compromised.
- General abdominal surgery care is performed:
  ◦ Pulmonary hygiene—cough, deep breathing.
  ◦ Monitor for complications: Bleeding, infection.
- Monitor for signs of complications of chemotherapy:
  ◦ Intestinal obstruction from adynamic ileus from vincristine, post-surgical adhesions, or edema.
  ◦ Nausea and vomiting, abdominal distention.

◐ Play therapy should include age-appropriate activities to entertain and distract child.

◐ Involve child and family in care planning.

◐ Because child is often left with one kidney, activity restrictions may include no contact sports or high-risk activity.

◐ Genitourinary care and hygiene taken to prevent infection, monitor for signs of infection.

Family-Centered Care

◐ Explain the symptoms that may result from preoperative radiation or chemotherapy:
- Discussion regarding hair loss can be postponed until after surgery because onset of alopecia occurs 2 weeks after onset of treatment.

◐ Support child and family through diagnosis, treatment/surgery, and follow-up care:
- Let family and child ventilate concerns and fears;, refer for counseling as needed.

✔ ROUTINE CHECKUP 3

1. Will Bason, age 3, was admitted with a parental complaint "problems peeing." The nurse would suspect a Wilms tumor if what assessment finding was noted?
   a. Pale yellow urine in urine bag
   b. Pallor and lethargy noted
   c. Pink oral mucosa
   d. Soft tender area on the left flank

Answer:

2. The nurse should provide _____ _____ including age- appropriate activities to entertain and distract the young child during cancer treatment.

Answer:

NEUROBLASTOMA

Neuroblastomas are the most common abdominal tumor in childhood. The tumors arise from greatly undifferentiated and invasive cells from the sympathetic nervous system. Tumors usually occur in the abdomen near the adrenal gland or spinal ganglia but may also be noted in the head, neck, chest, or pelvis. Neuroblastomas occur primarily in infants <2 years of age (50%) and preschool children (25%) and slightly more often in males than females. Metastasis is most commonly to the bone marrow, liver, and subcutaneous tissue.

Signs and Symptoms

- Common assessment findings:
  - Symptoms depend on the location and stage of the tumor (secondary to pressure on adjacent structures—respiratory distress from thoracic mass).
  - Cervical or supraclavicular lymphadenopathy may be noted.
  - Presents as a firm, irregular, painless mass in the abdomen that crosses the midline.
  - Urinary retention or frequency may be noted if kidney is compressed.
  - Periorbital edema, exophthalmos, and supraorbital ecchymosis are noted with metastasis to the retrobulbar tissue.
  - Weight loss and anorexia may be noted due to tumor pressure.
  - Difficulty swallowing and edema of the neck and face may occur from compression on the vena cava.
  - Jaundice from liver pressure may be noted and if metastasis to the skin has occurred, blue or purplish nodules may be noted on the arms or legs.
  - Flushed face, excessive sweating, and hypertension may result from adrenal pressure.
  - Symptoms of neurologic impairment, including paralysis from compressed nerves, may be noted, as well as neurologic changes from intracranial lesions.

Test Results

- Diagnosis by biopsy.
- Skeletal survey of skull, chest, abdomen, and bone marrow aspirates.
- Blood count, urinalysis (may reveal catecholamine excretion from adrenals).
- CT scan and bone scans to detect metastasis.
- Vanillylmandelic acid (VMA), homovanillic acid (HVA), dopamine in urine (breakdown products of catecholamines) may be noted with an adrenal tumor.
- Increased ferritin, neuron-specific enolase (NSE), and ganglioside(GD2) may be noted (isoenzymes from neurons).

Staging

- More than 70% of cases are found after metastasis has occurred (stage III or IV).
- Prognosis is poor because of late discovery.
- Survival inversely related to age with higher survival (75%) for infants <1 year of age and less (50%) if >1 year of age.
- Stage IV-S localized tumor with spread to liver, skin, and bone marrow but without metastasis to bone presented in very young infant may have good prognosis for cure.
- Spontaneous regression may be noted.

Treatments

- Surgical removal of tumor is treatment of choice.
- Chemotherapy to shrink tumor before surgery or as main treatment with metastasis.
  - Preferred agents:
    - Vincristine
    - Cisplatin
    - Teniposide
    - Cyclophosphamide
    - Carboplatin
    - Doxorubicin
    - Ifosfamide
    - Etoposide
- With addition of bone marrow transplant or peripheral stem cell rescue, survival rate to 10 to 20% in infants >2 years of age.
- Radiotherapy for late-stage tumor and for emergency management of spinal compression by large tumor; palliative treatment of bone, lungs, liver, or brain.

Nursing Interventions

- Support child during treatments:
  - Provide antiemetic and appetite stimulant.
  - Offer foods after antiemetic takes effect.
  - Allow to eat any food that is tolerated; avoid forcing food during nausea episode.
- Support parents and family with coping and with grieving process, when indicated:
  - Expect stages of grief, with anger expression.
  - Help parents work through feeling of guilt related to late diagnosis and feelings earlier action should have been taken.
- Assess for adequate nutritional intake:
  - No weight loss.
  - Lab work reveals protein levels within normal range.

✔ ROUTINE CHECKUP 4

1. There are _____ stages of _____ to be considered when planning with parents of children with a terminal cancer diagnosis.

Answer:

2. Neuroblastoma, neoplasm, retinoblastoma, and osteosarcoma are all examples of solid tumors. True or false?

Answer:

RHABDOMYOSARCOMA

What Went Wrong?

A **rhabdomyosarcoma** is the fourth most common solid tumor. It arises from the embryonic mesenchyme tissue that forms connective, vascular, muscle, and connective tissue. The primary sites of occurrence are the ocular orbit, paranasal sinuses, uterus, prostate, bladder, retroperitoneum, arms, or legs. Metastasis into the CNS occurs in addition to distant metastasis commonly to the lungs, bone, or the bone marrow. Rhabdomyosarcoma may occur at any age but occurs primarily in children <5 years of age with a second peak incidence during puberty.

Signs and Symptoms

- Common assessment findings:
  - Symptoms depend on the site and stage of the tumor:
    - Unilateral proptosis (exophthalmos), strabismus, and conjunctival ecchymosis are noted with metastasis to the eye orbit.
    - Palpable nontender, firm, hard mass in head and neck area.
    - Stuffy nose, nasal obstruction (dysphagia, nasal voice, and otitis media due to eustachian tube obstruction) with nasopharynx or paranasal tumor or middle ear tumor (pain, purulent drainage, and facial nerve palsy).
    - Abdominal mass (retroperitoneal) or superficial perineal mass with pain, or signs of bowel or bladder obstruction: Intestinal (nausea/vomiting) or genitourinary (urinary retention or frequency).

Test Results

- Diagnosis by biopsy to confirm histologic type.
- Bone scan, chest radiograph, CT scan, MRI, and bone marrow aspirations done to rule out metastasis.

◐ Lumbar puncture may be used for head and neck tumors with examination of cerebrospinal fluid for malignant cells.

Staging

◐ Metastasis has usually occurred by the time of diagnosis.
◐ Five-year survival rate is near 65%, as high as 80%; tumor will not recur if totally removed by surgery.
◐ Children disease free for 2 years are likely cured; prognosis is poor with relapse.

Treatment

◐ Multimodal therapy is the treatment of choice.
◐ Complete removal of primary tumor done when possible, however surgical removal of tumors is used less frequently.
◐ High-dose irradiation for tumors stages II through IV.
◐ Intrathecal chemotherapy may be included in the regimen.
◐ Chemotherapy as part of multimodal treatment with metastasis.
  • Preferred chemotherapeutic agents:
    ◦ Vincristine
    ◦ Cisplatin
    ◦ VP-16
    ◦ Actinomycin D
    ◦ Cyclophosphamide
    ◦ Carboplatin
    ◦ Topotecan
    ◦ Melphalan
    ◦ Doxorubicin
    ◦ Ifosfamide
    ◦ Etoposide
    ◦ Adriamycin

Nursing Interventions

◐ Same as with solid tumors with additions as follows:
  • Assess for signs of tumor:
    ◦ Inspect nasopharynx and oropharynx for visible mass.
  • Prepare child and family for extensive diagnostic testing.
  • Support child and family during diagnosis, procedures, and treatments.

RETINOBLASTOMA

What Went Wrong?

Retinoblastoma is a rare malignant tumor of the retina of the eye accounting for <3% of childhood cancers. It usually occurs in children <5 years of age with most cases occurring at the average age of 17 months. The majority of cases of retinoblastoma are spontaneous, but a few cases are associated with an autosomal-dominant pattern of inheritance with survivors of the disease at risk for being carriers to their children.

Signs and Symptoms

- Common assessment findings:
  - History of trauma to leg (client related pain to trauma and delayed trip to doctor)
  - Taller than average height due to rapid bone growth
  - Pain, warmth, and swelling at the tumor site
  - Pathologic fracture of the bone—as tumor invades and weakens bone

Test Results

- Refer child to ophthalmologist for evaluation.
- Indirect ophthalmoscopy performed with scleral indentation for diagnosis.

Staging

- Few cases have metastasis.
- Classification by Reese-Ellsworth used.
  - Group I: Very favorable with solitary tumor <4 disc diameters (DD) at or behind the equator or multiple tumors at or behind the equator all <4 DD.
  - Group II: Favorable with solitary tumor 4 to 10 DD at or behind the equator, or multiple tumors at or behind the equator 4 to 10 DD.
  - Group III: Doubtful with solitary tumor >10 DD behind the equator, or any tumors anterior to the equator.
  - Group IV: Unfavorable with multiple tumors some larger than 10 DD at or any tumors anterior to the ora serrata.
  - Group V: Very unfavorable: Massive tumors involving more than half the retina and vitreous seeding.
- Metastasis is seldom noted; invasive staging procedures such as aspiration or biopsy not performed.

Treatments

- Localized tumor treatment:
  - Plaque brachytherapy (implantation of a radiation applicator on sclera (iodine-125) until maximum dose delivered to the tumor.
  - Photocoagulation (laser beam used to destroy blood supply to tumor).
  - Cryotherapy (freezing of the tumor to destroy microcirculation to and cells of the tumor).
- With advanced tumor growth with involvement of the optic nerve, enucleation of the affected eye is treatment of choice.

◑ Chemotherapy in advance disease is controversial, but drugs of choice are:
  • Vincristine
  • Cisplatin
  • Cyclophosphamide
  • Adriamycin
  • Etoposide
◑ Intrathecal chemotherapy may be used if central nervous system involvement.
◑ If bilateral eye involvement, radiotherapy to both eyes is performed.

◢ Nursing Interventions

◑ Prepare infant/child and family for diagnostic and treatment procedures.
◑ Explain to parents that child's vision may be less focused after treatment and the eyes may be sensitive to light.
◑ If enucleation is performed, prepare parents for sight of empty eye socket and show pictures of postoperative child to show prosthesis in place.
◑ Instruct parents on care of prosthesis with return demonstration.
◑ Discuss possible hereditary aspect of disease and import of genetic testing and counseling.
◑ Encourage family to schedule follow-up visits and maintain regular checkups.

✔ ROUTINE CHECKUP 5

1. Tumor stages III and IV reveal benign tumors that can be completely removed. True or false?

Answer:

2. Hair-loss, constipation and numbness of the extremities may all result from the neurotoxic effects of _____.

Answer:

CONCLUSION

Cancer conditions in children cause many common concerns, and family-centered care is required to address these concerns. Maintaining growth and development is important for all pediatric clients, from infancy through adolescence. Support for adequate nutrition during the early stage of diagnosis through treatment is critical to helping the client and family cope with the physical stress of the condition. Emotional support for the client and the family is important in promoting coping skills during all stages of the condition and treatment. Key information covered in this chapter includes the following:

- Both the child and family may undergo a grieving process with the diagnosis of cancer and become depressed, overly protective, withdrawn, and angry. Teaching and support by the nurse is needed to correct misconceptions and keep the child and parents updated on the child's progress.
- Emotional support is needed to encourage the child to continue to function to the maximum within limitations.
- Cancer conditions affect multiple systems and require a multisystem plan of action.
- A thorough history and physical can provide critical data for diagnosis and treatment planning.
- Possible causes of cancer include exposure to carcinogens, in utero, or after birth and including an oncogenic virus, gene theory, or familial predisposition for cell mutation or predisposition due to previous cancer, or deficient tumor suppressor cell deficit.
- Leukemia is the most frequent type of cancer in children.
- Physical assessment of a child with cancer may reveal cardinal symptoms of cancer:
  - Unusual lump or swelling (i.e., abdominal mass or swollen lymph glands)
  - Unexplained fatigue or pallor (due to anemia)
  - Easy bruising (ecchymosis and petechiae)
  - Persistent pain or limping gait
  - Prolonged unexplained fever or illness
  - Sudden changes in eye or vision
  - Rapid or excessive weight loss
- Test results will often include low red blood cell count (anemia) secondary to the cancer (if bone marrow is involved) or as a complication of chemotherapy.
- Bleeding may be noted if platelets are reduced.
- Diagnostic tests may include serum analysis, biopsy, and imaging studies.
- Treatment for cancer requires biopsy to obtain a specimen for staging to determine the extent to which the cancer has spread.
- Radiotherapy in combination with surgery or chemotherapy may be used to treat cancer.
- Nutritional deficit may result from the increased metabolism or from difficulty eating due to fatigue, discomfort with chewing or swallowing, or nausea from the cancer invasion or cancer treatment.
- Immune deficiency can result from the bone marrow invasion or from cancer treatment.

○ Alopecia (patchy baldness) may be noted with chemotherapy or radio-therapy, so prepare child and family in advance when possible to allow preparation for hair cover.

○ Refer family for counseling and provide referral to community agencies to address resource needs for information or emotional or financial problems.

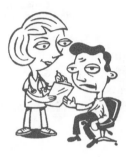

CASE STUDY

Adam, age 7, was admitted to the hospital with symptoms of fatigue and fever and a "cold that keeps hanging on." His mother states that Adam has not been eating or drinking much and is unable to tolerate school activities. He has had to stay home for the past 3 days. In the admission history the nurse learns that Adam lives alone with his mom. A diagnosis of leukemia was made after lab results were reviewed.

Assessment data: Laboratory values reveal below normal levels of red blood cells (2.5 million/mm^3), platelets (70,000 mm^3), and white blood cells (4000 mm^3). Immature lymphocytes are noted. What type of leukemia would that indicate?

Additional lab values reveal a protein level below normal (5.4 g/dL to 54g/L), and hematocrit of 40%, and Adam reveals a dry tongue and mucous membranes, and poor skin turgor when the skin over the forehead is pinched. The sample obtained for admission urinalysis is small in amount (50 mL) and golden.

Interpretation: What conditions should the nurse suspect from the history and lab value?

Nursing intervention: Provide small high calorie meals every 3 hours, after a rest during waking hours. Provide vitamins as ordered to stimulate appetite. Weigh Adam every 24 hours using the same scale. Food and oral fluids are offered (120 mL/hour) and within 24 hours Adam begins to show increased energy. The sodium level was noted as 160 mEq/L (160 mmol/L) in the admission labs, and the level was decreased to 142 mEq/L (142 mmol/L) after hydration. The nurse monitors intake and output and continues to offer fluids between meals but with lesser frequency (60 mL every 2 to 3 hours).

Further exploration: Assess client's vital signs along with what other elements daily?

Follow-up assessments and monitoring: The nurse watches Adam closely for fluid balance including urine output (becoming lighter gold in color with hydration, 30 cc/hour), weight (4.4 kg below is normal range on admission, but now only 3 kg below normal range), and continues intake and outputs. The nurse also watches for signs of anemia (realizing the hematocrit was within range because the client was hemoconcentrated and after rehydration the level will likely drop).

Evaluation and continued care: The nurses perform full assessments every 12 hours. Daily weights reveal weight gain of 1 pound after 1 week of treatment with six small high-calorie meals. Chemotherapy is tolerated well without nausea and vomiting and with administration of antiemetic. Adam moves into a remission of the leukemia. Skin is warm to touch with capillary refill in extremities <3 seconds. Mucous membranes begin to look moist, and urine color becomes clear and pale yellow with fluid intake of 8 ounces every 2 hours. The nurse instructs the mother to stop pushing fluid between meals and provide drink as requested by child because dehydration seems to have resolved. After further teaching, the mother voiced understanding of follow-up visits after discharge to monitor for condition change or continued remission.

Answers for the Case Study

1. Immature lymphocytes are noted, indicating acute lymphoid leukemia (ALL).
2. **Interpretation:** The nurse suspects malnourishment and dehydration because of the low protein and poor skin turgor and dehydration because of the dry tongue and mucous membrane and concentrated urine. The low RBCs, platelet, and WBC levels indicate anemia and reduced blood cell production from the leukemia.
3. **Follow-up:** Daily weight, skin turgor, and activity tolerance, note daily lab results, particularly hematocrit, protein, as well as blood cells—RBC, WBC—to determine hydration, nutrition, and anemia status.

? FINAL CHECKUP

1. **To remain aware of client needs and advocate for the client nurses must do which of the following?**
   a. Monitor lab results
   b. Note side effects from medications
   c. Explore historical data
   d. All of the above

2. **What is the most frequent type of cancer in children other than immature blood cell overgrowth?**
   a. Lymphomas
   b. Leukemia
   c. Rhabdomyosarcoma
   d. Gliomas

3. **The oncogenic virus theory states which of the following?**
   a. There is a familial predisposition for cell mutation
   b. Previous cancer produces high risk for cancer
   c. Cancer development is caused by exposure to carcinogenic organisms
   d. All of the above

4. **An assessment of a child with cancer includes but is not limited to which of the following?**
   a. Determining religious philosophy
   b. Assessing political views
   c. Reviewing diagnostic test findings
   d. None of the above

5. **Bone marrow aspiration is also known as which of the following?**
   a. Biopsy
   b. Metastasis
   c. Cachexia
   d. Ewing sarcoma

6. **What is Osteogenic sarcoma?**
   a. Malignant long-bone tumor
   b. Malignant tumor of the spine
   c. Malignant tumor in the bone marrow
   d. Benign tumor of the knee

7. **When caring for children with cancer and their families, what should the nurse do?**
   a. Explain procedures in terms only the parent will understand to protect the child.
   b. Do not contact families and allow them their privacy after discharge.
   c. Reinforce physician's explanations of diagnosis and treatment plans.
   d. None of the above.

8. **When explaining treatment protocol to parents, what should the nurse stress?**
   a. Child should be included as age and maturity permits.
   b. Parents should be told to continue with regular immunizations.
   c. Parents should push the child to eat favorite foods when feeling nauseated.
   d. b and c only.

9. **The care needs of families of children with cancer include the following:**
   a. Stabilization of child's weight during chemotherapy
   b. Referral for family counseling
   c. A maintenance of activity within the child's tolerance
   d. All of the above

10. **Soft, bland diets, and saltwater rinses are used to relieve the pain of which of the following?**
    a. Toothaches
    b. Malignant tumors
    c. Mucosal ulcerations
    d. Hemorrhagic cystitis

ANSWERS

Routine checkup 1
1. Headache, fatigue, nosebleeds, and excessive weight loss.
2. a.
3. Gene theory, in utero or secondary exposure to carcinogens, oncogenic virus, tumor suppressor cell deficit.

Routine checkup 2
1. d
2. Any of the following is accurate: Bleeding, infection—fever, nausea/vomiting.
3. False

Routine checkup 3
1. b
2. Play therapy

Routine checkup 4
1. Five, grief
2. False

Routine checkup 5
1. False
2. Chemotherapy

Final checkup

1. d	2. b	3. c	4. c
5. a	6. a	7. c	8. a
9. d	10. c		

CHAPTER 9

Endocrine and Metabolic Conditions

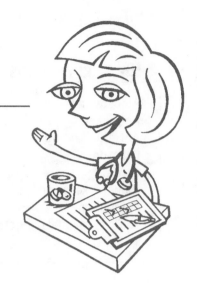

Learning Objectives

At the end of the chapter, the student will be able to

1. Understand the importance of early treatment of congenital hypothyroidism.

2. Identify the symptoms of Cushing syndrome.

3. Know the interventions for diabetes mellitus.

4. Explain the treatment for galactosemia.

5. Care for a patient who is diagnosed with Graves disease.

6. Assess a patient who has maple syrup urine disease.

7. Teach families about phenylketonuria.

KEY WORDS

Aldosterone
Androgens
Antidiuretic hormone (ADH)
Calcitonin
Cortisol
Diabetic ketoacidosis
Epinephrine
Follicle-stimulating hormone
    (FSH)

Glucagon
Growth hormone (GH)
Insulin
Insulin-dependent diabetes
    mellitus (IDDM)
Luteinizing hormone (LH)
Noninsulin-dependent
    diabetes mellitus (NIDDM)
Norepinephrine

Oxytocin hormone
Parathyroid hormone (PTH)
Prolactin hormone
Somatostatin
Thyroid-stimulating
    hormone (TSH)
Thyrotoxicosis
Thyroxine (T4)
Triiodothyronine (T3)

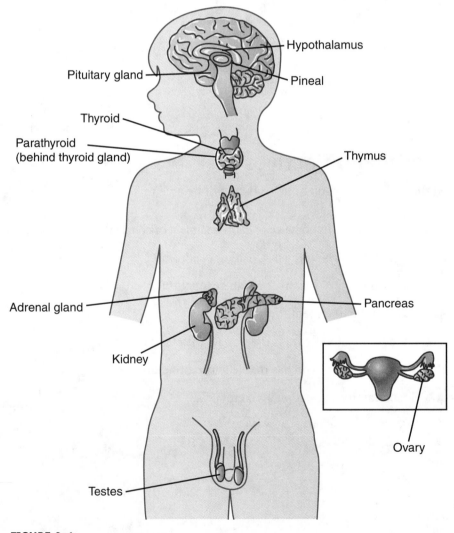

FIGURE 9-1

OVERVIEW

The endocrine system is comprised of several glands throughout the body. Glands release chemical messengers called hormones that control and regulate the activity of target cells and organs. Hormones influence growth, development, and digestion and regulate metabolism and reproduction.

Glands release the hormones into the blood to a stimulus, another hormone, or a threshold. Glands stop releasing hormones when they receive the signal to turn off the hormone production by a process called direct feedback.

The endocrine system maintains homeostasis. Feedback tells a gland to increase or decrease the hormone production so the body returns to homeostasis. When the concentration of a hormone reaches a threshold, hormone production is turned off.

THYROID GLAND

The thyroid gland is located in the anterior neck, overlying the trachea. The thyroid gland makes

- **Thyroxine (T4):** Regulates carbohydrate metabolism, lipids, proteins, and growth and development.
- **Triiodothyronine (T3):** Regulates carbohydrate metabolism, lipids, proteins, and growth and development.
- **Calcitonin:** Regulates blood calcium and phosphate release from the bones.

PITUITARY GLANDS

The pituitary gland is a pea-sized gland connected with the hypothalamus and divided into two parts:

- Anterior pituitary that produces
  - **Thyroid-stimulating hormone (TSH):** Stimulates the thyroid gland to produce hormones.
  - **Growth hormone (GH):** Increases protein synthesis, increases fat mobilization, and decreases the use of carbohydrate, all of which encourages tissue growth.
  - **Follicle-stimulating hormone (FSH):** Stimulates graafian follicles to mature and secrete estrogen (female) and stimulates the seminiferous tubules development (males).
  - **Luteinizing hormone (LH):** Causes the rupture of the follicle resulting in the release of the ovum (female). Stimulates production of testosterone (males).
  - **Prolactin hormone:** Simulates the secretion of breast milk.
- Posterior pituitary that produces
  - **Oxytocin hormone:** Stimulates uterus contraction and the letdown lactating reflex.

• **Antidiuretic hormone (ADH):** Regulates the concentration of fluids in the body by altering the permeability of the collecting ducts and distal convoluted tubules in the kidneys.

ADRENAL GLANDS

Adrenal glands are located at the top of each kidney in the retro peritoneum. Adrenal glands are comprised of two parts:

- ◑ Adrenal cortex:
  - **Aldosterone:** Responsible for renal reabsorption of sodium and excretion of potassium.
  - **Cortisol:** Maintains glucose control, increases hepatic gluconeogenesis (the making of glucose), and manages the body's stress response.
  - **Androgens:** Male sex hormones that promote secondary sex characteristics.
- ◑ Adrenal medulla:
  - Catecholamines:
    - **Epinephrine:** Increases heart and respiratory rate, and blood pressure and dilates airways and an increase in the metabolic rate.
    - **Norepinephrine:** Increases heart and respiratory rate, and blood pressure and dilates airways and an increase in the metabolic rate.

PARATHYROID GLANDS

Parathyroid glands are composed of usually four or more small glands located on the posterior side of the thyroid gland. Parathyroid glands produce:

- ◑ **Parathyroid hormone (PTH):** Maintains the calcium level in the blood and inhibits phosphorus. If the serum calcium level falls, PTH is released causing bones to break down, releasing calcium into the blood and kidneys to retain calcium and increase phosphate excretion.

PANCREAS

The pancreas contains a cluster of cells called the islets of Langerhans. These cells produce:

- ◑ **Insulin:** Produced by the beta cells, insulin increases the cellular use of glucose.
- ◑ **Glucagon:** Produced by the alpha cells, glucagon increases glucose when the blood level of glucose is low.
- ◑ **Somatostatin:** Produced by the delta cells, somatostatin inhibits the release of corticotrophin and growth hormone.

GONADS

Gonads are sex glands and include:

- ◑ Ovaries (female) are located on the uterus and produce eggs and also produce

- Estrogen: Promotes secondary female characteristics, regulates menstrual cycle.
- Progesterone: Supports pregnancy and prepares the breasts for lactation.
- ◐ Testes (male) are located in the scrotum and produce
  - Testosterone: Stimulates production of spermatozoa and maintains the secondary male sex characteristics.

CONGENITAL HYPOTHYROIDISM

What Went Wrong?

Congenital hypothyroidism is a lack of, or too little, thyroid hormone during fetal development or following birth resulting from an underdeveloped or absent thyroid gland caused by the mother's iodine deficiency or taking antithyroid medication during pregnancy or from autoimmune thyroiditis. Congenital hypothyroidism affects growth of the nervous system and bone and affects mental development if left untreated.

Nursing alert **Treatment must begin within 3 months of age to ensure normal development.**

Signs and Symptoms

- ◐ Fatigue due to slow metabolism
- ◐ Noisy respiration due to an enlarged tongue
- ◐ Hypothermia due to slow metabolism
- ◐ Short, thick extremities and neck
- ◐ Brittle nails due to low levels of thyroid hormone that helps growth and development
- ◐ Thin dry hair from lack of thyroid hormone
- ◐ Dry skin from lack of thyroid hormone
- ◐ Slow cognitive function due to slow metabolism
- ◐ Weight gain due to low levels of thyroid hormone that causes fatigue, sluggishness
- ◐ Cognitive impairment due to untreated condition

Test Results

- ◐ Thyroid scan: Decreased uptake of iodine or absence of thyroid.
- ◐ Serum TSH: Increase TSH unless the cause is due to a decrease production of TSH by the pituitary gland.
- ◐ Serum thyroid hormone: Decrease T3, T4.
- ◐ Radiograph: Absence of tibial or femoral epiphyseal line.
- ◐ Electrocardiogram: Flat or inverted T waves and bradycardia.

Treatment

- Replacement hormone (levothyroxine, liothyronine).
- Serum measurements of T3 and T4 will need to be performed after 6 to 8 weeks to determine if the patient is taking the correct dose.
- The patient needs to be aware this is lifetime replacement.
- Vitamin D supplement to prevent rickets that might result from rapid bone growth.

Nursing Intervention

- Ensure that the newborn is screened for congenital hypothyroidism so that treatment can begin within 3 months of birth.
- Monitor vital signs because treatment may cause tachycardia and hypertension.
- Monitor for irritability, sweating, and fever that indicate the dose is too high.
- Monitor for lethargy, constipation, decreased appetite, and fatigue that indicates the dose is too low.
- Provide a warm environment.
- Low-calorie diet.
- Increase fluids and fiber to prevent constipation.
- Take thyroid replacement hormone each morning to avoid insomnia.
- Monitor for signs of **thyrotoxicosis** (an increase in T3) (nausea, vomiting, diarrhea, sweating, tachycardia).
- Explain to the family the side effects of thyroid hormone replacement and review the signs of hyperthyroidism and hypothyroidism. Also teach the family that treatment is lifelong.

CUSHING SYNDROME

What Went Wrong?

Cushing syndrome occurs when the adrenal cortex secretes an excess of glucocorticoids or an excess secretion of adrenocorticotropic hormone (ACTH) by the pituitary gland as a result of either a pituitary tumor or adrenal tumor or from ongoing glucocorticoid therapy.

Signs and Symptoms

- Moon face during excess cortisol production
- Weight gain
- Buffalo hump (fat pad located in the upper back) from excessive corticosteroids
- Osteoporosis from an excess of corticosteroids, which weaken the bones
- Changes in mental status from excessive steroids

- ◐ Bruising
- ◐ Delayed wound healing
- ◐ Sleep disturbance
- ◐ Reddish purple striae on the abdomen

Test Results

- ◐ Dexamethasone suppression test: A dose of glucocorticoid is given to test the hypothalamus-pituitary-adrenal axis. If there is suppression of cortisol with the dose, it indicates a pituitary origin of the excess cortisol. If no suppression occurs, the etiology is an adrenal or ectopic tumor.
- ◐ A 24-hour urine collection: Increase in cortisol from excess production.
- ◐ Computed tomograph (CT) scan: Presence of a pituitary tumor or adrenal tumor.
- ◐ Serum: Increase blood glucose due to overproduction of steroids.
- ◐ Serum: Increase sodium due to excess fluid loss.
- ◐ Serum: Decrease potassium.

Treatment

- ◐ Surgical removal of the pituitary tumor or adrenal tumor

Nursing Intervention

- ◐ Weigh daily to monitor fluid status.
- ◐ Monitor input and output to ensure adequate hydration.
- ◐ Monitor for glucose and acetone in urine because elevated levels of corticosteroids may produce hyperglycemia.
- ◐ Allow for adequate rest to allow the body to stabilize.
- ◐ Avoid skin because elevated levels of corticosteroids can delay wound healing.
- ◐ Bone densitometry to assess for osteoporosis because corticosteroids can leech calcium from the bone.
- ◐ Following surgery:
  - Assist in early ambulation, deep breathing, coughing to facilitate mucus mobilization, decrease risk for emboli.
  - Monitor incision site for drainage, erythema, signs of infection.
  - Elevate the head of bed 30 degrees to reduce intracranial pressure.
- ◐ Explain to the family to maintain a high-calcium, high-protein, high-potassium, low-carbohydrate, low-sodium, and low-calorie diet to aid in wound repair and replace calcium.
- ◐ Administer pain medication as needed.

Nursing alert **The child is highly susceptible to infections; therefore it is critical to prevent the child from being exposed to infections.**

✔ ROUTINE CHECKUP 1

1. A parent of a child who is diagnosed with congenital hypothyroidism asks why her child is fatigued and cold. What is the best response?
   a. Explain that the thyroid controls metabolism and reduced thyroid hormones lowered the child's metabolism.
   b. Ask the parent to bring the child to the health-care provider immediately so that the health-care provider can increase the child's replacement hormone.
   c. Ask the parent to bring the child to the health-care provider immediately so that the health-care provider can decrease the child's replacement hormone.
   d. Ask the parent to take the child's temperature.

Answer:

2. The patient is administered the dexamethasone suppression test. Cortisol is not suppressed based on the test results. What does this indicate?
   a. The patient has a hypothalamus tumor.
   b. The patient has a pituitary tumor.
   c. The patient has an adrenal or ectopic tumor.
   d. The patient has a thalamus tumor.

Answer:

DIABETES MELLITUS

What Went Wrong?

Certain foods are converted into glucose, which is the primary energy supply. Insulin from beta cells of the pancreas transports glucose into cells for cell metabolism.

Diabetes mellitus occurs when beta cells either are unable to produce insulin (type 1 diabetes mellitus) or produces an insufficient amount of insulin (type 2 diabetes mellitus). As a result, glucose doesn't enter cells and remains in the blood.

Increased glucose levels in the blood signal the body to increase the intake of fluid to flush glucose out of the body in urine, resulting in increased thirst and increased urination in the patient. Cells become starved for energy because of the lack of glucose and signal the body to eat causing the patient to experience an increase in hunger.

There are three types of diabetes mellitus:
   1. Type 1: Known as **insulin dependent diabetes mellitus (IDDM).**
      Beta cells are destroyed by an autoimmune process. There is a

genetic predisposition, although coxsackie B, mumps, and congenital rubella viruses injure beta cells and can result in type 1 diabetes.

2. Type 2: Known as noninsulin dependent **diabetes mellitus (NIDDM).** Beta cells produce insufficient insulin.

3. Gestational diabetes mellitus: Insufficient insulin is produced by the mother during pregnancy. Patients with gestational diabetes mellitus recover following pregnancy; however, they are at risk for developing type 2 diabetes mellitus later in life.

Nursing alert **Patients with type 1 and type 2 diabetes mellitus are at risk for vision loss (diabetic retinopathy), damaged blood vessels and nerves (diabetic neuropathy), and kidney damage (nephropathy). However, complications can be minimized by maintaining a normal blood glucose level through consistent monitoring, administering insulin, and dieting.**

Signs and Symptoms

- ◑ Type 1:
  - Fast onset because no insulin is being produced.
  - Increased appetite (polyphagia) because cells are starved for energy and are signaling a need for more food.
  - Increased thirst (polydipsia) from the body attempting to rid itself of glucose.
  - Increased urination (polyuria) from the body attempting to rid itself of glucose.
  - Weight loss because glucose is unable to enter cells.
  - Frequent infections as bacteria feeds on the excess glucose.
  - Delayed healing because elevated glucose levels in the blood hinder healing process.
- ◑ Type 2:
  - Slow onset because some insulin is being produced.
  - Increased thirst (polydipsia) from the body attempting to rid itself of glucose.
  - Increased urination (polyuria) from the body attempting to rid itself of glucose.
  - Candidal infection as bacteria feeds on the excess glucose.
  - Delayed healing because elevated glucose levels in the blood hinder healing process.

Test Results

- ◑ Urine test: Increase glucose in urine (glucosuria).
- ◑ Fasting plasma blood glucose test: A plasma glucose level of ≥126 mg/dL (or 7.0 mmol/L) on three different tests.

◐ Oral glucose tolerance Test (OGTT): A plasma glucose of ≥200 mg/dL (or 11.1 mmol/L) 2 hours after ingesting 75 g oral glucose.

◐ Random plasma glucose test: A plasma of ≥200 mg/dL or 11.1 mmol/L.

◐ Glycosylated hemoglobin A1C: ≥6.0%.

Treatment

◐ ❸ Type 1:
- Regular monitoring of blood glucose.
- Administer insulin to maintain normal blood glucose levels (see Table 9-1).
- Maintain a diabetic diet.
- Administer:
  ○ Rapid acting:
    - Aspart
    - Lispro
    - Glulisine
  ○ Short acting:
    - Regular insulin
  ○ Intermediate:
    - Human insulin
      □ NPH
    - Human insulin
      □ Zinc
      □ Lente
  ○ Long acting:
    - Human insulin
      □ Zinc
      □ Ultralente
    - Glargine
    - Lantus
  ○ Inhaled insulin
  ○ Exubera: A short-acting insulin for before-meal control

TABLE 9–1 • Insulin Guide						
Insulin Drug	**Synonym**	**Appearance**	**Onset**	**Peak**	**Duration**	**Compatibility**
Rapid acting	Regular	Clear	0.5–1 h	2–4 h	6–8 h	All insulin except lente
Intermediate acting	NPH	Cloudy	1–1.5 h	8–12 h	18–24 h	Regular insulin
Long acting	Ultralente	Cloudy	4–6 h	16–20 h	30–36 h	Regular

◐ Type 2:
- Maintain ideal body weight through diet and exercise.
- Regular monitoring of blood glucose.
- Administer oral sulfonylureas to stimulate secretion of insulin from the pancreas (see Table 9-2).
- Administer oral Biguanides to reduce blood glucose production by the liver:
  ○ Metformin
- Administer thiazolidinediones to sensitize peripheral tissues to insulin:
  ○ Rosiglitazone
  ○ Pioglitazone
- Administer meglitinide analogs to stimulate section of insulin from the pancreas:
  ○ Repaglinide
- Administer D-phenylalanine derivative to stimulate insulin production:
  ○ Nateglinide
- Administer alpha-glucosidase inhibitors to delay absorption of carbohydrates in the intestine:
  ○ Acarbose
  ○ Miglitol
- Administer DPP4 (dipeptidyl peptidase 4) inhibitors to slow the inactivation of incretin hormones; GLP-I that assists insulin product in the pancreas:
  ○ Sitagliptin

TABLE 9–2 • Oral Hypoglycemic Agents

Oral Hypoglycemic Agents	Onset	Peak	Duration	Comments
Oral sulfonylureas				
Dymelor	1 h	4–6 h	12–24 h	
Diabinese	1 h	4–6 h	40–60 h	
Micronase, DiaBeta	15 min–1 h	2–8 h	10–24 h	
Oral biguanides				
Glucophage	2–2.5 h		10–16 h	Decreases glucose production in liver, decreases intestinal absorption of glucose, and improves insulin sensitivity
Oral α-glucosidase inhibitor		1 h		Delays glucose absorption and digestion of carbohydrates, lowers blood sugar, reduces plasma glucose and insulin
Precose	Rapid	2–3 h		
Glyset		2–3 h		

- Administer incretin mimetics to assist insulin production in the pancreas and help regulate liver production of glucose. It also decreases appetite and increases the time glucose remains in the stomach before entering the small intestine for absorption.
- Administer amylin analog that causes glucose to enter the bloodstream slowly and can cause weight loss:
  - Pramlintide

Nursing Intervention

- ◑ Educate the family and child about the disease and the importance of maintaining normal glucose levels.
- ◑ Demonstrate blood glucose monitoring.
- ◑ Review diet and food choices, including portion sizes.
- ◑ Encourage exercise.
- ◑ Discuss coping skills to reduce stress.
- ◑ Teach self-injection of insulin (type 1).
- ◑ Teach importance of daily medications and self-care including insulin injection. Explain to the family and patient the signs and symptoms and intervention for hypoglycemia, diabetic ketoacidosis, and hyperglycemia.

Nursing alert **For hypoglycemia (sweating, lethargy, confusion, hunger, dizziness, weakness), administer 4 ounces of fruit juice, several hard candies, glucose tablets, a small amount of carbohydrate or glucagon injection (causes the liver to release glucose) to increase glucose levels. For hyperglycemia (fatigue, headache, blurry vision, dry itchy skin), adjust the dose or type of medication; adjust meal planning. For diabetic ketoacidosis (DKA) (fruity smell of acetone, constant urination, hyperventilation, agitation, sluggishness), administer insulin. Symptoms of DKA are similar to alcohol intoxication.**

GALACTOSEMIA

What Went Wrong?

Galactosemia is the inability of the patient to metabolize galactose in carbohydrate to glucose due to the missing hepatic enzyme GALT, resulting in the buildup of galactose in the blood and causing liver dysfunction.

Signs and Symptoms

- ◑ Vomiting following intake of milk
- ◑ Weight loss
- ◑ Diarrhea
- ◑ Jaundice
- ◑ Lethargy

Test Results

- Serum: Increased galactose.
- Blood: Decreased or absent GALT activity in erythrocytes.
- Urine: Increased galactose.

Treatment

- Galactose (lactose)-free diet (avoid dairy products, canned and frozen foods that contain lactose, cakes, cookies, pies, food coloring)

Nursing Intervention

- Explain to the family and child the importance of avoiding dietary galactose.

✔ ROUTINE CHECKUP 2

1. A 15-year-old was brought to the Emergency Department by the police. He was agitated, sluggish, and slurring his speech. The police said they found him holding on to a tree urinating. They suspect he is drunk. What would you do?
   a. Prepare for a toxicology (tox) screen.
   b. Tell the police you need a parent or guardian's permission before drawing blood for a tox screen.
   c. Smell the child's breath for the smell of acetone; ask the child if he has diabetes, and look for a medical ID bracelet identifying him as a diabetic.
   d. Recognize that the child has diabetic ketoacidosis and inject glucagon per protocol.

Answer:

2. The parents of 7-year-old boy who is diagnosed with type 1 diabetes mellitus asks why he is thirsty and has an increased appetite. What is the best response?
   a. The child is thirsty because his body is signaling the need to flush glucose from blood vessels into the cells.
   b. The child is thirsty because his body is signaling the need to flush excess glucose from the body because there is too much glucose in the cells. Because cells are in need of glucose, the body is signaling the child to eat in order to ingest more glucose.
   c. The child is thirsty because his body is signaling the need to flush excess glucose from the body because glucose is not entering cells for metabolism. Because cells are in need of glucose, the body is signaling the child to eat in order to ingest more glucose.
   d. The child is hungry because his body is signaling the need to eat in order to ingest more glucose for cells.

Answer:

GRAVES DISEASE (HYPERTHYROIDISM)

What Went Wrong?

Graves disease is an overproduction of T3 and T4 by the thyroid gland that can be caused by an autoimmune disease, a benign tumor (adenomas) resulting in an enlarged thyroid gland (goiter), or an overproduction of TSH by the pituitary gland caused by a pituitary tumor.

The prognosis is good if the cause is treated; however, this is a chronic disease. Signs such as bulging eyes (exophthalmos) are not reversible. Furthermore, thyroid surgery may result in complications.

Signs and Symptoms

- Enlarged thyroid gland (goiter) caused by tumor.
- Protrusion of the eyeballs (exophthalmos) due to lymphocytic infiltration that pushes out the eyeball.
- Irritability.
- Sweating (diaphoresis): Excess thyroid hormone raises the metabolic rate.
- Increased appetite due to increased metabolism.
- Hyperactivity due to high levels of thyroid hormone.
- Weight loss due to increased metabolism.
- Insomnia due to increased metabolism.

Test Results

- Serum: Increased serum T3 and T4.
- Radioimmunoassay: Increased T4.
- Serum: Increased TRH and TSH if pituitary gland is the cause of hyperthyroidism.
- Serum: Presence of antibodies if cause is Graves disease.
- Thyroid scan: Enlarged thyroid.

Treatment

- For mild cases and for young patients, administer antithyroid medication such as propylthiouracil (PTU) and methimazole (Tapazole) to block synthesis of T3 and T4.
- For severe cases where the size of the thyroid gland interferes with swallowing or breathing, the thyroid gland is surgically reduced in size or removed. The patient must be on lifelong thyroid replacement therapy.

Nursing alert Medication might result in leucopenia and thrombocytopenia. The medication is stopped until the blood count returns to normal.

Nursing Intervention

- ❶ Monitor vital signs.
- ❶ Provide cool environment.
- ❶ Provide a quiet environment.
- ❶ Protect the patient's eyes with dark glasses and artificial tears if the patient has exophthalmos.
- ❶ Provide a diet high in carbohydrates, protein, calories, vitamins, and minerals.
- ❶ After surgery:
  - • Monitor for laryngeal edema following surgery (hoarseness or inability to speak clearly).
  - • Keep oxygen, suction, and a tracheotomy set near bed in case the neck swells and breathing is impaired.
  - • Keep calcium gluconate near the patient's bed following surgery, which is the treatment for tetany, to maintain the serum calcium level in normal range.
  - • Place the patient in a semi-Fowler position to decrease tension on the neck following surgery.
  - • Support the patient's head and neck with pillows following surgery.
  - • Monitor for muscle spasms and tremors (tetany) caused by manipulation of the parathyroid glands during surgery.
  - • Check drainage and hemorrhage from incision line. Red flags are frank hemorrhage and purulent, foul-smelling drainage.
  - • Monitor signs of hypocalcemia (tingling of hands and fingers).
  - • Check for Chvostek sign (tapping of the facial nerve causes twitching of the facial muscles). These signs are positive when the parathyroid glands have been manipulated during thyroid surgery, in which case they secrete too much phosphorus and not enough calcium. Because muscles and the heart need calcium for work, a low calcium level may cause spasms of muscle, which is easily detected by Chvostek sign and Trousseau sign. The treatment is intravenous calcium, administered quickly.
  - • Check for Trousseau sign (inflate blood pressure cuff on the arm and muscles contract).

MAPLE SYRUP URINE DISEASE

What Went Wrong?

In maple syrup urine disease the branched-chain amino acids are defective or absent due to a genetic disorder resulting in an increase in branched-chain amino acids and ketoacids (by-products), causing a burnt sugar smell in urine.

Signs and Symptoms

- ❶ ❻ Maple syrup odor from urine
- ❶ Seizures

- Difficulty feeding
- Moro reflex absent
- Abnormal respirations

Test Results

- Serum: Increased branched-chain amino acids.
- Urine: Increased branched-chain amino acids.
- Blood gases: Acidosis.

Treatment

- Increase dietary thiamine.
- Avoid dietary isoleucine, valine, and leucine.
- Hemodialysis to remove branched-chain amino acids from the body.

Nursing Intervention

- Perform urine and blood test following the first day of feeding.
- Assess diapers for maple syrup odor.
- Teach parents the importance of avoiding foods that contain isoleucine, valine, and leucine.

PHENYLKETONURIA

What Went Wrong?

Phenylketonuria (PKU) is a genetic disorder that occurs because of a dysfunctional phenylalanine hydroxylase enzyme that is used to convert phenylalanine to tyrosine, resulting in an accumulation of phenylalanine in the body that can cause mental retardation.

Nursing alert **The child has normal blood phenylalanine levels at birth; however levels increase after birth and can result in irreversible damage by 2 years of age if not detected and treated.**

Signs and Symptoms

- Family history of PKU
- Mental retardation as early as 4 months of age
- Dry skin
- Macrocephaly
- Irritable
- Hyperactive
- Musty skin odor
- Seizures (later years)

Test Results
- Guthrie screening test: Increased level in blood of phenylalanine 4 days after birth.
- Chromatography: Increased level in blood of phenylalanine 4 days after birth.

Treatment
- Maintain blood levels of phenylalanine between 3 mg/dL and 9 mg/dL by restricting dietary phenylalanine (protein-rich foods).
- Administer enzymatic hydrolysate of casein (Lofenalac, Pregestimil) in place of milk.

Nursing Intervention
- Explain to the family that the child should avoid eggs, meat, fish, poultry, breads, aspartame, and cheese for the child's entire life.
- The blood level of phenylalanine must be tested throughout the child's life to ensure that it remains within the desired level.

 Nursing alert **Be alert for signs of phenylalanine deficiency (anorexia, skin rashes, anemia, diarrhea, lethargy) that might occur from too little phenylalanine in the diet.**

CONCLUSION

The endocrine system is comprised of glands that release chemical messages called hormones that regulate activities of target cells and organs using a feedback mechanism. A high level of a hormone causes a gland to decrease secretion of that hormone, and a low level causes the hormone's secretion to increase in an effort to maintain homeostasis.

There are times when a disorder results in an abnormal increase or decrease in a hormone causing the body out of homeostasis. Once such disorder is congenital hypothyroidism where the thyroid gland is not secreting sufficient levels of thyroid hormones, resulting in a decrease in the body's metabolism.

Too much thyroid hormones causes hyperthyroidism, commonly called Graves disease, which increases metabolism and causes the patient to become hyperactive, irritable, and lose weight. This condition is characterized by protrusion of the eyeballs (exophthalmos) and an enlarged thyroid gland (goiter).

Abnormal tissue growth can also increase hormonal secretion as in the case of Cushing syndrome where excess glucocorticoids are secreted by the adrenal gland or the pituitary gland secretes excess ACTH. This results in weight gain, moon face, and delayed wound healing.

A very common endocrine disorder is diabetes mellitus. Diabetes mellitus is the absences (type 1) of or low production (type 2) of insulin by the pancreas, resulting in the inability of glucose to enter cells for metabolism.

Three relatively rare metabolism disorders are galactosemia, maple syrup urine disease, and phenylketonuria. Galactosemia is the inability of the patient to metabolize galactose, which is necessary to convert carbohydrates into glucose for energy because the patient is missing the GALT hepatic enzyme.

Maple syrup urine disease is a defective or absence of the branched-chain amino acid, causing a buildup of the amino acid and ketoacids in urine resulting in urine smelling like burnt sugar.

Phenylketonuria is a disorder that is the result of a dysfunctional phenylalanine hydroxylase, leading to a buildup of phenylalanine in the body that can cause mental retardation.

? FINAL CHECKUP

1. **Why would a patient diagnosed with Cushing syndrome experience delayed wound healing?**
   a. Excessive corticosteroids reduce the inflammation process.
   b. Decreased corticosteroids reduce the inflammation process.
   c. Frequent bruising.
   d. Changes in mental status.

2. **A parent of a child who is recently diagnosed with type 1 diabetes mellitus is concerned that her child still exhibits hyperglycemic and hypoglycemic symptoms. What is your best response?**
   a. You must carefully monitor your child's blood glucose level.
   b. The health-care provider adjusts the insulin dose based on the child's activities and diet.
   c. The health-care provider is still in the process of adjusting your child's insulin dose and diet to determine the proper balance for your child.
   d. You must carefully monitor your child's urine glucose level.

3. **The mother of a child who has been diagnosed with type 1 diabetes mellitus asks what effect a glucagon injection has on her child. What is the best response?**
   a. Glucagon transports glucose into the cell where glucose is metabolized.
   b. Glucagon causes the liver to release glucose.
   c. Glucagon is used for signs of hyperglycemia.
   d. Glucagon is a form of long-lasting insulin.

4. **What test should frequently be performed on a child who is being treated for Graves disease?**
   a. A urine test to determine if the patient has developed type 1 diabetes mellitus.
   b. A urine test to determine if the patient has developed type 2 diabetes mellitus.
   c. A blood test to determine if the patient has developed type 1 diabetes mellitus.
   d. A blood count because the treatment may result in leucopenia and thrombocytopenia.

5. **A patient being treated for phenylketonuria becomes lethargic, has diarrhea, and a skin rash. What would you expect the health-care provider to order?**
   a. Administer glucagon.
   b. Adjustment in the patient's diet to include less phenylalanine.
   c. Adjustment in the patient's diet to include more phenylalanine.
   d. Administer insulin.

6. **Why would you place a child who is diagnosed with Graves disease in a quiet environment?**
   a. To reduce unnecessary stimuli that might increase the hyperactivity already caused by high levels of thyroid hormone.
   b. To reduce unnecessary stimuli that might increase the hyperactivity already caused by low levels of thyroid hormone.
   c. To enable the family to have private time with their child.
   d. To prevent the patient from annoying other patients.

7. **A parent of a child who is diagnosed with galactosemia asks why her child has a yellow tint on his skin. What is the best response?**
   a. This is jaundice and is a side effect of medication used to treat the disorder.
   b. This is jaundice and is an adverse effect of medication used to treat the disorder.
   c. The child is unable to metabolize galactose resulting in the buildup of galactose in the blood causing liver dysfunction. The liver is unable to convert bilirubin, which is a by-product of old hemoglobin, to bile, and therefore bilirubin builds up in the body giving it a yellow tint called jaundice.
   d. The child is unable to metabolize galactose resulting in the buildup of galactose in the blood causing liver dysfunction.

8. **A parent whose child is recently diagnosed with type 1 diabetes mellitus tells you that her father was just diagnosed with it also. How would you respond?**
   a. Explain that her father probably was diagnosed with type 2 diabetes mellitus, which is common in the older population because the beta cells in the pancreas can no longer produce a sufficient amount of insulin.
   b. Explain that her father probably was diagnosed with type 2 diabetes mellitus, which is common in the older population because the alpha cells in the pancreas can no longer produce a sufficient amount of insulin.
   c. Explain that her father probably was diagnosed with type 2 diabetes mellitus, which is common in the older population because the beta cells in the pancreas can no longer produce a sufficient amount of glucagon.
   d. Explain that her father probably was diagnosed with type 2 diabetes mellitus, which is common in the older population because the alpha cells in the pancreas can no longer produce a sufficient amount of glucagon.

9. **A parent of a type 1 diabetic adolescent asks why she shouldn't wear sandals. What is the best response?**
   a. Sandals expose the feet to a fungus infection that increase the need for insulin.
   b. People with type 1 diabetes may develop diabetic neuropathy where nerves are damaged, making it difficult for patients to detect when they have an open wound. Therefore, it is best to protect the feet at all times with shoes.
   c. People with type 1 diabetes may develop diabetic neuropathy where nerves are damaged, making it difficult for the patient to detect when they have an open wound.
   d. People with type 1 diabetes may develop diabetic neuropathy where nerves are damaged, making it difficult for the patient to detect when they have an open wound. Therefore, it is best to go barefoot when possible.

10. **What is the risk of not treating congenital hypothyroidism within the first 3 months following birth?**
    a. To ensure normal growth
    b. To prevent cognitive impairment
    c. To prevent mental retardation
    d. All of the above

ANSWERS

Routine checkup 1
   1. b
   2. c

Routine checkup 2
   1. c
   2. c

Final checkup

1. a	2. c	3. b	4. d
5. c	6. a	7. c	8. a
9. b	10. d		

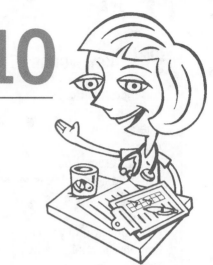

CHAPTER 10

Neurologic Conditions

Learning Objectives

At the end of the chapter, the student will be able to

1 Understand seizures.

2 Identify the symptoms of meningitis.

3 Know the interventions for encephalitis.

4 Explain the stages of Reye syndrome.

5 Recognize neural tube defects.

6 Teach families about brain tumors.

7 Care for a patient who is diagnosed with cerebral palsy.

8 Assess a patient who has Down syndrome.

9 Explain the test for Duchenne muscular dystrophy.

10 Intervene with a Guillain-Barré syndrome patient.

11 Explain the different types of hydrocephalus.

KEY WORDS

Absence seizure	Encephalocele	Noncommunicating
Akinetic seizure	Febrile seizure	hydrocephalus
Anencephaly	Glasgow Coma Scale	Petit mal seizure
Astrocytoma	Gliomas	Simple partial seizure
Ataxic cerebral palsy	Grand mal seizure	Spastic cerebral palsy
Athetoid cerebral palsy	Infantile spasms	Spinal bifida cystica
Bacterial meningitis	Meningiomas	Spinal bifida occulta
Clonic seizure	Meningocele	Status epilepticus
Communicating hydrocephalus	Myelomeningocele	Tonic seizure
Complex partial seizures	Myoclonic seizure	Viral meningitis
Demyelination		

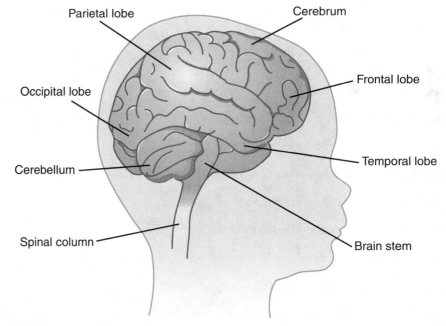

FIGURE 10-1

OVERVIEW

The neurologic system is divided into three categories: central nervous system (CNS), peripheral nervous system, and the autonomic nervous system (ANS).

CENTRAL NERVOUS SYSTEM

The CNS is comprised of the brain and spinal cord. The brain is contained in the skull. Anterior and posterior fontanels of the skull are separated allowing the brain to increase in size. After 8 weeks of age, the posterior fontanel closes, and the anterior fontanel closes by 18 months of age.

The portion of the skull that encloses the brain is called the cranium. The brain and the spinal cord are covered by a three-layer membrane called the meninges. Collectively they protect the brain and the spinal cord. The layers of the meninges are as follows:

- Dura mater: This is the outer membrane that folds the brain into compartments.
- Arachnoid mater: This is the inner membrane of fibrous and elastic tissue that contains a spongy structure of subarachnoid fluid.
- Pia mater: This is the third layer of a fine membrane that contains small blood vessels.

CEREBRAL SPINAL FLUID

Blood in the capillary network called the choroid plexuses form a clear liquid called cerebral spinal fluid (CSF). CSF contains water, glucose, protein, and minerals. CSF surrounds the brain helping to absorb shock and reduces forces that might be applied to the brain.

CSF also fills four cavities within the brain called ventricles. Each cerebral hemisphere (see cerebrum) contains a ventricle. A third ventricle is located midbrain (see brain stem), and a fourth is located at the posterior brain fossa at the base of the brain.

CSF is reabsorbed in blood vessels in the arachnoid villi.

BRAIN

The brain is divided into three areas. These are the cerebrum, cerebellum, and brainstem.

Cerebrum

The cerebrum is the nerve center that controls motor activities, sensory information, and intelligence. The outside layer of the cerebrum is called the cerebral cortex and consists of neuron cells commonly referred to as the gray matter. The inner layer of the cerebrum contains axons and basal ganglia. Axons are referred to as white matter. Basal ganglia controls balance and motor coordination.

Fissures divide the cerebrum longitudinal into two hemispheres. The hemispheres are connected by nerve fibers called the corpus callosum, which is used to transmit impulses between hemispheres. The left hemisphere controls the right side of the body, and the right hemisphere controls the right side of the body.

Below the corpus callosum is the thalamus. The thalamus is a relay station that passes perceptual data from other areas of the brain to the cerebral cortex, helping the cerebral cortex manage information.

Beneath the thalamus is the hypothalamus, which regulates blood pressure, temperature, appetite, breathing, and sleep.

Other fissures divide the cerebral cortex into four lobes. The fissure of Sylvius separates the frontal and parietal lobes from the temporal lobe. The fissure of Rolando separates the parietal lobe from the frontal lobes. The parieto-occipital fissure separates the parietal lobes from the occipital lobe. Each of the four lobes controls a function:

- Frontal lobe: Moving voluntary muscles, speech (Broca area), personality, behavior, judgment, problem solving, memory, intelligence, autonomic functions, emotional response, and cardiac response.
- Temporal lobe: Interprets spoken language, smell, taste, and hearing.
- Parietal lobe: Interprets sensory information.
- Occipital lobe: Interprets visual stimuli.

Cerebellum

The cerebellum is at the base of the brain and is responsible for maintaining muscle tone, equilibrium, smooth muscles, and coordinating impulses to muscles.

Brainstem

The brainstem connects the spinal cord to other parts of the brain. The brainstem is divided into three parts:

- Midbrain: The reflex center for the eye.
- Pons: Regulates chewing, saliva secretion, taste, and helps respirations, equilibrium, and hearing.
- Medulla oblongata: Helps vasomotor function, cardiac and respiratory functions.

SPINAL CORD

The spinal cord leads from the brainstem through the second lumbar vertebra. The spinal cord has 31 pairs of spinal nerves that carry sensory impulses from parts of the body to the brain and motor impulses from the brain to the peripheral nervous system. The spinal cord generates reflex impulses such as deep tendon reflexes that are outside of the brain control.

Peripheral Nervous System

The peripheral nervous system is portion of the neurologic system that is outside the CNS and divided into two subsystems:

- Somatic nervous system: Responsible for voluntary function and for reflex actions, and conscious and subconscious mental processes.
- Autonomic nervous system: Responsible for involuntary function.

The autonomic nervous system is divided into two opposing systems:

- Sympathetic nervous system: Expends energy by releasing adrenergic catecholamines.
- Parasympathetic nervous system: Conserves energy by absorbing cholinergic neurohormone acetylcholine.

The peripheral nervous system also consists of 31 spinal nerves and 12 pairs of cranial nerves. Spinal nerves extend from the spinal cord forming a network of overlapping nerves that transmit nerve impulses from nerve endings to the brain and from the brain to nerve endings.

Spinal nerves are identified by its origination point in the vertebra:

- Cervical (C1 to C8)
- Thoracic (T1 to T12)
- Lumbar (L1 to L5)
- Coccygeal

Cranial nerves transmit motor and sensory impulses between the brainstem and the neck. The cranial nerves are labeled as follows:

- I Olfactory nerve—sensory: Smell
- II Optic nerve—sensory: Vision
- III Oculomotor nerve—motor: Extraocular eye movement
- IV Trochlear nerve—motor: Extraocular eye movement
- V Trigeminal nerve—sensory: Corneal reflex, face and head senses; motor: Biting and jaw movement.
- VI Abducens nerve—motor: Extraocular eye movement
- VII Facial nerve—sensory: Taste; motor: Facial expression
- VIII Vestibulocochlear nerve—sensory: Hearing and balance
- X Vagus nerve—sensory: Larynx, thoracici, throat, lungs, heart, and digestive tract; motor: Swallowing peristalsis, heart rate, gag reflex
- XI Accessory nerve—motor: Head rotation, shoulder
- XII Hypoglossal nerve—motor: Tongue

SEIZURES

What Went Wrong?

1 Abnormal discharge of neurons in the CNS causes sudden involuntary movement for a limited time commonly called a seizure that is caused by birth injury, infections, or congenital defects.

There are 12 types of seizures. Recurring seizures is considered epilepsy. These are defined as follows:

- **Tonic seizure:** Unconsciousness, continuous muscle contraction, and sustained stiffness.
- **Clonic seizure:** Alternating muscle contract in a rhythmic repetitive jerking motion.

- **Tonic-clonic (grand mal):** Abnormal electrical activity simultaneously occurs in both hemispheres of the brain and then moves from the cortex to the brainstem. It begins with the tonic phase expressed as unconsciousness, continuous muscle contraction, and sustained stiffness. This is followed by the clonic phase, which is expressed as alternating muscle contractions in a rhythmic repetitive jerking motion.
- **Simple partial seizure:** Abnormal electrical activity occurs in one hemisphere of the brain or from an area of the cerebral cortex. There is no loss of consciousness and lasts <30 seconds.
- **Complex partial seizures:** Abnormal electrical activity occurs in one hemisphere of the brain or from an area of the cerebral cortex resulting in impaired consciousness lasting up to 5 minutes and postseizure confusion.
- **Absence seizure (petit mal):** Brief loss of consciousness lasting <30 seconds with no postseizure confusion and minimal or no loss of postural tone.
- **Atonic seizure:** Loss of posture tone causing a drop-and-fall action.
- **Myoclonic seizure:** Involuntary jerking and loss of body tone resulting in falling forward, often occurring when falling asleep or awakening. There is no loss of consciousness or postseizure confusion.
- **Akinetic seizure:** Brief loss of muscle tone and brief loss of consciousness.
- **Infantile spasms:** Delays in neurologic development or neurologic abnormalities result in abrupt jerking and contracting of the head and neck that begin at 2 months of age and resolve by 2 years of age.
- **Febrile seizure:** Rapid rise in body temperature of >102.2° F (39°C) in children 6 months to 6 years of age might result in tonic/clonic seizures lasting <15 minutes.
- **Status epilepticus:** Continuous seizure or a series of seizures lasting for >30 minutes during which there is a loss of consciousness. Postseizure period can last for up to 2 hours.

Signs and Symptoms

- Tonic:
  - Unconsciousness
  - Continuous muscle contraction
  - Sustained stiffness
- Clonic:
  - Alternating muscle contract in a rhythmic repetitive jerking motion
  - Syncope
  - Incontinence
  - Biting of the tongue
  - Holding breath
- Tonic-clonic:
  - Unconsciousness
  - Continuous muscle contraction
  - Sustained stiffness

- Alternating muscle contract in a rhythmic repetitive jerking motion
- Syncope
- Incontinence
- Biting of the tongue
- Holding breath

○ **Simple partial seizure:**
- Continuous muscle contraction and stiffness and jerking motion of the face, neck, and extremities
- Deviations of the eyes
- Head turning

○ Complex partial seizures:
- Impaired consciousness
- Blinking
- Staring
- Lip smacking
- Sleepwalking
- Chewing
- Night terrors
- Sucking

○ Absence seizure:
- Brief loss of consciousness
- No or minimal loss of postural tone
- Eye blinking
- Rolling of the eyes
- Drooping eyelid

○ Atonic:
- Loss of posture tone
- Drop-and-fall action

○ Myoclonic seizure:
- Involuntary jerking
- Loss of body tone
- Falling forward
- Flexing the upper chest
- Infantile spasms
- Pallor

○ Akinetic:
- Brief loss of consciousness
- Brief loss of muscle tone

○ Abrupt jerking:
- Contraction of the head and neck
- Cyanosis
- Altered consciousness
- Eye rolling

- ◑ Febrile seizure:
  - >102.2°F (39°C)
  - Unconsciousness
  - Continuous muscle contraction
  - Sustained stiffness
  - Alternating muscle contract in a rhythmic repetitive jerking motion
  - Syncope
  - Incontinence
  - Biting of the tongue
  - Holding breath
- ◑ Status epilepticus
  - Unconsciousness
  - Continuous muscle contraction
  - Sustained stiffness
  - Alternating muscle contract in a rhythmic repetitive jerking motion
  - Syncope
  - Incontinence
  - Biting of the tongue
  - Holding breath

Test Results

- ◑ Blood glucose level because a low glucose level might precipitate a seizure.
- ◑ Electrolytes level because an abnormal sodium level might precipitate a seizure.
- ◑ Blood level of anticonvulsant medication to determine if medication is at a therapeutic level and not nearing the toxic level.
- ◑ Computed tomography (CT) scan to identify lesions on brain that might be causes of the seizure.
- ◑ Magnetic resonance imaging (MRI) scan to identify lesions on brain that might be causes of the seizure.
- ◑ Lumbar puncture to rule out meningitis.
- ◑ Electroencephalogram (EEG) to differentiate between nonepileptic and epileptic seizures.

Treatment

- ◑ Seizures lasting 5 minutes are self-limiting.
- ◑ Seizures lasting 5 to 10 minutes: administer Ativan (lorazepam), Dilantin (phenytoin), or Fosphenytoin as ordered.
- ◑ Administer single medication to reduce adverse effects of multiple medications.
- ◑ Transfer the patient to the intensive care unit after 45 minutes.
- ◑ Surgery might be necessary to remove portion of the brain that is causing the seizure.

Nursing Intervention

- ◐ Maintain airway.
- ◐ Place patient in a side laying position to prevent aspiration.
- ◐ Slightly elevate the head of bed to prevent aspiration.
- ◐ Administer 100% oxygen using a face mask if the patient is hypoxic.
- ◐ Monitor for depressed respiratory rate because this might indicate increase intracranial pressure.
- ◐ Monitor vital signs.
- ◐ Monitor pulse oximetry continuously.
- ◐ Monitor level of consciousness.
- ◐ Pad the side rails of the bed or crib to prevent injury.
- ◐ Document seizure activity.
- ◐ Determine the child's weight because the dose of medication is calculated by the patient's weight.
- ◐ Explain to parents that the child should wear a medical identification bracelet stating that the child is prone to seizures. Parents should also tell the school and caregivers about the child's seizures and explain that they should lay the child on his side, protect him from injuring himself during the seizure, and not place anything in the child's mouth.

 Nursing alert **Never place anything in the patient's mouth during a seizure. Maintain airway by placing the patient on his side.**

MENINGITIS

What Went Wrong?

The meningeal covering of the brain and spinal cord becomes inflamed, which is commonly caused by bacteria or a virus but can also be caused by fungus, protozoa, or toxic exposure.

Bacterial meningitis is most common and typically due to *Streptococcus pneumoniae* (pneumococcal), *Neisseria meningitides* (meningococcal), or *Haemophilus influenzae*. The incidence of *H. influenzae* meningitis infections has decreased since the routine use of vaccine against *H. influenzae* began to be used in infants in the early 1990s. Other organisms that can cause bacterial meningitis include *Staphylococcus aureus, Escherichia coli,* and *Pseudomonas.*

Organisms typically travel through the bloodstream to the CNS or enter by direct contamination (skull fracture, extension from sinus infections).

Bacterial meningitis is more common in colder months when upper respiratory tract infections are more common. People living in close living conditions, such as prisons, military barracks, or college dorms, are at greater risk for outbreaks of bacterial meningitis due to the likelihood of transmission.

Viral meningitis may follow other viral infections such as mumps, herpes simplex or zoster, enterovirus, or measles. Viral meningitis is often a self-limiting illness.

Patients with immunocompromise have an increased risk for contracting a fungal meningitis. This may travel from the bloodstream to the CNS or by direct contamination. *Cryptococcus neoformans* may be the causative organism in these patients.

Bacterial meningitis still has a significant mortality rate, and these patients need to be managed in the hospital. Some patients will have permanent neurologic effects following the acute episode. Viral meningitis is typically self-limited. Fungal meningitis often occurs in patients who are immunocompromised.

Nursing alert **Always isolate a patient who is suspected of having bacterial meningitis until bacterial meningitis is ruled out.**

Signs and Symptoms

- Stiff neck due to meningeal irritation and irritation of the spinal nerves.
- Nuchal rigidity (pain when flexing chin toward chest) due to meningeal irritation and irritation of the spinal nerves.
- Headache due to increased intracranial pressure.
- Nausea and vomiting due to increased intracranial pressure.
- Photophobia (sensitivity to light) due to irritation of the cranial nerves.
- Fever due to infection.
- Malaise and fatigue due to infection.
- Myalgia (muscle aches) due to viral infection.
- Petechial rash on skin and mucous membranes with meningococcal infection.
- Seizures due to irritation of brain from increased intracranial pressure.
- Bulging anterior fontanel in infants.
- Kerning sign where the child lies flat with legs flexed at hips and knees. The child resists positioning and experiences pain indicating a positive Kerning sign.
- Brudzinski sign where the head is flexed while in the supine position. A positive sign is if the child experiences pain or if the child's hips and knees are flexed.

Test Results

- Lumbar puncture for CSF analysis, glucose (bacterial low), protein (bacterial elevated), cell counts (bacterial elevated neutrophils), and culture.
- Increased CSF pressure noted.
- Polymerase chain reaction (PCR) test of CSF to test for organisms: Results within a few hours (not all labs).

◐ Culture and sensitivity: Results may take up to 72 hours.
◐ Blood cultures to identify the microorganism that is causing the infection.
◐ CT brain to rule out space-occupying lesion as cause of symptoms.

Treatment

◐ Administer antibiotics as soon as possible to improve outcome for bacterial meningitis:
  • Penicillin G
  • Ceftriaxone
  • Cefotaxime
  • Vancomycin plus ceftriaxone or cefotaxime
  • Ceftazidime
◐ Fungal infections are typically treated with
  • Amphotericin B
  • Fluconazole
  • Flucytosine
◐ Administer corticosteroid to decrease inflammation in pneumococcal infection:
  • Dexamethasone
◐ Administer osmotic diuretic for cerebral edema:
  • Mannitol
◐ Administer analgesics for headache if needed:
  • Acetaminophen
◐ Administer anticonvulsant if necessary:
  • Phenytoin, phenobarbital
◐ Administer Decadron (IV) every 6 hours for 4 days to reduce hearing loss and severe neurologic damage.
◐ Bed rest until neurologic irritation improves.
◐ Administer D5/0.22 NSS IV plus potassium (two thirds of maintenance fluids requirements) to reduce intracranial pressure.
◐ No oral fluids.
◐ Fluid restriction.

Nursing Intervention

◐ Monitor intake and output to check fluid balance.
◐ Keep room darkened due to photophobia.
◐ Keep room quiet. Place Quiet sign on the door.
◐ Monitor neurologic function at least every 2 to 4 hours, changes in mental status, level of consciousness, pupil reactions, speech, facial movement symmetry, signs of increased intracranial pressure.
◐ Seizure precautions per institution policy.
◐ Isolation per policy depending on organism (meningococcal).
◐ Cluster care activities.

- Elevate head of bed 30 degrees to decrease intracranial pressure.
- Keep suction and oxygen available at bedside.
- Administer cooling blanket if the patient's temperature rises >101.3°F (38.5°C).
- Assess the anterior fontanel in infant to determine if it is bulging due to increase intracranial pressure.
- Measure the patient's head circumference per shift to detect increase intracranial pressure.
- Assess motor skills.
- Assess vital signs for indication of increase intracranial pressure.
- Assess the patient's level of consciousness.
- Explain to the patient why restrictions such as bed rest are necessary and that a vaccine is available for meningococcal meningitis. The two different types are meningococcal polysaccharide vaccine (MPSV4) and conjugate vaccine (MCV4).

✔ ROUTINE CHECKUP 1

You are the triage RN in the Emergency Department (ED). A parent and 5-year old walk into the ED. The parent says that the child has a fever and a stiff neck. What would you do?

a. Ask the parent to sign in and take a seat until they are called since the child is ambulatory.
b. Take the child immediately to an isolation room.
c. Ask the parent how long the child has had the fever.
d. Ask the parent to take the child to his family health-care provider.

Answer:

ENCEPHALITIS

What Went Wrong?

Encephalitis is the inflammation of the brain tissue most often caused by a virus but also can be caused by bacteria, fungus, or protozoa. In viral encephalitis, the patient typically has had viral symptoms prior to the current illness because the virus enters the CNS via the bloodstream and begins to reproduce. Inflammation in the area follows, causing damage to the neurons.

Demyelination of the nerve fibers in the affected area and hemorrhage, edema, and necrosis occur, which creates small cavities within the brain tissue. Herpes simplex virus 1, cytomegalovirus, echovirus, coxsackie virus, and herpes zoster can all cause encephalitis. Some causes of encephalitis can be transmitted by insects (such as mosquitoes or ticks) to humans, such as West Nile virus, St. Louis encephalitis, or equine encephalitis.

Identification of the organism is important to individualize the treatment for the patient. The earlier symptoms are recognized and the patient enters the health-care system, the better. Some patients incur permanent disability from the irreversible damage that occurs to the brain. These patients may be in need of long-term custodial care.

Signs and Symptoms

- Fever due to infection
- Nausea and vomiting due to increased intracranial pressure
- Stiff neck due to meningeal irritation
- Drowsiness, lethargy, or stupor due to increased intracranial pressure
- Altered mental status: irritability, confusion, disorientation, personality change
- Headache due to increased intracranial pressure
- Seizure activity possible due to irritation of brain tissue
- Bulging fontanels in infant

Test Results

- Blood cultures used to help identify organism when patient febrile
- CT scan
- MRI
- Analysis of CSF for microorganism that is causing the infection

Treatment

- Monitor respiratory status for compromise.
- Monitor vital signs for widened pulse pressure and bradycardia, signs of increased intracranial pressure.
- Monitor neurologic function for change.
- Administer corticosteroid to decrease inflammation:
  - Dexamethasone
- Administer antipyretics to reduce fever:
  - Acetaminophen
- Administer anticonvulsants to decrease chance of seizure activity:
  - Phenytoin, phenobarbital
- Administer diuretics to decrease cerebral edema if indicated:
  - Furosemide
  - Mannitol

Nursing Intervention

- ◐ ❸ Range of motion exercises—active or passive.
- ◐ Turn and position patient.
- ◐ Monitor neurologic status for changes; typically use the **Glasgow Coma Scale** or similar tool to grade response to stimuli (highest score: 15):
  - Eye opening response:
    - ○ Spontaneous   4
    - ○ To sound   3
    - ○ To pain   2
    - ○ None   1
  - Motor responses:
    - ○ Obeys commands   6
    - ○ Localizes pain   5
    - ○ Withdrawal (normal) 4
    - ○ Abnormal flexion   3
    - ○ Extension   2
    - ○ None   1
  - Verbal responses:
    - ○ Oriented   5
    - ○ Confused conversation 4
    - ○ Inappropriate words 3
    - ○ Incomprehensible sounds 2
    - ○ None   1
- ◐ Provide a quiet environment to decrease unnecessary stimulation.
- ◐ Monitor fluid input and output.
- ◐ Explain to the family that home care is needed and that the patient must be turned and positioned every 2 hours. Also alert the family to adverse reactions and side effects of medication and interactions with other medications.

REYE SYNDROME

What Went Wrong?

During the urea cycle, ammonia is changed to urea in the liver. Urea is then excreted by the kidneys. In Reye syndrome, there is a disruption in the urea cycle resulting in an increase in ammonia levels in the blood and increased fatty acids that infiltrate the kidneys, muscles, and neuronal cells. Reye syndrome occurs within 3 days from a viral infection and is linked to the use of aspirin in children.

Recovery is related to the degree of cerebral edema. If the patient is diagnosed and treated in the early stages, recovery is excellent; otherwise the patient may die within a few days. The prognosis is poor for a patient who has lapsed into a coma.

There are five stages of Reye syndrome:
1. Viral infection
2. Recovery period
3. Intractable vomiting, confusion, agitation
4. Coma
5. Seizures, decreased respiration, decreased tendon reflexes

Nursing alert **Children <15 years who exhibit fever and flulike symptoms should be administered acetaminophen rather than aspirin. Alka Seltzer, Anacin, Ascriptin, Bufferin, Pamprin, Pepto-Bismol, and Vanquish all contain aspirin.**

Signs and Symptoms

- Stage 1:
  - Fever
  - Flulike symptoms
- Stage 2:
  - No symptoms
- Stage 3:
  - Persistent and recurring nausea and vomiting
  - Listlessness
  - Irritability
  - Combativeness
  - Disorientation
  - Confusion
  - Increased blood pressure
  - Increased pulse
  - Hyperactive reflexes
- Stage 4:
  - Loss of consciousness
- Stage 5:
  - Decreased tendon reflexes
  - Respiratory failure
  - Delirium
  - Convulsions
  - Seizures

Test Results

- Increased serum liver enzyme
- Increased serum ammonia levels
- Decreased serum glucose level
- Liver biopsy to confirm liver damage

Treatment

- Administer Dextrose IV for hypoglycemia.
- Place patient on mechanical ventilation, if comatose.
- Monitor electrolytes, blood chemistry, and blood pH.

Nursing Intervention

- Assess the level of consciousness and report changes immediately to the health-care provider.
- Monitor signs of increased cranial pressure as a result of cerebral edema.
- Monitor vital signs.
- Monitor for dehydration.
- Strict intake and output.
- Explain to the family the nature of the disorder and the treatment plan.

 ROUTINE CHECKUP 2

A parent called saying that her child has flulike symptoms and an upset stomach. What should you tell the parent?
  a. Give the child an aspirin.
  b. Give the child acetaminophen.
  c. Give the child Children's Alka Seltzer.
  d. Give the child Anacin.

Answer:

NEURAL TUBE DEFECTS

What Went Wrong?

The neural tube develops into the brain and the spinal cord. A neural tube defect is the failure of the neural tube to close within 28 days after conception in an area of the neural tube or the entire length of the neural tube resulting in a neurologic disorder in the fetus.

5 The cause of neural tube defects is unknown; however, there is a link between inadequate intake of folic acid prior to pregnancy and during the first trimester. The most common neural tube defects are as follows:

- **Spinal bifida occulta:** This is the incomplete closure without the spinal cord or meninges protruding. This patient usually doesn't experience neurologic dysfunction, although there might be bladder or bowel disturbances or weakness in the foot.

- **Spinal bifida cystica:** This is the incomplete closure with the spinal cord or meninges protruding in a sac. There are two types of spinal bifida cystica:
    - **Myelomeningocele:** The sac contains the spinal cord, CSF, and meninges. This patient usually experiences neurologic dysfunction.
    - **Meningocele:** The sac contains CSF and meninges. This patient rarely experiences neurologic dysfunction.
- **Anencephaly:** Cerebral hemispheres of the brain and the top portion of the skull. The brainstem is intact, enabling the infant to have cardiopulmonary functions; however, the infant is likely to die of respiratory failure a few weeks after birth.
- **Encephalocele:** Portions of the brain and meninges protrude in the sac. This patient usually experiences neurologic dysfunction.

Signs and Symptoms

- Spinal bifida occulta:
    - Tuft of hair in the lumbar or sacral area
    - Depression in the lumbar or sacral area
    - Hemangioma in the lumbar or sacral area
- Spinal bifida cystica meningocele:
    - Presence of sac
- Spinal bifida cystica myelomeningocele:
    - Presence of sac
    - Bowel incontinence
    - Bladder incontinence
    - Hydrocephalus
    - Spastic paralysis
    - Club foot
    - Knee contractures
    - Curvature of the spine
    - Arnold-Chiari malformation
- Anencephaly:
    - The top portion of the skull is missing
- Encephalocele:
    - Mental retardation
    - Paralysis
    - Hydrocephalus

Test Results

- Alpha-fetoprotein (AFP): Measure the alpha-fetoprotein between 16 and 18 weeks of gestation.
- Amniocentesis: Assess if alpha-fetoprotein is in amniotic fluid. This test is performed if the alpha-fetoprotein test is abnormal.
- Ultrasound: Assess if there is a neural tube defect or defect in the ventral wall. This test is performed if the alpha-fetoprotein test is abnormal.

- Transillumination of the sac: Differentiates between myelomeningocele and meningocele. A meningocele sac does not transilluminate. This test is performed if the sac is present after birth.
- CT scan: Assess the presence of a neural tube defect after birth.
- Radiograph: Assess the presence of a neural tube defect after birth.

Treatment

- Surgery within 48 hours of birth to close the opening to decrease the risk of infection and prevent spinal cord damage.
- Insert a shunt to relieve hydrocephalus.

Nursing alert **Surgery does not reverse the disorder.**

Nursing Intervention

- Prenatal:
    - Encourage the mother to take adequate amounts of folic acid during childbearing years.
    - Explain the disorder and treatment following birth.
- After birth:
    - Lay the infant on his side to prevent pressure on the sac.
    - Keep the sac covered with a sterile dressing soaked in warmed saline solution to keep the sac moist.
    - Place a strip of plastic below the sac to prevent contamination from urine and stool to prevent infection.
    - Measure head circumference to determine if hydrocephalus develops.
    - Monitor for infection.
    - Assess for leakage around the sac.
    - Assess bladder and bowel function.
    - Assess neurologic signs.
    - Reposition the patient every 2 hours to prevent pressure ulcers and contractures.
    - Explain to the family that surgery will be performed to close the opening within 48 hours following birth.
- After surgery:
    - Monitor vital signs.
    - Monitor for signs of infection.
    - Reposition the patient every 2 hours to prevent pressure ulcers from developing.
    - Monitor bowel and bladder function to assess for changes from the preoperative period.
    - Assess neurologic signs.

- Measure head circumference to determine if hydrocephalus develops.
- Be prepared to insert a straight urinary catheter if the infant is not urinating adequately.
- Perform range-of-motion exercises to maintain muscle tone.

BRAIN TUMORS

What Went Wrong?

A brain tumor is a growth of abnormal cells within the brain tissue. The tumor may be a primary site that originated in the brain or a secondary site that has metastasized from a cancer site elsewhere in the body.

Because the tumor is growing within the confined space of the skull, the patient will eventually develop signs of increased intracranial pressure. Some cell types grow faster than others, and patients with the more aggressive, fast-growing cancers develop symptoms more quickly.

Meningiomas are typically benign tumors that begin from the meninges (covering of the brain). Meningiomas are typically benign tumors that begin from the meninges (covering of the brain). They are more common in women and more common as people age. Treatment is surgical removal, but the growth tends to recur.

Gliomas are a malignant brain tumor of the neuroglial cells that tends to be rapidly growing. Patients have nonspecific symptoms of increased intracranial pressure. Treatment typically includes surgical debulking of the tumor; complete removal is often not possible at the time of diagnosis. Surgery is followed by radiation and chemotherapy.

Astrocytoma is the most common glioma and has a variable prognosis. Oligodendroglioma is slow growing and may be calcified. Glioblastoma is a poorly differentiated glioma with a poor prognosis.

Signs and Symptoms

- Cerebellum or brainstem:
  - Lack of coordination: Cerebellum help coordinate gross movements.
  - Hypotonia of limbs.
  - Ataxia.
- Frontal lobe:
  - Inability to speak (expressive aphasia)
  - Slowing of mental activity
  - Personality changes
  - Anosmia (loss of sense of smell)
- Occipital lobe:
  - Impaired vision: Defect in visual fields; patient may deny or be unaware of defect.
  - Prosopagnosia (patient is unable to recognize familiar faces).
  - Change in color perception.

ⓞ Parietal lobe:
  • Seizures.
  • Sight disturbances result in visual field defect.
  • Sensory loss: Unable to identify object placed in hand without looking.
ⓞ Temporal lobe:
  • Seizures
  • Taste or smell hallucinations
  • Auditory hallucinations
  • Depersonalization
  • Emotional changes
  • Visual field defects
  • Receptive aphasia
  • Altered perception of music

Test Results

ⓞ MRI with gadolinium (contrast) defines tumor location, size.
ⓞ CT shows characteristic appearance of meningioma.
ⓞ Angiography shows blood flow to the area; some tumors displace vessels as they grow.

Treatment

ⓞ Chemotherapeutic agents alone, in combination with radiation and surgery. May be given orally, intravenously, or through an Ommaya reservoir. Drugs are chosen based on cell type:
  • Carmustine, lomustine, procarbazine, vincristine, temozolomide, erlotinib, gefitinib
ⓞ Irradiation of the area to decrease tumor size.
ⓞ Craniotomy to remove the tumor, if appropriate, depends on location, size, primary site of cancer, and number of tumors. Some patients may have several small, scattered tumors, making surgery impractical.
ⓞ Administer glucocorticoid to reduce swelling or inflammatory response within confined space inside skull (no room to expand; bone does not give):
  • Dexamethasone
ⓞ Administer osmotic diuretic to reduce cerebral edema:
  • Mannitol
ⓞ Administer anticonvulsant to reduce chance of seizure activity:
  • Phenytoin, phenobarbital, carbamazepine, divalproex sodium, valproic acid, levetiracetam, lamotrigine, clonazepam, topiramate, ethosuximide
ⓞ Administer mucosal barrier fortifier to reduce risk of gastric irritation:
  • Sucralfate
ⓞ Administer H_2 receptor antagonists to reduce risk of gastric irritation:
  • Ranitidine, famotidine, nizatidine, cimetidine

○ Administer proton pump inhibitors (PPIs) to reduce risk of gastric irritation:
        • Lansoprazole, omeprazole, esomeprazole, rabeprazole, pantoprazole

Nursing Intervention
○ Monitor neurologic function.
○ Check for side effects to medications.
○ Seizure precautions per institution protocol.
○ Assess for pain control.
○ Explain to the family that home care is necessary and there is a possible need for hospice depending on prognosis.

CEREBRAL PALSY

What Went Wrong?
Cerebral palsy is the dysfunction of the portion of the brain that controls motor function resulting in partial paralysis and uncontrolled movement. The dysfunction might be caused by hemorrhage, anoxia, rubella during pregnancy, malnutrition, or other conditions that might affect normal development of the brain.

    The dysfunction might be caused during pregnancy by the mother contracting rubella or other infection, malnutrition, abnormal attachment of the placenta, toxemia, radiation, or medication. Cerebral palsy could also be caused by a difficult birth, prolapsed umbilical cord, or multiple births. An infant might develop cerebral palsy if the infant becomes infected or as a result of trauma and result in prolonged anoxia or decreased circulation to the brain.

    There are three types of cerebral palsy:
○ **Spastic** (most common): The cortex is affected resulting in the child having a scissor-like gait where one foot crosses in front of the other foot.
○ **Athetoid:** The basal ganglia are affected resulting in uncoordinated involuntary motion.
○ **Ataxic:** The cerebellum is affected resulting in poor balance and difficulty with muscle coordination.

Nursing alert **The patient has normal intelligence regardless of the patient's uncontrollable movements.**

Signs and Symptoms
○ Possible seizures
○ Poor sucking
○ Difficulty feeding

- Spastic:
  - Scissor-like gait
  - Underdeveloped limbs
  - Increased deep tendon reflexes
  - Contractures
  - Involuntary muscle contraction and relaxation
  - Flexion
- Athetoid:
  - Uncontrolled, involuntary movements
  - Drooling
  - Writhing
  - All extremities move with voluntary movement
  - Difficulty swallowing
  - Facial grimacing
- Ataxic:
  - Wide-based gait
  - Unsteadiness
  - Clumsiness
  - Poor balance
  - Unnatural muscle coordination

Test Results

- EEG: Identifies the site in the brain that is causing seizures
- CT scan: Identifies the site of the disorder in the brain
- MRI: Identifies the site of the disorder in the brain
- Metabolic labs: To rule out metabolic disorders
- Delayed developmental milestones

Treatment

- Administer skeletal muscle relaxant (baclofen [Lioresal]) using a pump to relax skeletal muscles and reduce spasticity.
- Administer anticonvulsants (phenytoin [Dilantin], phenobarbital [Bellatal]) to control seizures.
- Surgery to correct contractures.

Nursing Intervention

- Perform range-of-motion exercises to prevent contractures.
- Use special appliances to help the child perform activities of daily living.
- Provide protective head gear and bed pads to prevent injury.
- Provide a high-calorie diet because the child will have a high metabolism rate due to high motor function.
- Explain the disorder and treatment to the family and that efforts should be made to ensure that the child reaches the optimal developmental level possible.

DOWN SYNDROME

What Went Wrong?

Down syndrome is a genetic disorder resulting in retardation most commonly caused by three instead of two chromosomes 21. Down syndrome can also be caused by translocation of chromosome 21 where a portion breaks off and attaches to another chromosome.

Abnormal chromosomes might occur because the mother is >34 years of age or the father is >41 at the time of conception. It might also occur because of a virus or radiation.

The degree of mental retardation varies. Some patients are fully dependent on their caregivers. Other patients can function with little assistance.

Signs and Symptoms

- Broad flat forehead
- Small oral cavity
- Protruding tongue
- Speckling of the irises (Brushfield spots)
- Eyes slanting upward
- Low-set ears
- A single crease across the palm (simian crease)
- Hypotonia
- Mental retardation apparent in older infants

Test Results

- Pregnancy-associated plasma protein A serum test (PAPP-A): Performed during the first trimester to detect the level of plasma protein A that is covering the fertilized egg. A low level is linked to Down syndrome.
- Inhibit A serum test: Inhibit A inhibits the pituitary gland from producing the follicle-stimulating hormone (FSH) hormone. An increase level of inhibit A is linked to Down syndrome.
- Human chorionic gonadotropin (HCG) hormone serum test: The placenta produces the human chorionic gonadotropin hormone, which is used to determine pregnancy. An increase in the beta subunit of the human chorionic gonadotropin hormone is linked to Down syndrome.
- Alpha-fetoprotein (AFP) serum test: A decrease in alpha-fetoprotein is linked to Down syndrome.
- Amniocentesis: Identifies the chromosome abnormality and is performed if the mother is >34 years of age or if the father carries a translocated chromosome.

Treatment

- There is no cure for Down syndrome.
- Provide occupational therapy to help the child master the skills of independent living when possible.

- Provide speech therapy to help the child develop communications skills.
- Treatment is focused on treating complications of Down syndrome such as trauma and infection.

Nursing Intervention

- Explain the disorder to the family and suggest they plan activities based on the child's abilities rather than based on the child's age and to involve the child in success-oriented activities.
- Maintain a routine to reduce the child's frustration.
- Arrange for a social worker to help the family deal with the challenges that face the child and the family.

ROUTINE CHECKUP 3

A parent of a Down syndrome child calls saying that she has doubts about the diagnosis because her 2-month-old seems to act like her other child when she was 2 months old. What is the best response?
   a. Call your health-care provider and ask her to retest your child.
   b. You child has Down syndrome according to the child's test results.
   c. Behavioral differences are not easily noticeable until later in the infant's development.
   d. Your child has the facial characteristics of a child who has Down syndrome; therefore your child has the disorder.

Answer:

DUCHENNE MUSCULAR DYSTROPHY

What Went Wrong?

Duchenne muscular dystrophy is a sex-linked recessive genetic degenerative muscular disease caused by the absence of dystrophin, which is a muscle protein used in muscle fibers. Muscle fibers are replaced by connective tissue and fat. The mother carries the gene and passes it to a son who contracts the disease. Early signs occur between 3 and 5 years of age.

Signs and Symptoms

- Calves have normal appearance but are weak.
- Weak pelvic muscles.
- Wide stance.
- Waddling gait.

○ Difficulty climbing and running.
○ Gowers sign where the child uses upper body to move from a prone to upright position
○ Posture changes.
○ Scapular flaring due to weakened thoracic muscles.
○ Muscle atrophy.
○ Contractures.

Test Results

○ Electromyography (EMG): Decreased electrical impulses in muscles.
○ Serum creatine kinase: Increase indicates early sign of muscular dystrophy.
○ Nerve conduction velocity: Abnormal nerve response to electrical stimulus.
○ Muscle biopsy: Identifies degenerative muscle fibers, fat, and connective tissues.

Treatment

○ There is no cure for Duchenne muscular dystrophy.
○ Provide physical therapy to help maintain muscle tone.
○ Provide occupational therapy to help the child master the skills of independent living when possible.
○ Treatment is focused on treating complications of Duchenne muscular dystrophy such as trauma and infection.
○ Surgery for contractures.

Nursing Intervention

○ Prevent infection.
○ Monitor vital signs.
○ Provide a balanced diet to prevent obesity.
○ Perform range-of-motion exercises.
○ Change position every 2 hours.
○ Arrange for a social worker to help the family deal with the challenges that face the child and the family.

GUILLAIN-BARRÉ SYNDROME

What Went Wrong?

Guillain-Barré syndrome is an acute, progressive autoimmune condition that affects the peripheral nerves. Symptoms occur as the myelin surrounding the axon on the peripheral nerves is damaged from the autoimmune effect. The disease typically follows a viral infection, surgery, other acute illness, or immunization by a couple of weeks.

Ascending Guillain-Barré exhibits muscle weakness and/or paralysis that begins in the distal lower extremities and travels upward. Patient may also experience altered sensory perception in the same areas, such as the sensation of crawling, tingling, burning, or pain. The progression of symptoms may take hours or days.

Descending Guillain-Barré begins with muscles in the face, jaw, or throat and travels downward. Respiratory compromise is a concern as the paralysis reaches the level of the intercostal muscles and diaphragm. Breathing can become compromised more quickly in patients with descending disease. Level of consciousness, mental status, personality, and pupil size is not affected.

Patient support and monitoring are important during symptom progression. Involvement of respiratory muscles may result in respiratory compromise or failure. Involvement of ocular areas may cause blindness.

If the nerve cell body is damaged during the acute phase, there may be permanent deficits for the patient in the involved area. Otherwise, the axons of the nerves may be able to repair the damage over several months.

Signs and Symptoms

- Burning or pickling feeling due to demyelination of the nerve axons.
- Symmetric weakness or flaccid paralysis, typically ascending in pattern.
- Absence of deep tendon reflexes due to changes within the nerves: Reflexes are a sensory-motor response that happen at the spinal level, not the brain.
- Recent infection or other acute illness.
- Facial weakness, dysphagia, visual changes in descending disease.
- Labile blood pressure and cardiac dysrhythmias due to autonomic nervous system response.

Test Results

- Lumbar puncture shows CSF with increased protein; may not be present initially.
- Nerve conduction studies show slowed velocity.
- Pulmonary function tests show diminished tidal volume and vital capacity.

Treatment

- Monitor respirations and support ventilation if necessary.
- Plasmapheresis for plasma exchange to remove the antibodies in the circulation.
- Administer immunoglobulin IV after drawing labs for serum immunoglobulin A.
- Nasogastric tube feeding if swallowing is a problem.

Nursing Intervention

- 10 Monitor for progression of change of sensation.
- Monitor respiratory status for change in effort or rate, use of accessory muscles, cyanosis, change in breath sounds, breathlessness when talking, irritability, decreased cognitive awareness.

- ◐ Call physician for respiratory changes or decrease in pulse oximeter reading.
- ◐ Monitor gag reflex.
- ◐ Monitor for visual changes.
- ◐ Monitor for communication ability; may need special method to communicate with staff; may not be able to use call bell system.
- ◐ Turn and reposition.
- ◐ Consult with social worker or chaplain for support services available to patient.
- ◐ Explain to the family the importance of turning and positioning the patient every 2 hours and the proper care of the plasmapheresis access site. Also explain that the patient will require home care.

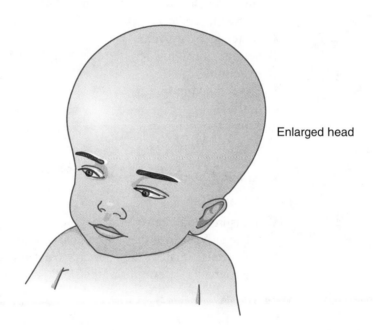

Enlarged head

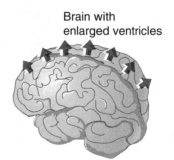

Brain with normal ventricles

Brain with enlarged ventricles

FIGURE 10-2

HYDROCEPHALUS

What Went Wrong?

Hydrocephalus occurs when there is disruption of circulation and absorption of CSF resulting in an accumulation of CSF in ventricles of the brain causing ventricles to dilate and increase intracranial pressure. There are two types of hydrocephalus:

- **Noncommunicating hydrocephalus:** Caused by an obstruction of CSF flow.
- **Communicating hydrocephalus:** Caused by disruption of CSF absorption.

Signs and Symptoms

- Rapidly increasing head circumference in infants
- Bulging and widening of fontanels in infants
- Underdeveloped neck muscles
- Shiny thin scalp
- Distended scalp veins
- Setting-sun sign where the sclera is above the iris
- Irritability
- Projectile vomiting
- Shrill cry
- Anorexia
- Weak sucking
- Nuchal rigidity
- Arnold-Chiari malformation

Test Results

- Measure head circumference to detect enlargement.
- CT scan: Visualizes the ventricles to determine if the ventricles are dilated.
- MRI scan: Visualizes the ventricles to determine if the ventricles are dilated.
- Radiograph: Determines if the skull is thinning or widening

Treatment

- Surgical removal of or bypass the obstruction using a ventriculoperitoneal (VP) shunt that connects the ventricles to the peritoneal cavity or to the right atrium of the heart.
- Administer Tylenol as needed for postoperative pain.
- VP shunt infection or malfunction:
  - Administer vancomycin IV.
  - Administer Tylenol if the temperature is >101.3°F (38.5°C).

Nursing Intervention

- Before surgery:
  - Measure the head circumference daily and report increases of 0.5 cm to the health-care provider.
  - Monitor for increase intracranial pressure.

- Monitor vital signs every 4 hours.
- Maintain strict intake and output measurement.
- Provide small feedings due to the risk of vomiting.
- Burp frequently during feedings.
- Support the child's head during feedings.

◐ After surgery:
- Position the patient flat on the nonoperative side to prevent the CSF from rapidly draining.
- Assess the level of consciousness.
- Monitor for vomiting.
- Assess for infection and VP shut malfunction:
  ○ Severe headaches
  ○ Irritability
  ○ Vomiting
  ○ Redness along the shunt
  ○ Fluid around the VP shunt valve
  ○ Fever
  ○ Lethargy
- Assess for abdominal distention resulting from paralytic ileus due to the VP shunt.
- The child should not participate in contact sports.
- Explain the disorder and treatment to the family and explain that VP shunt may have to be replaced periodically to accommodate the child's growth. Also explain how to identify infection or malfunctioning of the VP shunt and to call the health-care provider immediately if it should occur.

CONCLUSION

There are three divisions of the neurologic system. These are the central nervous system (CNS), peripheral nervous system, and the autonomic nervous system (ANS).

When an abnormal discharge of neurons in the CNS occurs, the patient experiences involuntary movement referred to as a seizure.

The brain and spinal cord is covered by a meningeal covering that can become inflamed by invading bacterial, virus, fungus, or other microorganism. This is called meningitis. A microorganism can also infect the brain tissue that results in inflammation called encephalitis. Encephalitis can lead to the demyelination of nerve fibers in the affected brain tissue.

The brain is surrounded by cerebral spinal fluid (CSF). CSF circulates throughout the brain and becomes absorbed to maintain balance pressure. A disruption of this circulation or absorption results in a buildup of CSF referred to as hydrocephalus.

The brain can also be adversely affected by the disruption of the urea cycle in the liver. The liver changes ammonia to urea that is excreted in urine. The disruption causes ammonia levels to build in the blood and cross the blood-brain barrier, causing neurologic problems and problems with muscles and kidneys. This disorder is called Reye syndrome.

Neurologic disorders can stem from genetic and development abnormalities such as neural tube defects. A neural tube defect occurs when the neural tube, which later develops into the brain and spinal cord, fails to close within 28 days after conception.

Cerebral palsy is another disorder that can occur during fetal development, a difficult birth, or trauma. This is where the portion of the brain that controls motor functions becomes disabled, resulting in partial paralysis and uncontrolled movement.

Down syndrome and Duchenne muscular dystrophy are both genetic disorders that affect children. Down syndrome is a genetic disorder resulting in retardation most commonly caused by three instead of two chromosomes 21. Duchenne muscular dystrophy is a sex-linked recessive genetic degenerative muscular disease where muscle fibers are replaced by connective tissue and fat.

A child might develop Guillain-Barré syndrome following a viral infection, surgery, or from immunization. This disorder is an acute, progressive autoimmune condition that affects the peripheral nerves where the myelin surrounding the axon on the peripheral nerves is damaged.

An abnormal growth of cells in the brain might develop. This called a brain tumor. A brain tumor might consist of brain tissue or tissues from a secondary site that has metastasized to the brain. As a result, the brain tumor can interfere with normal neurologic activities and might increase intracranial pressure.

FINAL CHECKUP

1. **What is the disorder called where there is a brief loss of consciousness lasting <30 seconds with no postseizure confusion and minimal or no loss of postural tone?**
   a. Myoclonic seizure
   b. Complex partial seizure
   c. Absence seizure
   d. Tonic-clonic seizure

2. **What would you do for a patient diagnosed with encephalitis?**
   a. Monitor for increased intracranial pressure.
   b. Encourage family and friends to visit at all times a day and night to support the child.
   c. Avoid administering corticosteroid.
   d. All of the above.

3. **What stage of Reye syndrome would you suspect if the patient lost consciousness?**
   a. Stage 2
   b. Stage 3
   c. Stage 4
   d. Stage 5

4. **How would you care for the sac in a patient who has spinal bifida occulta?**
   a. Keep the patient on his side to remove pressure from the sac.
   b. Place a sterile dress soaked in warm saline solution to prevent the sac from dehydration.
   c. Place a strip of plastic below the sac to prevent contamination from urine and stool.
   d. None of the above.

5. **You notice a child having a scissor-like gait. What disorder would you suspect?**
   a. Cerebral palsy spastic
   b. Cerebral palsy athetoid
   c. Cerebral palsy ataxic
   d. Duchenne muscular dystrophy

6. **A patient diagnosed with Guillain-Barré syndrome has difficulty swallowing. What would you expect the health-care provider to order?**
   a. Peg tube feeding
   b. Nasogastric tube feeding
   c. Nothing by mouth (NPO)
   d. Only fluids by mouth

7. **The parent of a 3-year-old who has been treated for hydrocephalus at birth calls saying that the child has severe headaches and is irritable and vomiting. What would you tell the parent?**
   a. Bring the child to the health-care provider's office immediately.
   b. Give the child an aspirin.
   c. Give the child acetaminophen.
   d. This is a reaction to the medication administered for hydrocephalus.

8. **What would you do if the health-care provider diagnosed a newborn with anencephaly?**
   a. Teach the family how to care for infant's sac.
   b. Make an appointment with the social worker to explain services that are available to parents of a child who is paralyzed.
   c. Explain to the family that the child will likely develop hydrocephalus.
   d. Prepare the family for the child's death.

9. **Increased intracranial pressure can cause which of the following?**
   a. Seizure
   b. Nausea
   c. Vomiting
   d. All of the above

10. What could occur if the child's temperature is 103°F?
   a. Falling forward
   b. Drop-and-fall action
   c. Febrile seizure
   d. Night terror

ANSWERS

Routine checkup 1
   1. b

Routine checkup 2
   1. b

Routine checkup 3
   1. c

Final checkup

1. c	2. a	3. c	4. d
5. a	6. b	7. a	8. d
9. d	10. c		

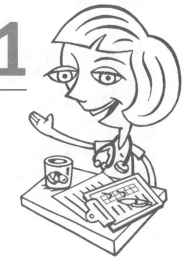

CHAPTER 11

Gastrointestinal Conditions

Learning Objectives

At the end of the chapter, the student will be able to

1. Understand the effects of a ruptured appendix.

2. Identify signs of celiac disease.

3. Know the interventions for a cleft palate and cleft lip.

4. Explain the treatment for Crohn disease.

5. Care for a patient who is diagnosed with hepatitis.

6. Assess a patient who has Hirschsprung disease.

7. Teach families about intussusception.

8. Intervene with a patient who has pyloric stenosis.

9. Discuss transmission tracheoesophageal fistula and esophageal atresia.

10. Recognize a patient who has ulcerative colitis.

11. Respond to a patient who has volvulus.

KEY WORDS

Borborygmi	Lower esophageal	Pyloric sphincter
Cardiac sphincter	sphincter (LES)	Radiopaque catheter
Cheiloplasty	McBurney point	Rebound pain
Gluten	Megacolon	Upper esophageal
Ileocecal valve	Palatoplasty	sphincter (UES)

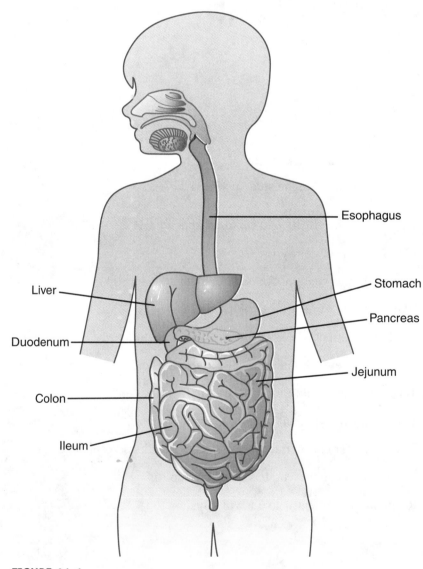

FIGURE 11-1

OVERVIEW

The two major components of the gastrointestinal (GI) system are the alimentary canal and the accessory organs. The alimentary canal is commonly referred to as the GI tract and consists of the following

- Oral cavity
- Pharynx
- Esophagus
- Stomach
- Small intestine
- Large intestine

THE ESOPHAGUS

Digestion involves mechanical and chemical processes, both of which begin in the mouth. Chewing, movement through the GI tract, and churning within the stomach are parts of the mechanical process. Saliva, hydrochloric acid, bile, and other digestive enzymes all contribute to the chemical process of digestion.

The esophagus extends from the oropharynx to the stomach. At the top of the esophagus is the **upper esophageal sphincter (UES)** to prevent the influx of air into the esophagus during respiration. At the bottom of the esophagus is the **lower esophageal sphincter (LES)** that prevents the reflux of acid from the stomach into the esophagus.

THE STOMACH

The contents of the esophagus empty into the stomach through the **cardiac sphincter.** The stomach has three parts: the fundus, body, and pylorus. The fundus is the upper portion of the stomach that connects to the lower end of the esophagus. The body is the middle portion of the stomach where gastrin secretes. Gastrin promotes secretion of pepsinogen and hydrochloric acid, pepsin, and lipase, all of which aid digestion, and mucus formation, which helps protect the stomach lining. The pylorus is the lower portion of the stomach that connects to the duodenum by the **pyloric sphincter.**

THE LIVER

The liver is a very vascular organ located in the right upper quadrant of the abdomen under the diaphragm. It has two main lobes that are comprised of smaller lobules. The liver stores a variety of vitamins and minerals. It metabolizes proteins; synthesizes plasma proteins, fatty acids, and triglycerides; and stores and releases glycogen. The liver detoxifies foreign substances such as alcohol, drugs, or chemicals.

The liver forms and secretes bile to aid in digestion of fat. Bile will release into the gallbladder for storage or into the duodenum if needed for digestion if the sphincter of Oddi is open due to the secretion of the digestive enzymes secretin, cholecystokinin, and gastrin. The gallbladder is a small receptacle that holds bile until it is needed. It is located on the inferior aspect of the liver.

THE PANCREAS

The pancreas is located retroperitoneally in the upper abdomen near the stomach and extends from just right of midline to the left toward the spleen.

The pancreas has both endocrine and exocrine functions. The endocrine functions include secretion of insulin in response to elevations in blood glucose from the beta cells of the islets of Langerhans and glucagon in response to decrease in blood glucose from the alpha cells. The exocrine function includes secretion of trypsin, lipase, amylase, and chymotrypsin to aid in digestion.

THE INTESTINES

The small intestine is comprised of the duodenum, jejunum, and the ileum. The duodenum attaches to the stomach, is about a foot long and C-shaped, and it curves to the left around the pancreas.

The common bile duct and pancreatic duct enter here. The jejunum is between the duodenum and ileum and is about 8 feet long. The last portion of the small intestine is the ileum, which is up to 12 feet long, depending on the size of the patient.

The **ileocecal valve** separates the ileum from the large intestine. The appendix is found at this juncture. The large intestine can be broken down into the ascending colon, transverse colon, descending colon, and sigmoid colon. The sigmoid colon joins the rectum and ultimately the anal canal.

Food moves through the GI tract through a process called peristalsis. Peristalsis is the pushing of food through pulsating muscle action.

APPENDICITIS

What Went Wrong?

Appendicitis is the inflammation of the vermiform appendix, which is a blind pouch located near the ileocecal valve in the right lower quadrant of the abdomen that may be obstructed by stool.

The mucosal lining of the appendix continues to secrete fluid, which will increase the pressure within the lumen of appendix, causing a restriction of the blood supply to the appendix. This decrease in blood supply may result in gangrene or perforation as the pressure continues to build.

Pain localizes at the **McBurney point,** located midway between the umbilicus and right anterior iliac crest. Appendicitis may occur at any age, but the peak occurrence is from the teenage years to age 30.

Nursing alert **Rupture of the appendix is more likely to occur in acute appendicitis within the first 36 to 48 hours and can result in peritonitis, which is inflammation of the peritoneum, the membrane lining the abdominal cavity. Rapid diagnosis and surgical intervention are necessary to avoid rupture of the appendix.**

Signs and Symptoms

- Abdominal pain begins periumbilical and travels to right lower quadrant.
- **Rebound pain,** pain when pressure on the abdomen is quickly removed, occurs with peritoneal inflammation.
- Guarding, protecting the abdomen from painful exam.
- Rigidity of the abdomen (abdomen feels more firm when palpating).
- Fever due to infection.
- Nausea.
- Vomiting.
- Loss of appetite.

Nursing alert **Right lower quadrant pain that improves with flexing the right hip suggests perforation.**

Test Results

- Serum: Elevated white blood cell count.
- Computed tomography (CT) scan: Shows enlarged appendix.
- Ultrasound: May show enlarged appendix.

Treatment

- Surgical removal of the appendix (appendectomy).
- Intravenous fluids until diet resumed.
- Pain medications after surgery as needed; pain medication is used cautiously preoperatively to maintain awareness of increase in pain due to possible rupture of appendix.
- Antibiotics postoperatively if needed.

Nursing alert **Nothing by mouth to avoid further irritation of the intestinal area and to prepare for surgery.**

Nursing Intervention

- Monitor vital signs.
- Assess pain level for changes.
- Monitor surgical site for appearance of wound, drainage.

- Monitor abdomen for distention, presence of bowel sounds.
- Monitor intake and output.
- Monitor bowel function.
- Explain the disorder and treatment to the family.

CELIAC DISEASE

What Went Wrong?

Celiac disease occurs when enzymes in the intestinal mucosal cells are damaged when they are in contact with **gluten,** resulting in decreased absorption by the small intestines. Gluten is a protein found in wheat, rye, oats, and barley. Celiac disease is detected in infants when they are introduced to gluten-containing foods.

Signs and Symptoms

- Diarrhea
- Fatty, foul-smelling stool
- Distention
- Vomiting
- Irritability
- Abdominal pain

Nursing alert **The child may be malnourished and experience coagulation problems due to the malabsorption of fat-soluble vitamins.**

Test Results

- Glucose tolerance test: Poor absorption of glucose
- Serum: Decreased level of albumin, potassium, cholesterol, calcium, and sodium
- Blood count: Decreased platelets, white blood cells (WBC), and hematocrit
- Stool: High fat content
- Biopsy: Positive for celiac disease

Treatment

- Diet free from wheat, rye, oats, and barley.
- Increase dietary protein, calories.
- Decrease dietary fat.
- Administer water-soluble vitamins A and D.
- Administer iron supplements.
- Administer folic acid.

Nursing Intervention

- Teach the family about the disorder and treatment and inform them that dietary changes are for the child's entire life.

ROUTINE CHECKUP 1

1. A 16-year-old was taken to the Emergency Department (ED) complaining about abdominal pain on the lower right quadrant, nausea, and vomiting. He guards the area when you palpating it. Fifteen minutes after you assessed the child, he reports feeling much better now that the pain went away. What is your best response?
   a. Notify the health-care provider immediately and prepare to take the patient to surgery.
   b. Notify the health-care provider and prepare to discharge the patient.
   c. Tell the patient that he'll need to stay in the ED for a few hours for observation.
   d. Tell the patient that the pain will likely reoccur and that he'll need to stay in the ED until the results of the lab tests are returned.

Answer:

2. The mother of a 7-month-old tells you that her child acts strangely when she is given oatmeal for breakfast. What is your best response?
   a. Tell the mother that the child has celiac disease.
   b. Tell the mother to change brands of oatmeal.
   c. Ask the mother if the child's stools are foul-smelling and if the child has diarrhea and is vomiting after breakfast.
   d. Tell the mother that the child is simply fussing.

Answer:

CLEFT PALATE AND CLEFT LIP

What Went Wrong?

A cleft palate and cleft lip is a birth defect caused by chromosomal abnormalities or exposure to alcohol, anticonvulsant medication, and other teratogens resulting in the upper jaw and palate bone and tissue not fusing together properly in the second month of pregnancy.

 Nursing alert **A cleft palate may not be detected until feeding problems develop or until the first-month examination of the infant if the infant's lip is normal.**

Signs and Symptoms
- ◗ Distended abdominal due to swallowing air
- ◗ Abnormal formation of the lip
- ◗ Abnormal formation of the palate

Test Results

- Prenatal ultrasonograph: Shows cleft lip

Treatment

- **Cheiloplasty** to surgically repair the cleft lip within the first 3 months after birth to provide adequate sucking.
- **Palatoplasty** to surgically repair the cleft palate between 12 months and 18 months of age before the child begins speaking.

Nursing alert **The infant who has a cleft palate must be able to drink from a cup before the palatoplasty can be performed.**

Nursing Intervention

- Elevate the infant when feeding.
- Use an oversized nipple.
- Stimulate the sucking reflex because this helps with speech.
- Give the infant time to swallow to prevent choking.
- Feed slowly giving the infant a rest period after swallowing.
- Burp frequently to expel swallowed air and prevent vomiting.
- Provide small, frequent feedings to prevent the infant from getting tired.
- Give water following feedings to flush food from the mouth and thereby preventing the growth of microorganisms.
- Cleft palate:
  - Feed using a cleft palate nipple.
  - Use a Teflon implant for feeding.
  - Assess for abdominal distention.
  - Strict intake and output.
  - Assess the ability to suck.
  - Monitor the vital signs.
- Postoperative care:
  - Maintain airway.
  - Monitor for respiratory distress.
  - Restrain the infant from accessing the site.
  - Clean the site after feeding.
  - Place the infant on the right side after feedings to prevent aspiration.
  - Cleft palate:
    - Don't use a pacifier.
    - Use a cup rather than a nipple for feeding.
    - Don't brush teeth for 2 weeks following surgery.
    - Don't use pointed objects near the infant's mouth.
- Explain the disorder and treatment to the family.

Nursing alert **Monitor for failure to thrive and aspiration during and after feedings.**

CROHN DISEASE

What Went Wrong?

Crohn disease is the inflammation of any portion of the GI tract. The majority of cases involve the small and large intestine, often in the right lower quadrant at the point where the terminal ileum and the ascending colon meet.

Patients typically have an insidious onset of intermittent symptoms. The disease causes transmural inflammation, going deeper than the superficial mucosal layer of the tissue to affect all layers. Over time the inflammatory changes within the GI tract can lead to strictures or the formation of fistulas. The affected tissue develops granulomas and takes on a mottled appearance interspersed with normal tissue.

There is a genetic predisposition and a bimodal peak of onset. Crohn disease is a chronic disorder with periods of exacerbation and remission. Many patients ultimately need surgery to deal with bowel obstruction, development of strictures, or fistula formation.

Nursing alert **Healed lesions can lead to strictures.**

Signs and Symptoms

- Fever
- Right lower quadrant pain
- Diarrhea (nonbloody)
- Abdominal mass
- Weight loss (unintentional)
- Fatigue
- Bloating after meals
- Abdominal cramping due to spasm
- **Borborygmi:** Loud, frequent bowel sounds
- Aphthous ulcers (oral ulcerations)

Test Results

- Erythrocyte sedimentation rate: Elevated during exacerbations.
- Blood count: Decreased hemoglobin level (anemia) due to both vitamin B_{12} and folic acid deficiency.
- Serum: Decreased albumin level.
- Blood chemistry: Abnormal due to loss from diarrhea and malabsorption.
- Barium studies: Show "apple core" in area of stricture formation, narrowing due to inflammation, and fistula formation.

- CT scan: Shows abscess formation and thickening of bowel wall due to inflammation.
- Sigmoidoscopy: Inflamed tissue visualized.
- Colonoscopy: Inflamed tissue visualized.

Treatment

- Dietary restriction: Limit fiber such as nuts and popcorn during flare-ups.
- Nutritional supplementation.
- Administer vitamin B_{12} and folic acid.
- Administer aminosalicylates to induce or maintain remission:
  - Mesalamine
  - Sulfasalazine
  - Olsalazine
  - Balsalazide
- Administer glucocorticoids to reduce inflammation:
  - Hydrocortisone
  - Budesonide
- Administer purine analogs to induce or maintain remission:
  - Azathioprine
  - 6-mercaptopurine
- Administer methotrexate to induce or maintain remission.
- Administer antidiarrheal medications (with caution) to decrease fluid loss:
  - Diphenoxylate hydrochloride
  - Atropine sulfate
- Intravenous fluids to maintain hydration.
- Surgical correction of intestinal obstruction, fistula, perforation.

Nursing Intervention

- Monitor vital signs for temperature increase, pulse increase, and change in blood pressure.
- Monitor intake and output.
- Assess abdomen for bowel sounds, tenderness, and masses.
- Assess postoperative wound for signs of infection, drainage.
- Wound care postoperatively:
  - Proper skin care if bowel-skin fistula:
    - Use of drainable pouch with skin wafer.
    - Cleaning skin promptly if drainage comes in contact with skin.
  - Nutritional supplementation:
    - Ensure
    - Sustacal
    - Vivonex
- Explain the disorder and treatment to the family and about home care needs.

Nursing alert **Be alert for signs of toxic megacolon (spiking fever, abdominal distention, and acute abdominal pain), which can lead to peritonitis and hemorrhage.**

 # ROUTINE CHECKUP 2

1. A father of an 8-month-old daughter who has been diagnosed with a cleft palate asks why he has to give her water following every feeding. What is your best response?
   a. The water stimulates the sucking reflex and helps develop her speech.
   b. Food can become stuck in her mouth due to her cleft palate and become a breeding ground for bacteria. The water flushes any food that remains in her mouth.
   c. The water helps prevent her from swallowing air and thereby reducing vomiting and the risk of aspiration.
   d. It prevents choking.

   Answer:

2. The mother of a child diagnosed with Crohn disease asks why her child is being administered hydrocortisone. What is your best response?
   a. Crohn disease is an inflammation of the GI tract. Hydrocortisone decreases the body's inflammation process and therefore reduces inflammation of the GI tract.
   b. Hydrocortisone decreases the inflammation process and is given to prevent secondary inflammation of organs that assist in digestion.
   c. Hydrocortisone decreases the inflammation process, thereby enabling strictures to form to enhance digestion.
   d. Hydrocortisone decreases the inflammation process, thereby enabling a fistula to form to enhance digestion.

   Answer:

HEPATITIS

What Went Wrong?

Hepatitis is an inflammation of the liver cells commonly caused by a virus and can be an acute or chronic illness. Hepatitis may also be due to exposure to drugs or toxins. There are seven types of hepatitis:

- Hepatitis A is transmitted via an oral route, often due to contaminated water or poor sanitation when traveling; it is also transmitted in daycare settings and residential institutions. It can be prevented by vaccine.

◑ Hepatitis B is transmitted via a percutaneous route, often due to sexual contact, intravenous (IV) drug use, mother-to-neonate transmission, or possibly blood transfusion. It can be prevented by vaccine.

◑ Hepatitis C is transmitted via a percutaneous route, often due to IV drug use or, less commonly, sexual contact. There is currently no vaccine available.

◑ Hepatitis D is transmitted via a percutaneous route and needs hepatitis B to spread cell to cell. There is no vaccine available for hepatitis D.

◑ Hepatitis E is transmitted via an oral route and is associated with water contamination. There is no known chronic state of hepatitis E and no current vaccine available.

◑ Hepatitis G is transmitted via a percutaneous route and is associated with chronic infection but not significant liver disease.

Exposure to medications (even at therapeutic doses), drugs, or chemicals can also cause hepatitis. Onset is usually within the first couple of days of use, and it may be within the first couple of doses. Hepatotoxic substances include acetaminophen, carbon tetrachloride, benzenes, and valproic acid.

Hepatitis may occur as an acute infection (viral type A, E) or become a chronic state. The patient with chronic disease may be unaware of the illness until testing of liver function shows abnormalities and further testing reveals presence of hepatitis.

The chronic (viral type B, C) disease state creates the potential development of progressive liver disease. Some patients with chronic disease will need liver transplantation. Recurrence rate posttransplantation is high. Liver cancer may develop in those with chronic disease states.

Nursing alert **Decrease in the size of an enlarged liver is a sign of tissue necrosis.**

Signs and Symptoms

◑ Acute hepatitis:
- Malaise
- Nausea and vomiting
- Diarrhea or constipation
- Low-grade fever
- Dark urine due to change in liver function
- Jaundice due to liver compromise
- Tenderness in right upper quadrant of abdomen
- Hepatomegaly
- Arthritis, glomerulonephritis, polyarteritis nodosa in hepatitis B

◑ Chronic hepatitis:
- Asymptomatic with elevated liver enzymes
- Symptoms as acute hepatitis

- Cirrhosis due to altered liver function
- Ascites due to decrease in liver function, increased portal hypertension
- Bleeding from esophageal varices
- Encephalopathy due to diminished liver function
- Bleeding due to clotting disorders
- Enlargement of spleen

Test Results

- ◑ Serums: Elevated aspartate aminotransferase (AST), alanine aminotransferase (ALT)
- ◑ Immunoglobulin (Ig)M anti-HAV: Presence in acute or early convalescent stage of hepatitis A
- ◑ IgG anti-HAV: Presence in later convalescent stage of hepatitis A.
- ◑ HBeAg: Presence of current viral replication of hepatitis B and infectivity.
- ◑ HBsAg: Presence of the surface antigen, either current or past infection with hepatitis B.
- ◑ IgM anti-HBc: Presence of acute or recent infection with hepatitis B.
- ◑ IgG anti-HBc: Presence of past infection with hepatitis B.
- ◑ HBV DNA: Shows presence of hepatitis B DNA, most sensitive.
- ◑ Anti-HCV: Presence of hepatitis C infection.
- ◑ HCV RNA: Presence of hepatitis C infection.
- ◑ Anti HDV: Presence of hepatitis D infection.
- ◑ Blood count: Normal to low WBC.
- ◑ Liver biopsy: Shows hepatocellular necrosis.
- ◑ Urinalysis: Presence of protein and bilirubin.

Treatment

- ◑ Avoid medications metabolized in the liver.
- ◑ Avoid alcohol.
- ◑ Remove or discontinue causative agent if drug induced or toxic hepatitis.
- ◑ IV hydration if vomiting during acute hepatitis.
- ◑ Activity as tolerated.
- ◑ High-calorie diet; breakfast is usually the best tolerated meal.
- ◑ Administer interferon or lamivudine for chronic hepatitis B.
- ◑ Administer interferon and ribavirin for hepatitis C.
- ◑ Administer prednisone in autoimmune hepatitis.
- ◑ Liver transplantation.

Nursing Intervention

- ◑ Monitor vital signs.
- ◑ Assess abdomen for bowel sounds, tenderness, ascites.
- ◑ Plan appropriate rest for patient in acute phase.

- Monitor intake and output.
- Assist patient to plan palatable meals; remember that breakfast is generally the best tolerated meal.
- Avoid smoking areas—intolerance to smoking.
- Assess mental status for changes due to encephalopathy.
- Explain the disorder and treatment to the family.

HIRSCHSPRUNG DISEASE

What Went Wrong?

Hirschsprung disease is a congenital condition where there is the lack of nerve cells in the colon causing a lack of peristalsis, resulting in stool being unable to be pushed through the colon.

Nursing alert **Hirschsprung disease is common in Down syndrome.**

Signs and Symptoms

- Failure to pass meconium within the first 48 hours following birth
- Failure to pass stool within the first 48 hours following birth
- Abdominal distention
- Abdominal mass
- Ribbon-like or liquid stool
- Sunken eyes
- Pallor
- Dehydration
- Irritable
- Weight loss
- Lethargic

Nursing alert **Monitor for fecal vomiting.**

Test Results

- Abdominal radiograph: Shows distended colon
- Rectal biopsy: Absence of ganglion cells in the colon
- Full-thickness surgical biopsy: Absence of ganglion cells in the colon
- Suction aspiration of rectum: Absence of ganglion cells in the colon

Treatment

- Surgery: After 9 months of age, the affected portion of the colon is removed.

Nursing alert **If the colon is obstructed, a temporary colostomy or ileostomy is performed to decompress the colon. Once decompressed, a second surgery is performed to remove the affected portion of the colon and remove the colostomy or ileostomy.**

Nursing Intervention

- ○ Preoperative care:
  - Nothing by mouth.
  - Administer IV fluids as ordered to prevent maintain fluid and electrolyte balance.
  - Insert an nasogastric (NG) tube to decompress the upper GI tract.
  - Administer normal saline or mineral oil enemas to clean the bowel.
  - Administer antibiotics as ordered.
- ○ Postoperative care:
  - Strict input and output.
  - Provide care for the colostomy or ileostomy, if necessary.
  - Monitor bowel sounds.
  - Begin feeding by mouth when bowel sounds are present.
  - Nothing should be placed in the rectum.
  - Monitor for constipation.
- ○ Explain the disorder and treatment to the family and instruct them on proper care for the wound and how to care for the colostomy or ileostomy, if necessary. Tell the family to call the health-care provider at the first signs of constipation, dehydration, fever, vomiting, and diarrhea.

Nursing alert **Don't use tap water in the enema because this can induce water intoxication. Return of anal sphincter control and complete continence can take months to develop.**

INTUSSUSCEPTION

What Went Wrong?

Intussusception is a disorder where the intestine telescopes and causes inflammation and edema resulting in blood vessel occlusion leading to necrosis. Intussusception occurs between 6 months and 3 years of age and is common in children who have cystic fibrosis (See Figure 11-2).

Signs and Symptoms

- ○ Colicky
- ○ Knees drawn to chest

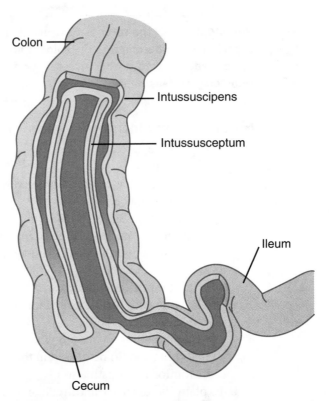

FIGURE 11-2

- Grunting
- Fecal material in vomit
- Sweating
- Red currant jelly-like stool
- Dehydration
- Distended abdomen
- Fever
- Shallow respiration
- Sausage-shaped abdominal mass

Test Results

- Abdominal radiograph: Shows mass.
- Barium enema: Shows intussusception.
- Complete blood count—elevated WBC (leukocytosis):
  - 10,000 to 15,000 μL is a sign of bowel obstruction.
  - 15,000 to 20,000 μL is a sign of bowel strangulation.
  - >20,000 μL is a sign of bowel infarction.

Treatment

- ☾ Insert an NG tube to reduce vomiting and decompress the GI tract.
- ☾ Hydrostatic reduction of bowel: The bowel is moved back into position using a barium solution, water-soluble contrast solution, or air pressure.
- ☾ Surgery: Pulling the intussusceptions back into position or resectioning the bowel if other treatments fail to resolve the intussusceptions.

Nursing alert **Treatment must begin within 24 hours.**

Nursing Intervention

- ☾ Monitor vital signs.
- ☾ Insert the NG tube as ordered and measure output.
- ☾ Administer the enema as ordered.
- ☾ Strict intake and output.
- ☾ Postoperative care:
  - • Administer antibiotics
  - • Monitor signs of infection
  - • Monitor bowel sounds
- ☾ Explain the disorder and treatment to the family.

Nursing alert **Intussusception is an emergency condition.**

PYLORIC STENOSIS

What Went Wrong?

Pyloric stenosis is spasms of the pylorus muscle in the pyloric sphincter that connects the stomach to the duodenum, causing the pyloric sphincter to become inflamed and swell, thus preventing the stomach from emptying into the duodenum. The cause is unknown and is seen in children between 1 and 6 months of age.

Signs and Symptoms

- ☾ Projectile vomiting caused by reverse peristaltic and gastritis
- ☾ No nausea
- ☾ Blood-stained vomit caused by gastritis
- ☾ Olive-shaped bulge below the right costal margin
- ☾ Malnutrition
- ☾ Poor weight gain
- ☾ Normal appetite
- ☾ Eats after vomiting

Test Results

- ⦿ Abdominal ultrasound: Increased size of pyloric sphincter
- ⦿ Endoscopy: Increased size of pyloric sphincter
- ⦿ Upper GI series: Delayed gastric emptying
- ⦿ Blood chemistry: Decreased calcium, sodium, potassium
- ⦿ Blood gases: Metabolic alkalosis

Treatment

- ⦿ Insert NG tube to decompress the GI tract.
- ⦿ Administer IV fluids and electrolytes to maintain fluid and electrolytes balance.
- ⦿ Surgery: Pyloromyotomy to repair the pyloric sphincter.

8 Nursing Intervention

- ⦿ Nothing by mouth.
- ⦿ Strict intake and output to assess for dehydration.
- ⦿ Daily weight.
- ⦿ Assess vomitus for character and frequency.
- ⦿ Monitor vital signs.
- ⦿ Postoperative care:
  - • Monitor intake and output.
  - • Elevate the child's head when feeding.
  - • Burp frequently.
  - • Small frequent feedings until the pyloric sphincter function returns to normal.
- ⦿ Explain the disorder and treatment to the family.

Nursing alert **Position the child on her right side to prevent aspiration and to use gravity to help emptying of the stomach.**

TRACHEOESOPHAGEAL FISTULA/ESOPHAGEAL ATRESIA

What Went Wrong?

9 A tracheoesophageal fistula is a congenital anomaly in which the trachea and the esophagus are connected. A child with a tracheoesophageal fistula is likely to have an esophageal atresia where the esophagus ends in a blind pouch preventing food from entering the stomach. These disorders occur approximately at 5 weeks of gestation when the foregut normally develops into the trachea and esophagus.

Nursing alert **Tracheoesophageal fistula and esophageal atresia are an emergency condition.**

Signs and Symptoms

- Frothy saliva
- Coughing due to excessive secretions
- Gagging when feeding
- Feedings exiting the mouth and nose
- Aspiration
- Difficulty breathing
- Distended stomach

Nursing alert **Monitor for aspiration when first feeding a newborn.**

Test Results

- **Radiopaque catheter** radiograph: A radiograph is taken after the radiopaque catheter is inserted into the esophagus to identify the fistula or blind pouch.
- Bronchoscopy: Shows the fistula.
- Chest radiograph: Shows pneumonia and air in the esophageal pouch.

Treatment

- Suction the contents of the blind pouch.
- Insert NG tube to decompress the stomach.
- Surgery: Repair the fistula and/or blind pouch.

Nursing Intervention

- Nothing by mouth:
    - Insert the NG tube as ordered.
    - Suction the contents of the blind pouch as ordered.
    - No pacifier because this increases saliva production.
    - Elevate the child's head.
- Postoperative care:
    - Monitor vital signs.
    - Place NG tube to low suction per order.
    - Monitor output of NG tube every 4 hours.
    - Provide gastrostomy feeding until esophagus returns to normal.
    - Monitor chest tube drain, if necessary.
    - Use pacifier.
    - Start feeding by mouth with sterile water and then advance diet as tolerated.
- Explain the disorder and treatment to the family.

Nursing alert **No pacifier prior to surgery because sucking increases saliva production. Saliva can enter the lungs through the fistula and/or accumulate in the blind pouch.**

ULCERATIVE COLITIS

What Went Wrong?

Ulcerative colitis is an inflammation of the large intestine affecting the mucosal layer beginning in the rectum and colon and spreading into the adjacent tissue. Ulcerations in the mucosal layer of the intestinal wall lead to inflammation and abscesses, resulting in bloody diarrhea with mucus, which is the primary symptom.

There are periods of exacerbations and remissions. Symptom severity may vary from mild to severe. The exact cause is unknown, but there is increased incidence in people with northern European, North American, or Ashkenazi Jewish origins. The peak incidences are from mid-teen to mid-20s and again from mid-50s to mid-60s.

Patients may have an increase in symptoms with each flare-up of the disease. Malabsorption of nutrients can cause weight loss and health problems. Some patients need surgery to resect the affected area of the large intestine, resulting in a colostomy, ileal reservoir, ileoanal anastomosis, or ileoanal reservoir. There is an increased risk of colon cancer in patients with ulcerative colitis. The patient is also at risk for developing toxic megacolon or perforating the area of ulceration.

Nursing alert **The patient is at risk for toxic megacolon, perforation of the intestine, and colon cancer.**

Signs and Symptoms

- Weight loss
- Abdominal pain
- Chronic bloody diarrhea with pus due to ulceration
- Electrolyte imbalance due to diarrhea
- Tenesmus, which is a persistent desire to empty bowel

Test Results

- Blood count: Decreased hemoglobin (anemia), hematocrit due to blood loss and chronic disease
- Erythrocyte sedimentation rate: Elevated due to inflammation
- Electrolytes: Abnormal due to diarrhea and poor absorbance of nutrients
- Double-contrast barium enema: Shows ulceration and inflammation.
- Sigmoidoscopy: Shows ulcerations and bleeding
- Colonoscopy: Shows ulcerations and bleeding

Treatment

- Keep stool diary to identify irritating foods.
- Low-fiber, high-protein, high-calorie diet.
- Administer antidiarrheal medications:
  - Loperamide
  - Diphenoxylate hydrochloride and atropine
- Administer salicylate medications to reduce inflammation within the intestinal mucosa:
  - Sulfasalazine
  - Mesalamine
  - Olsalazine
  - Balsalazide
- Administer corticosteroids during exacerbations to reduce inflammation:
  - Prednisone
  - Hydrocortisone
- Nothing by mouth to rest the bowel during exacerbations.
- Administer anticholinergics to reduce abdominal cramping and discomfort:
  - Dicyclomine
- Surgical resection of affected area of large intestine.

Nursing Intervention

- Monitor intake and output.
- Monitor stool output, frequency.
- Weigh patient regularly.
- Provide a sitz bath to soothe the skin.
- Administer A and D ointment or barrier cream to skin.
- Administer witch hazel to soothe sensitive skin.
- Teach:
  - Dietary modification, foods to avoid
  - Medication use, schedule, and side effects
  - Importance of follow-up care
  - Proper wound care for postoperative patients
  - Proper skin care of perianal area to avoid skin breakdown
  - Avoidance of fragrant products that can be irritating
  - Home care for new ostomy patients

Nursing alert **Monitor for toxic megacolon (distended and tender abdomen, fever, elevated WBC, elevated pulse, distended colon).**

VOLVULUS

What Went Wrong?

Volvulus is a disorder where the intestine twists around itself as a result of ingesting a foreign substance and adhesion or from unknown causes that result in blood vessels to compress and an ischemia to that can lead to necrosis.

Signs and Symptoms

- Abdominal pain
- Vomiting after feeding
- No bowel sounds
- Bloody stool
- Distended abdomen

Test Results

- Abdominal radiograph: Shows distended intestine loops and no gas in large intestine
- Upper GI series: Shows distended intestine loops and no gas in large intestine
- Barium enema: Shows distended intestine loops and no gas in large intestine
- Blood chemistry: Increased potassium and decreased calcium

Treatment

- Surgery: Untwisting the intestine and removal of any necrotic tissue.
- Administer total parenteral nutrition (TPN) to maintain nutrition until the intestine heals.
- Administer antibiotics to prevent infection.
- Administer IV fluids to maintain fluid and electrolyte balance.

Nursing Intervention

- Nothing by mouth.
- Insert NG tube to decompress the GI tract.
- Monitor bowel sounds.
- Monitor bowel movements.
- Postoperative care:
  - Increase dietary fiber and fluid and increase the child's activity to encourage normal bowel movements.
- Explain the disorder and treatment to the family.

Nursing alert **Administer stool softeners following surgery because opioid analgesics decrease GI motility.**

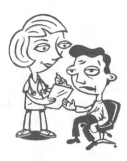

CASE STUDY

Vivian Hoffman, age 5, presented in the ED with his parents at 12:30 PM. His mother reported that he vomited a few minutes after eating and the vomit flew nearly across the table. She was fine afterward but the vomit had reddish tint so she thought to bring her into the ED.

Assessment data: There was no nausea. The child has a normal appetite and wants to eat after vomiting. The child's weight seems below the normal percentile for her age. She appears to have a bulge below the costal margin. Blood gases show an elevated pH and bicarbonate. Blood chemistry shows a decreased calcium, sodium, and potassium.

Interpretation: Blood-stained projectile vomiting without nausea is characteristic of pyloric stenosis. Further confirming this suspicion is the child's normal appetite and wanting to eat after vomiting. The low weight gain is probably caused by malnutrition because little food is passing through to the intestines. The bulge below the costal margin is also an indication of an obstruction in the area of the pyloric sphincter. Blood gases indicate metabolic alkalosis, which is consisted with severe vomiting, as is the results of the blood chemistry.

Nursing intervention: Give the child nothing by mouth because pyloric sphincter is either partially or fully obstructed. Prepare to insert an NG tube to decompress the GI tract and prepare to administer IV fluids to maintain fluid and electrolyte balance. Prepare the child for pyloromyotomy surgery to repair the pyloric sphincter. Strict intake and output. Monitor vital signs. Daily weight. After surgery, elevate the child's head when feeding. Burp frequently and provide small frequent feedings until the pyloric sphincter function returns to normal. Position the child on her right side to prevent aspiration and to use gravity to help emptying of the stomach.

Evaluation: Assess the surgical site for infection. Listen to determine if the child's bowel sounds return following surgery. Monitor the child's intake and output and weigh daily to determine if the child is receiving nutrition.

CONCLUSION

The GI system consists of the alimentary canal and accessory organs that are commonly referred to as the GI tract. Appendicitis is a common problem in the GI system. This occurs when the vermiform appendix, which is a blind pouch located near the ileocecal valve in the right lower quadrant of the abdomen, may be obstructed by stool. This decrease in blood supply may result in gangrene or perforation as the pressure continues to build.

Certain congenital disorders affect the GI system. One of these is celiac disease where enzymes in the intestinal mucosal cells are damaged when they are in contact with gluten. As a result, there is decreased absorption by the small intestines.

Another congenital disorder is a cleft palate and cleft lip. This occurs when the upper jaw and palate bone and tissue don't fuse together properly during the second month of pregnancy.

Hirschsprung disease is a congenital condition where stool is unable to be pushed through the colon due to lack of peristalsis caused by missing nerve cells in the colon.

Tracheoesophageal fistula and esophageal atresia are congenital anomalies that are an emergency. A tracheoesophageal fistula is a congenital anomaly in which the trachea and the esophagus are connected. A child with a tracheoesophageal fistula is likely to have an esophageal atresia where the esophagus ends in a blind pouch, preventing food from entering the stomach.

Children between 6 months and 3 years of age might experience intussusceptions, which is a disorder in which the intestine telescopes, causing inflammation and edema and resulting in occlusion of blood vessels and necrosis. Volvulus is also an intestinal disorder in which the intestine twists around itself as a result of ingesting a foreign substance or from adhesions. This can lead to compressed blood vessels and an ischemia leading to necrosis.

Infants can experience spasms of the pylorus muscle resulting in pyloric stenosis that prevents the pyloric sphincter from emptying stomach contents into the duodenum.

Any portion of the GI tract can become inflamed. Chronic inflammation of the GI tract is called Crohn disease. In most cases, the small and large intestine become inflamed and can lead to strictures or the formation of fistulas.

Another inflammatory disorder is ulcerative colitis. This occurs when the large intestine becomes inflamed and can lead to ulcerations and abscesses. Patients who have ulcerative colitis experience periods of exacerbations and remissions.

Hepatitis is another inflammation disorder of the GI system that affects liver cells commonly as a result of a virus infection or exposure to drugs or toxins. There are seven types of hepatitis.

? FINAL CHECKUP

1. **Your neighbor calls early Saturday morning asking you what is a good remedy for someone who drank too much the night before. She says that her 16-year-daughter awakened after coming home late last night complaining about abdominal pain and nausea. For the past hour she has been vomiting. Her daughter claims she wasn't drinking, but your neighbor thinks otherwise. What is your best response?**
   a. Give her several cups of black coffee once she stops vomiting.
   b. Call 911 and get her to the emergency department immediately
   c. Put her back to bed after she stops vomiting and let her sleep it off.
   d. You probably should call your health-care provider.

2. **A mother mentions in passing that her 6-month-old started to have foul-smelling stools. What is your best response?**
   a. What new foods have you introduced to him recently?
   b. He is probably getting teeth.
   c. Have you introduced him to foods that contain wheat, rye, oats, and barley?
   d. Give him more water.

3. **A parent of a child who is diagnosed with Crohn disease asks why her child can't have popcorn. What is your best response?**
   a. Your child can have popcorn except when there is a flare-up of Crohn disease. Limit fiber such as popcorn during a flare-up to reduce aggravating the intestine.
   b. Popcorn can cause appendicitis.
   c. Popcorn causes Crohn disease.
   d. Popcorn can lead to perforation of the intestine.

4. **A father of a 4-year-old is concerned that his son will contract hepatitis B while attending day care. What is your best response?**
   a. Children may contract Hepatitis A from an oral route due to poor sanitation, which could occur in day care. However, hepatitis A can be prevented with a vaccination.
   b. There isn't any chance that he will contract hepatitis B from a day-care facility.
   c. Hepatitis B is transmitted by sexual contact, from a blood transfusion, or passed to the fetus from his mother so it is unlike that your son will contact hepatitis B from the day-care facility.
   d. Day-care personnel are vaccinated against hepatitis B by law.

5. **A father of a child who is diagnosed with hepatitis calls you very excited, saying that his son is getting better because his enlarged liver has decreased in size. What is your best response?**
   a. That is not a good sign. This is a sign of tissue necrosis.
   b. Can you visit your health-care provider today?
   c. That is good news. Be sure to tell your health-care provider about this change.
   d. I'm sorry to hear about that.

6. **A new mother whose child is diagnosed with Hirschsprung disease is concerned how her daughter will deal with having a colostomy for the rest of her life. What is your best response?**
   a. As she grows older, we'll show her how to care for her colostomy.
   b. The child quickly adapts, and it really isn't a problem.
   c. The colostomy is temporary.
   d. The colostomy is temporary. Once the colon heals, she will undergo another surgery to reverse the colostomy. Afterward she'll be normal.

7. **A child who is diagnosed with cystic fibrosis is colicky and has his knees drawn to his chest and is producing currant jelly-like stool. What is your best response?**
   a. Wait and see if the episode passes.
   b. Call the health-care provider immediately.
   c. Assess for a sausage-shaped abdominal mass and take his vital signs.
   d. Suspect that the child has intussusceptions.

8. **The mother of a child who is diagnosed with pyloric stenosis asks what causes projectile vomiting. What is your best response?**
   a. Projectile vomiting is caused by muscles in the esophagus pushing the food up the esophagus because there is an obstruction at the bottom of the stomach.
   b. Projectile vomiting is caused by reverse peristaltic and gastritis.
   c. An upset stomach.
   d. Projectile vomiting is caused by muscles in the esophagus pushing the food down the esophagus because there is an obstruction at the bottom of the stomach.

9. **A child diagnosed with ulcerative colitis has a fever, distended colon and tender abdomen, and his pulse is elevated. What would you suspect?**
   a. Toxic megacolon
   b. Tenesmus
   c. Exacerbations of ulcerative colitis
   d. Sigmoidoscopy

10. **What is the most serious risk of not reversing volvulus?**
    a. Malnutrition
    b. Bowel obstruction
    c. Infection
    d. Blood vessels to compress and an ischemia to that can lead to necrosis

ANSWERS

Routine checkup 1
  1. a
  2. c

Routine checkup 2
   1. b
   2. a

Final checkup

1. b	2. c	3. a	4. c
5. b	6. d	7. c	8. a
9. a	10. d		

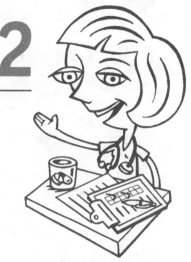

CHAPTER **12**

Genitourinary Conditions

Learning Objectives

At the end of the chapter, the student will be able to

1. Understand the difference between acute and chronic glomerulonephritis.

2. Identify urinary tract congenital anomalies.

3. Know the interventions for hemolytic uremic syndrome.

4. Explain the treatment for nephrotic syndrome.

5. Care for a patient who is diagnosed with renal failure.

6. Assess a patient who has Wilms tumor.

7. Teach families about pyelonephritis.

8. Intervene with a patient who has a urinary tract infection.

KEY WORDS

Albumin	Hypospadia	Proteinuria
Bladder	Micturition reflex	Renal stage
Duplicated ureter	Nephroblastoma	Renin
Exstrophy bladder	Nephrons	Ureterocele
Glomerulus	Nephron tubules	Ureters
Hematuria	Postrenal stage	Ureter stenosis
Hyperkalemia	Prerenal stage	Urethra

OVERVIEW

The urinary system consists of organs and structures involved in the production and transport of urine. These are the kidneys and the urinary tract.

The kidneys are found in the posterior part of the upper abdominal area protected by the lower ribs. The left kidney is higher than the right kidney due to the location of the liver within the abdomen. There are two divisions of the kidneys:

    ◐ Renal cortex: Outside surface of the kidney
    ◐ Renal medulla: Inside the kidney where nephrons are located

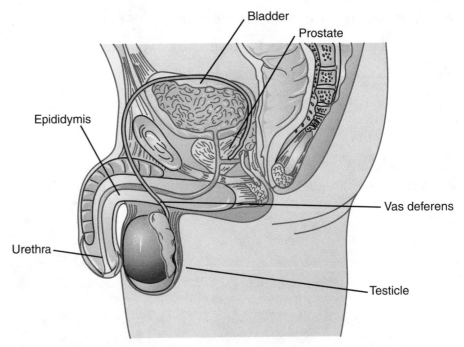

FIGURE 12-1

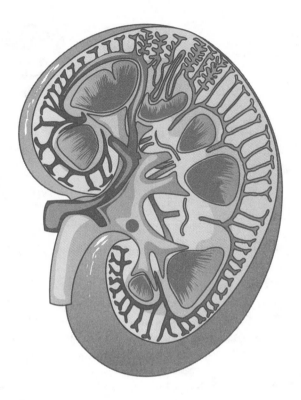

FIGURE 12-2

NEPHRONS

Nephrons are the site where urine is formed. A branch of the abdominal aorta called the renal artery transports blood inside the kidney to the **glomerulus.** The area that surrounds the glomerulus is called the Bowman capsule. The Bowman capsule narrows into a proximal convoluted tubule that eventually enters the loop of Henle and then through a network of small bloods that delivers blood to the nephron tubules in a process called glomerular filtration.

Nephron tubules filter waste fluid from blood. Waste fluid (urine) is secreted into the urinary tract while proteins, electrolytes, and blood cells are resorbed by the nephron tubules and returned to the bloodstream.

THE URINARY TRACT

The urinary tract has three components:

- **Ureters:** Tubes that connect each kidney to the bladder
- **Bladder:** A flexible muscular pouch used to store urine
- **Urethra:** The tube that connects the bladder to outside the body to excrete urine

As waste fluid is filtered by the kidney, it moves through the ureters through peristaltic contraction to the bladder. The ureters have valves that prevent urine from back flowing from the bladder to the kidneys.

TABLE 12–1 • 24-Hour Urine Output by Age	
Age	24-Hour Urine Output
Newborn	300 mL
1 month–1 year	550 mL
2–4 years	800 mL
5–12 years	1400 mL
13–18 years	1500 mL

As the bladder fills usually to about 300 mL, the **micturition reflex** occurs, triggering a signal to the brain that there is a need to urinate. The greater the volume of urine in the bladder, the higher the urge to urinate is received by the brain. The person can voluntarily inhibit the micturition reflex until he or she voluntarily releases the urethral sphincter allowing urine to exit the urethra.

A child's bladder holds 44.4 mL of urine for each year of the child's age. Table 12-1 lists the volume of urine that can be expected in 24 hours.

Nursing alert **Voluntarily inhibition of the micturition reflex, commonly referred to as toilet training, occurs by 3 years of age.**

REGULATOR

The kidneys regulate electrolytes, fluid volume, and blood pressure. Electrolytes are sodium, potassium, calcium, phosphorus, chloride, bicarbonate, and magnesium. Electrolytes must be balanced to ensure cell metabolism and muscle and nerve function. The kidneys help maintain this balance by excreting or retaining electrolytes.

Fluid volume is maintained by the kidneys excreting or retaining urine based on the volume of fluid in the body. When the body is dehydrated, the kidneys produce a low urine output to conserve fluid, and when the body is overhydrated, the kidneys increase urine output to reduce fluid volume in the body.

The kidneys produce the hormone erythropoietin (EPO), which stimulates the production of red blood cells in the bone marrow. Therefore, renal failure causes less production of EPO and thus decreases production of red blood cells, resulting in the patient becoming anemic.

The kidneys also produce the enzyme **renin,** which regulates blood pressure by stabilizing blood vessels. Decreased blood pressure signals the kidneys that there is insufficient blood for perfusion. In response, the kidneys increase renin production, which indirectly causes vasoconstriction and increases secretion of aldosterone to increase blood pressure.

GLOMERULONEPHRITIS

What Went Wrong?

Glomerulonephritis is an inflammation of the glomerulus. There are two types of glomerulonephritis:

- ○ Acute: This might occur up to 6 weeks following a respiratory tract streptococcal bacterial infection or from a skin infection as a result of antigen/antibody groups trapped in the tubules causing edema that decreases filtering and thus causes urine to be retained.
- ○ Chronic: An abnormal immune system, bacterial or viral infection, disease or toxin causes progressive dysfunction of the glomerulus over the years.

Signs and Symptoms

- ○ Acute:
  - Lower than normal urine output (oliguria)
  - Fever
  - Edema of the face and extremities
  - Hypertension
  - Lethargy
- ○ Chronic:
  - Lower than normal urine output (oliguria)
  - Hypertension
  - Does not respond to treatment for acute glomerulonephritis

Test Results

- ○ Acute:
  - Urine analysis: Blood in the urine (**hematuria**), cola-color urine, high specific gravity, and protein in the urine (**proteinuria**)
  - Serum: Elevated creatinine and blood urea nitrogen (BUN)
  - Antistreptolysin-O test: Positive for streptococcal bacteria
  - Throat culture: Positive for streptococcal bacteria
  - Renal ultrasound: Shows enlarged kidneys
  - Renal biopsy: Positive for glomerulonephritis
- ○ Chronic:
  - Urine analysis: Blood in the urine (hematuria), cola-color urine, high specific gravity, and protein in the urine (proteinuria)
  - Serum: Elevated potassium (**hyperkalemia**), creatinine, and BUN
  - Computed tomography (CT) scan: Shows decreased size of kidneys
  - Ultrasound: Shows decreased size of kidneys
  - Renal biopsy: Shows glomeruli scarring and tests positive for glomerulonephritis
  - Electrocardiogram (ECG): Abnormal; possibly indicating hyperkalemia

Treatment

- ◐ Acute:
    - • Administer antibiotics for 10 days.
    - • Administer diuretics to reduce edema.
    - • Administer corticosteroids to reduce the inflammatory response.
    - • Administer antihypertensive medication to reduce blood pressure.
    - • Low-sodium, low-protein diet to prevent fluid retention.
    - • Fluid restriction.
    - • Dialysis if the patient experiences renal failure.
- ◐ Chronic:
    - • Administer corticosteroids to reduce the inflammatory response.
    - • Administer antihypertensive medication to reduce blood pressure.
    - • Low-sodium, low-protein diet to prevent fluid retention.
    - • Fluid restriction.
    - • Dialysis or kidney transplant if the patient experiences renal failure.
    - • For hyperkalemia:
        - ○ For emergency reduction of potassium, administer insulin, hypertonic glucose, and calcium gluconate.
        - ○ To remove potassium, administer sodium polystyrene sulfonate (Kayexalate).

Nursing Intervention

- ◐ Strict intake and output
- ◐ Daily weights
- ◐ Acute:
    - • Provide a quiet environment.
    - • Monitor vital signs and report changes to the health-care provider.
    - • Explain to the family the importance of a low-salt, low-protein, and fluid-restricted diet, and teach the family not to stop administering antibiotics when the child's condition improves.
- ◐ Chronic:
    - • Monitor for signs of hyperkalemia (muscle weakness, paresthesia, anorexia, and malaise).
    - • Explain to the family the importance of a low-salt, low-protein, low-potassium, and fluid-restricted diet and the importance of ongoing monitoring of the child by their health-care provider.

Nursing alert **Monitor for renal failure where urine output <1 mL/kg per hour in infants and <0.5 mL/kg per hour in children, and creatinine, BUN, and urine creatinine clearance are elevated.**

URINARY TRACT CONGENITAL ANOMALIES

What Went Wrong?

Urinary tract congenital anomalies consist of abnormal ureter, bladder or urethra whose cause is unknown. The most common urinary tract congenital anomalies are

- **Duplicated ureter:** Either a complete duplication of the ureter or incomplete duplication where two duplicate ureters are joined together prior to entering the bladder.
- **Ureter stenosis:** Narrowing of the ureter.
- **Exstrophy bladder:** The bladder is inside out and exposed on the outside of the abdomen.
- **Ureterocele:** The ureter balloons into the bladder to form a pouch.
- **Hypospadia:** Abnormal position of the urinary meatus in boys.

Signs and Symptoms

- Signs and symptoms depend on the nature of the anomaly but might include
  - Fever
  - Chills
  - Reduced urine output
  - Flank pain
  - Burning on urination
  - Recurrent infection
  - Abnormal voiding pattern
  - Dark color urine

Test Results

- Urography: Shows anomaly
- Retrograde pyelography: Shows anomaly
- Cystoureterography: Shows anomaly

Treatment

- Administer antibiotic if there is a bacterial infection.
- Surgical repair of the anomaly.

Nursing Intervention

- Daily weights.
- Strict intake and output.
- Insert indwelling urinary catheter if ordered.
- Cover the exposed area (i.e., exstrophy bladder) with sterile saline dressing.
- Teach the family how to care for the child at home.

ROUTINE CHECKUP 1

1. A parent of a child who is diagnosed with acute glomerulonephritis asks why her child hasn't improved following 20 days of treatment. What is the best response?
   a. Explain that the health-care provider is likely to order another round of antibiotic treatment.
   b. Tell the parent to bring the child to see the health-care provider immediately.
   c. Tell the parent to give the child increased fluids to help flush the kidneys.
   d. Tell the parent to decrease fluids to protect the kidneys until the infection resolves.

Answer:

2. Your patient has an exstrophy bladder. Which of the following is the most important intervention to perform?
   a. Cover the exposed area with sterile saline dressing.
   b. Strict intake and output.
   c. Daily weights.
   d. Teach the family how to care for the child at home.

Answer:

HEMOLYTIC UREMIC SYNDROME

What Went Wrong?

Hemolytic uremic syndrome is a common cause of renal failure in children and is a result of damage to the glomerular arterioles secondary to a bacterial infection. Glomerular arterioles become blocked by lesions and thrombi causing enlargement of the kidneys and decreased filtering.

Signs and Symptoms

- Pallor
- Irritability
- Petechiae
- Decreased urination
- Hypertension
- Diarrhea

Test Results

- Urine analysis: Presence of protein and blood
- Serum: Decreased red blood cells (RBC), decreased platelet count, increased prothrombin time (PT) and partial thromboplastin time (PTT), elevated white blood cells (WBC), elevated BUN and creatinine

◐ Coombs test: Negative
   ◐ Stool culture: Positive for *Escherichia coli*

Treatment
   ◐ Administer corticosteroids to reduce inflammation.
   ◐ Maintain fluid and electrolyte balance to prevent seizures.
   ◐ Administer antihypertensive if patient has hypertension.
   ◐ Reduce fluid and salt intake if patient has hypertension.
   ◐ Dialysis if patient is in renal failure.

◢ Nursing Intervention
   ◐ Daily weights.
   ◐ Strict intake and output.
   ◐ Maintain hydration.
   ◐ Monitor vital signs every 4 hours.
   ◐ Monitor for renal failure.
   ◐ Explain the disorder and treatment to the family.

Nursing alert **Antibiotics are administered only if the underlying infection is caused by *Shigella dysenteriae*.**

NEPHROTIC SYNDROME

What Went Wrong?

Nephrotic syndrome occurs when **albumin** is released by the kidneys into the urine, resulting in decreased albumin in blood because the glomerular filtration membrane is injured, thus causing a fluid switch and edema because of the decreased albumin in the blood.

   A number of disorders can cause nephritic syndrome, including glomerulonephritis, diabetes mellitus, allergic reactions, toxins, and circulatory disease. Nephrotic syndrome occurs in children of preschool age.

Signs and Symptoms
   ◐ Weight gain
   ◐ Decreased urination
   ◐ Dark color urine
   ◐ Lethargy
   ◐ Irritability
   ◐ Activity intolerance
   ◐ Edema

Test Results
   ◐ Urine analysis: Presence of protein and blood and elevated specific gravity

- ◑ Serum: Elevated cholesterol, decreased albumin, and elevated platelet count
- ◑ Renal biopsy: Identifies type of nephritic syndrome

⬛ Treatment

- ◑ Administer prednisone (Deltasone) to reduce inflammation.
- ◑ Administer albumin (Albuminar) intravenously (IV) to replace serum albumin and return to normal fluid balance.
- ◑ Administer furosemide (Lasix) IV to increase urination.
- ◑ Administer antihypertensive medication if the child has hypertension.
- ◑ Administer antibiotics to prevent infection due to the administration of prednisone (Deltasone).
- ◑ Restrict dietary salt.

Nursing Intervention

- ◑ Daily weights.
- ◑ Strict intake and output.
- ◑ Monitor for pulmonary congestion.
- ◑ Monitor for signs of infection.
- ◑ Take precautions to avoid infection.
- ◑ Maintain adequate nutrition.
- ◑ Monitor for electrolyte imbalance.
- ◑ Explain the disorder and treatment to the family.

✔ ROUTINE CHECKUP 2

1. A parent of a child who was diagnosed with hemolytic uremic syndrome asks you why the child must be weighed every day. What is the best response?
   a. To measure the child's daily fluid intake
   b. To assess if the condition has negatively influenced the child's growth
   c. To assess if the child is retaining fluid
   d. To determine if the child is adhering to dietary restrictions

Answer:

2. What should you alert to if the patient is being given corticosteroids to reduce inflammation?
   a. Renal failure
   b. Infection because the immune system is surprised
   c. Hypertension
   d. Elevated sodium levels

Answer:

RENAL FAILURE

What Went Wrong?

Renal failure is the sudden or progressive decrease in renal function. The two types of renal failure are acute and chronic.

Acute renal failure is the sudden decrease in renal function. It is reversible following intensive treatment of the underlying condition. Acute renal failure is divided into three categories:

- **Prerenal stage:** Diminished renal perfusion is caused by a disorder occurring before blood reaches the kidneys such as fluid loss, third-spacing of fluids, congestive heart failure, or medication such as diuretics.
- **Renal stage:** Diminished renal perfusion is caused by tubular necrosis within the kidney related to pyelonephritis, glomerulonephritis, medication, or allergic reaction.
- **Postrenal stage:** Diminished renal perfusion is caused by a urinary tract obstruction due to a stone, tissue growth, or compressed ureter.

Chronic renal failure is the progressive decrease in renal function secondary to diabetes mellitus, hypertension, glomerulonephritis, HIV infection, polycystic kidney disease, or ischemic nephropathy. Chronic renal failure is an irreversible, permanent loss of kidney function.

Signs and Symptoms

- Abdominal bruit with ischemic nephropathy
- Peripheral edema with third spacing of fluids
- Decreased urinary output
- Uremic pruritus
- Prerenal stage:
  - Tachycardia
  - Orthostatic hypotension
  - Dry skin
  - Mucous membranes
- Chronic renal failure:
  - Anemia related to kidneys production of erythropoietin
  - Weight loss

Test Results

- Serum: Elevated BUN, creatinine, and BUN-to-creatinine ratio
- Urinalysis: Casts, RBC, WBC, proteinuria, glomerular filtration rate decreased in chronic disease, creatinine clearance decreased
- Renal ultrasound: Decrease in renal size in chronic renal failure; dilation and fluid buildup in postrenal failure

Treatment

- Resolve underlying cause.
- Administer IV fluids to replace hypovolemia (acute renal failure prerenal stage).

◑ Administer inotropic agents for patients with congestive heart failure (CHF) to enhance cardiac output.
◑ Administer antibiotics for pyelonephritis.
◑ Insert a stent or catheter (urethral, suprapubic, nephrostomy) to drain urine if there is a blockage.
◑ Dialysis.
◑ Administer erythropoietin to treat anemia.
◑ Restrict dietary potassium, phosphate, sodium, and protein.
◑ Administer phosphate binders to reduce phosphate levels.
◑ Administer sodium polystyrene sulfonate to reduce potassium levels.
◑ Monitor electrolyte levels.
◑ Administer antihypertensive medication to control blood pressure.
◑ Monitor and control blood glucose levels.

Nursing alert **Chronic renal failure is asymptomatic until kidney function declines 20% at which time the child becomes lethargic and fatigued.**

Nursing Intervention

◑ Monitor vital signs for changes in heart rate or blood pressure.
◑ Strict intake and output.
◑ Check dialysis access site for signs of infection.
◑ Check arteriovenous (AV) shunt for thrill and bruit.
◑ No contrast dye tests.
◑ No nephrotoxic medication.

WILMS TUMOR

What Went Wrong?

Wilms tumor, also referred to as **nephroblastoma,** is cancer of the kidney that begins in the womb that is linked to abnormal chromosomal and congenital renal abnormalities. The Wilms tumor is encapsulated but may begin to metastasize to the renal vein, vena cava, lymph nodes, lungs, and other organs when the child is 4 years of age. Prognosis is good if the tumor is removed before it metastasizes. The five stages of the Wilms tumor are

◑ Stage I: The tumor is contained in one kidney.
◑ Stage II: The tumor metastasized beyond the kidney; however, the tumor can be completely removed.
◑ Stage III: The tumor metastasized to lymph nodes and the abdomen.
◑ Stage IV: The tumor metastasized to the bone, liver, lung, and brain.
◑ Stage V: The tumor metastasized to both kidneys.

Signs and Symptoms

◑ Nontender abdominal mass confined to one side
◑ Enlarged abdomen

- ◖ Blood in urine
- ◖ Hypertension
- ◖ Vomiting
- ◖ Constipation
- ◖ Anemia

Test Results

- ◖ Ultrasound: Identifies the size of the mass and if the mass is solid
- ◖ CT scan: Identifies the location of the mass
- ◖ Magnetic resonance imaging (MRI): Identifies the location of the mass
- ◖ Chest radiograph: Identifies the location of the mass
- ◖ Urograph: Assesses kidney function

Treatment

- ◖ Biopsy to determine the type of tumor
- ◖ Surgical removal of the tumor and the kidney if necessary
- ◖ Chemotherapy (dactinomycin [Cosmegen], vincristine) to reduce the size of the tumor
- ◖ Radiation to reduce the size of the tumor

Nursing Intervention

- ◖ Handle the child carefully during transportation and repositioning to avoid rupturing the tumor capsule.
- ◖ Explain the disorder and treatment to the family.

Nursing alert **Don't palpate the site of the tumor. Palpation can rupture the tumor capsule resulting in the tumor metastasizing quickly.**

PYELONEPHRITIS

What Went Wrong?

Pyelonephritis is a kidney infection typically following a urinary tract infection commonly caused by *E. coli, Klebsiella, Enterobacter, Proteus, Pseudomonas,* and *Staphylococcus saprophyticus.* Inflammation may impair renal function.

Signs and Symptoms

- ◖ Flank pain
- ◖ Fever due to infection
- ◖ Chills
- ◖ Frequency, urgency, dysuria due to urinary tract infection
- ◖ Nausea, vomiting, and diarrhea due to infection
- ◖ Increased heart rate due to fever
- ◖ Costovertebral angle (CVA) tenderness

Test Results

- Urinalysis: Presence of bacteria, nitrites, RBC, and WBC.
- Urine culture and sensitivity: Identifies microorganism that causes the infection and the antibiotic that kills the microorganism.
- Complete blood count: Elevated WBC (leukocytosis).

Treatment

- Administer antibiotics to treat infection:
  - Nitrofurantoin
  - Ciprofloxacin
  - Levofloxacin
  - Ofloxacin
  - Trimethoprim-sulfamethoxazole
  - Ampicillin
  - Amoxicillin
- Administer antipyretics for fever.
- Administer fluids for dehydration due to vomiting and diarrhea.
- Administer phenazopyridine for relief of dysuria symptoms.
- Repeat urine culture after completion of antibiotic course.

Nursing Intervention

- Monitor vital signs.
- Monitor intake and output.
- Assess for side effects of medication.
- Teach patient that phenazopyridine will cause orange-colored urine.

URINARY TRACT INFECTION

What Went Wrong?

Urinary tract infection occurs when a microorganism, typically a gram-negative bacteria such as *E. coli,* enters the urinary tract. The microorganism is present in the genital area and enters through the urethral opening or during sexual contact. A nosocomial urinary tract infection can also develop in patients who have a urinary catheter in place or who have undergone procedures such as a cystoscopy where an instrument is placed in the urinary tract.

Nursing alert   **Urinary tract infections must be treated immediately to prevent pyelonephritis.**

Signs and Symptoms

- Dysuria due to irritation of mucosal lining
- Feeling of fullness in suprapubic area
- Low back pain

Test Results

- ◐ Urinalysis: Presence of WBC, RBC, and nitrites.
- ◐ Urine culture and sensitivity: Identifies microorganism and the antibiotic that kills the microorganism.

Treatment

- ◐ Administer antibiotics:
  - Nitrofurantoin
  - Ciprofloxacin
  - Levofloxacin
  - Ofloxacin
  - Trimethoprim-sulfamethoxazole
  - Ampicillin
  - Amoxicillin
- ◐ Encourage fluids, to make urine less concentrated.
- ◐ Administer phenazopyridine for symptoms of dysuria.
- ◐ Repeat urine testing after antibiotics are completed.

8️⃣ Nursing Intervention

- ◐ Monitor intake and output.
- ◐ Monitor vital signs for changes, signs of fever.
- ◐ Encourage fluid intake.
- ◐ Encourage cranberry juice to acidify urine.
- ◐ Teach patient that phenazopyridine will cause orange-colored urine.

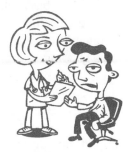

CASE STUDY

Judy Miller, age 6, arrived at the Emergency Department with her mother at 5 PM. Her mother reported that she had become lethargic in recent days. Her mother became concerned when she felt warm to the touch and hadn't urinated as much as she normally would. The mother reports that Judy had a strep throat 4 weeks ago, but she recovered and she was fine up to a few days ago.

Assessment data: Temperature 101.3°F +1 pitting edema bilaterally arms and legs. Slight edema around the eyes. Urine analysis showed hematuria, proteinuria, and specific gravity is 1.034 g/mL. Blood serum shows elevated creatinine and BUN. Urine culture and sensitivity is positive for streptococcal bacteria.

Interpretation: A streptococcal infection normally precedes acute glomerulonephritis by up to 6 weeks. During that time the bacteria infects the glomerulus, causing the kidneys to malfunction temporarily, resulting in hematuria, proteinuria, and elevated creatinine and BUN. Urine output is decreased, resulting in a high specific gravity of the urine. Proteinuria causes a fluid switch to the third space, resulting in edema.

Nursing intervention: Strict intake and output, daily weights, place the patient in a quiet environment. Place the patient on a low-salt, low-protein and fluid-restricted diet. Administer antibiotics to resolve the infection; diuretics to reduce edema, and corticosteroids to reduced inflammatory response as ordered. Monitor for renal failure. Instruct Mrs. Miller to administer the complete round of antibiotics and not to stop when Judy begins to feel better.

Evaluation: Assess Judy's temperature and urine output a week following treatment to determine the success of treatment.

CONCLUSION

The kidneys and the urinary tract comprise the urinary system. Contained within the kidneys are nephrons, which is the site where urine is formed. Nephron tubules filter waste fluid (urine) from blood and flows urine into the urinary tract.

The urinary tract consists of ureter (tubes connecting the kidney to the bladder), the bladder (a pouch to contain urine), and the urethra (the tube connecting the bladder to outside the body). Urine in the bladder causes the micturition reflex, which signals the brain that it is time to voluntarily urinate. The micturition reflex develops around 3 years of age.

The kidneys also regulate the production of red blood cells, electrolytes, fluid volume, and blood pressure.

Microorganisms can enter the urinary tract causing a urinary tract infection, which if left untreated can cause glomerulonephritis, inflammation of the glomerulus, or pyelonephritis, which is a kidney infection.

Bacterial infections can also cause hemolytic uremic syndrome where glomerular arterioles are damaged that can lead to renal failure. Renal failure is a sudden or progressive decrease in renal function. There are two types of renal failure. Acute renal failure is reversible once the underlying condition is treated. Chronic renal failure is irreversible because the underlying condition damaged the kidney.

Damage to the glomerular filtration membrane can result in nephritic syndrome where the kidneys release albumin into the urine, resulting in edema due to a fluid switch in the body.

The urinary tract can also be affected by congenital anomalies, resulting in abnormal structure of components of the urinary tract. These are typically resolved by surgery.

Wilms tumor is another congenital disorder. Wilms tumor is a cancerous growth that can go unnoticed until the child reaches 4 years of age. At first the tumor is encapsulated, but the capsule can rupture, resulting in the tumor metastasizing to other areas of the body.

? FINAL CHECKUP

1. **The mother of a child diagnosed with Wilms tumor asks why they must be careful when touching their child's abdomen. What is the best response?**
   a. To prevent unnecessary pain to the child.
   b. They might inadvertently injure the child.
   c. The tumor is soft and encapsulated. Pressure on or near the tumor might rupture the capsule.
   d. The tumor may metastasize to the lung.

2. **A parent of a child who is recently diagnosed with a urinary tract infection frantically calls saying that her daughter's infection has worsened since she started treatment. Her urine is orange when before it was cloudy. What is your best response?**
   a. This is a normal side effect of phenazopyridine.
   b. Go to the Emergency Department immediately.
   c. Bring the child to the health-care provider immediately.
   d. This is a tinge of blood that will resolve itself in 7 to 10 days.

3. **The mother of a child who has been diagnosed with ureter stenosis asks for you to explain this disorder. What is your best response?**
   a. Ureters are tubes that connect each kidney to the bladder. These tubes are narrower than normal.
   b. Ureters are tubes that connect each kidney to the bladder. These tubes did not exist at birth; however, they can be restored surgically.
   c. Ureters are tubes that connect each kidney to the bladder. There is a duplication of these tubes.
   d. Ureters are tubes that connect each kidney to the bladder. Two ureters are joined together prior to entering the bladder.

4. **A patient experiences a sudden decrease in renal function as a result of pyelonephritis. What category acute of renal failure is the patient experiencing?**
   a. Prerenal
   b. Renal
   c. Postrenal
   d. None of the above

5. **A patient being treated for glomerulonephritis is prescribed Kayexalate. His mother asks why this medication is prescribed. What is the best response?**
   a. Increases potassium that has decreased due to chronic glomerulonephritis
   b. Increases potassium that has decreased due to acute glomerulonephritis
   c. Removes potassium that has increased due to acute glomerulonephritis
   d. Removes potassium that has increased due to chronic glomerulonephritis

6. **The parents of a child with a recently diagnosed with Wilms tumor asks why must the health-care provider stage the tumor. What is your best response?**
   a. To assess if the tumor has metastasized and if so where it has metastasized
   b. To determine the child's level of discomfort
   c. To determine the best course of treatment
   d. To prevent the tumor from spreading

7. **A parent of a child who is diagnosed with hemolytic uremic syndrome asks why her child's kidney became enlarged. What is your best response?**
   a. A tumor developed on the kidney
   b. Blood vessels within the kidneys became blocked by lesions
   c. The child has a bacterial infection
   d. The child has injected too much fluid

8. **The health-care provider asks the patient's mother to collect a urine sample from the patient so the sample can be sent for a culture and sensitivity study. The mother asks you why this is done. How would you respond?**
   a. Explain that the culture and sensitivity study identifies microorganism that causes the infection
   b. Explain that the culture and sensitivity study identifies RBC and WBC in the urine
   c. Explain that the culture and sensitivity study identifies microorganism that causes the infection and the antibiotic that kills the microorganism
   d. Explain that the culture and sensitivity study identifies nitrites in the urine

9. **A parent of a child diagnosed with renal failure overhears the health-care provider saying that the child has signs of third spacing of fluids. She asks you what this means. What is your best response?**
   a. I'll ask the health-care provider to explain this to you.
   b. There is a backup of fluid because the kidneys are not working properly.
   c. Extracellular fluids are contained either in the interstitial compartment or the intravascular compartment. Renal failure causes fluids to move into a third compartment within the body.
   d. Fluid that is outside the cell is stored in tissue or in the vascular system. Renal failure causes fluid to enter other areas of the body other than tissue or the vascular system, resulting in edema.

10. **Why could insertion of a urinary catheter cause a nosocomial urinary tract infection?**

    a. The urinary catheter provides a pathway for microorganisms to enter the urinary tract.

    b. The health-care provider used poor aseptic technique when inserting the urinary catheter.

    c. The patient was not administered prophylactic antibiotics.

    d. All of the above.

ANSWERS

Routine checkup 1
   1. b
   2. a

Routine checkup 2
   1. c
   2. b

Final checkup

1. c	2. a	3. a	4. b
5. d	6. a	7. b	8. c
9. d	10. d		

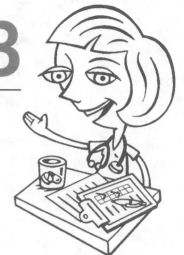

CHAPTER 13

Musculoskeletal Conditions

Learning Objectives

At the end of the chapter, the student will be able to

1. Understand the structure and function of the musculoskeletal system.

2. Treat soft tissue injury.

3. Know how traction is used realign fractures.

4. Assess for compartment syndrome.

5. Explain hip dysplasia.

6. Identify scoliosis.

7. Care for a child with juvenile rheumatoid arthritis.

8. Teach parents about the treatment for a clubfoot.

Cartilage	Ligaments
Comminuted fracture	Pavlik harness
Compartment syndrome	Periosteum
Contusion	RICE
Epiphyseal line	Sprain
Epiphyseal plate	Strain
Fascia	Synovial joints
Greenstick fracture	Tendons
Hairline fracture	Traction

OVERVIEW

The musculoskeletal system consists of bones, muscles, tendons, ligaments, and fascia and provides support for soft tissue and protection for organs within the body. The musculoskeletal system is also a reservoir for calcium and phosphorus and the site where red blood cells are produced.

Bones provide the rigid framework for the body and are moved when skeletal muscles contract. Skeletal muscles are connected to bones by bands of fibrous connective tissue called **tendons.** Bones are connected to each other to form a joint by fibrous connective tissue called a **ligament.**

🔒 Bones, muscles, and other structures in the body are covered by an uninterrupted web of tissues called **fascia** that maintains the body's structural integrity.

BONES

Bones are covered by the **periosteum,** a double layer of connective tissue that covers all bone except for joints. The periosteum nourishes the bone. Children have a thick vascular periosteum that provides nourishment for bone growth and faster healing.

Bones develop from tissues during the ossification process where osteoblasts provide the structure for bone cells. Deposits of calcium and phosphorus, regulated by the thyroid and parathyroid glands, form salt that strengthens the framework for new bone. Placing bones under stress results in increased deposits in bone; periods of no stress results in resorption of deposits by the body.

Long bones have a growth end called the epiphysis. At the epiphysis there is the **epiphyseal plate** commonly referred to as the growth plate. The epiphyseal plate is composed of **cartilage,** dense connective tissue that does not contain blood vessels. As the child grows, the epiphyseal plate is replaced by

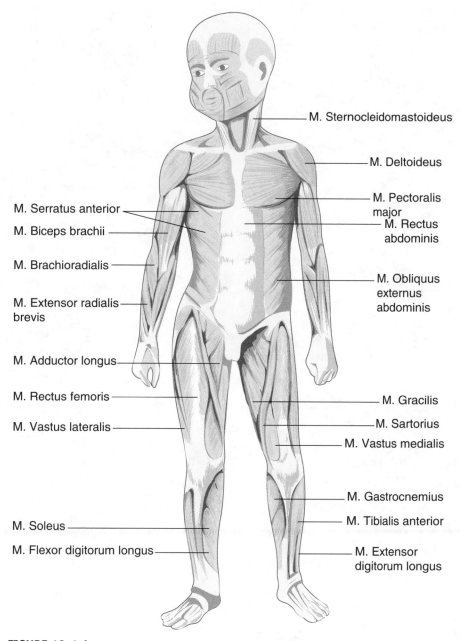

M. Sternocleidomastoideus

M. Deltoideus

M. Pectoralis major

M. Rectus abdominis

M. Obliquus externus abdominis

M. Serratus anterior

M. Biceps brachii

M. Brachioradialis

M. Extensor radialis brevis

M. Adductor longus

M. Rectus femoris

M. Vastus lateralis

M. Gracilis

M. Sartorius

M. Vastus medialis

M. Gastrocnemius

M. Tibialis anterior

M. Soleus

M. Flexor digitorum longus

M. Extensor digitorum longus

FIGURE 13-1 A

bone. Once the child stops growing, the epiphyseal plate transforms into the **epiphyseal line,** which provides a smooth surface for articulating bones.

Nursing alert **Damage to a child's epiphysis might impede the child's growth.**

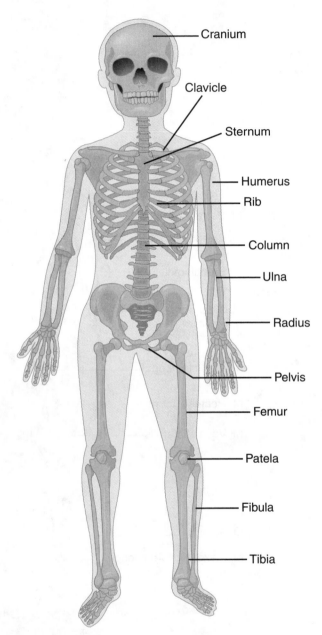

FIGURE 13-1 B

JOINTS

A joint is where two articulated bones come together. Joints are held together by ligaments, and cartilage cushions the surface area between each bone.

    Joints are classified by movement:

◐ Synarthrodial: Immovable such as the skull.
◐ Amphidiarthrodial: Semimovable such as between the vertebras.
◐ Diarthrodial (**synovial joints**): Freely movable such as the knees. These are encapsulated joints that contain synovial fluid to lubricate the joint.

SKELETAL MUSCLES

Skeletal muscles are striated fibrous bundles covered with connective tissue that contract when stimulated by an electrical impulse. During a contraction, the muscle shortens, called flexing, causing the attached bone to be pulled in the direction of the contraction.

Sets of opposing muscles are used to articulate a bone. One set of muscles contracts while the opposing muscles relax, called extending, resulting in bone movement. The opposing muscle contracts to return the bone to the original position.

ROUTINE CHECKUP 1

Which of the following takes longer to heal if damaged?
    a. Muscles
    b. Tendons
    c. Ligaments
    d. Cartilage
Answer:

SOFT TISSUE INJURY

What Went Wrong?

Soft tissue injury is a sprain, strain, or contusion that affects the soft tissue of the musculoskeletal system.
    ◐ A **strain** is the tearing, twisting, or stretching of a muscle or tendon.
    ◐ A **sprain** is injury to a ligament as a result of stretching or tearing the ligament and is commonly the result of an automobile accident, fall, or sports injury.
    ◐ A **contusion,** commonly known as a bruise or hematoma, occurs when a blood vessel ruptures beneath the skin and bleeds into the tissue and causes discoloration.

Nursing alert **Most ankle injuries in children are sprains.**

Signs and Symptoms

- ◑ Strain:
  - Pain.
  - Localized swelling.
  - Possibly muscle weakness.
  - Severe strain is disabling.
- ◑ Sprain:
  - Edema
  - Pain
  - Joint immobility
- ◑ Contusion:
  - Purple discoloration of the tissue.
  - Discoloration fades to brown, yellow, and green as coagulated blood rises to the upper layers of the skin.

Nursing alert **The area of discoloration should decrease as blood coagulates. Blood disorders and medication may decrease blood coagulation, resulting in ongoing bleeding from a contusion.**

Test Results

- ◑ Radiograph: Health-care providers typically order a radiograph to rule out a fracture.

Treatment

- ◑ **RICE** (rest, ice, compression, and elevation) for 24 to 36 hours following the injury. Ice, compression, and elevation reduce inflammation that causes swelling. Resting the injury reduces pain caused by movement, encourages healing, and prevents further injury.
- ◑ Support the injured extremity to reduce pain caused by movement and to prevent further injury.

Nursing Intervention

- ◑ Contusion:
  - Encircle the area of the contusion with a pen and label it with the date and time to document the size of the contusion.
  - Monitor the contusion frequently during the first hour to assess if the blood has coagulated.
- ◑ Assist patient with activities of daily life to reduce pain caused by movement and to prevent further injury.
- ◑ Teach the patient and parents:
  - The nature of the injury.
  - How the treatment will help heal the injury.

ROUTINE CHECKUP 2

Why is ice placed on the site of a soft tissue injury?
 a. Decreased temperature from the ice causes blood vessels to dilate, increasing blood flow to the site and increasing edema and swelling.
 b. Decreased temperature from the ice causes blood vessels to contract, reducing blood flow to the site and decreasing edema and swelling.
 c. Decreased temperature from the ice causes blood vessels to dilate, decreasing blood flow to the site and decreasing edema and swelling.
 d. Decreased temperature from the ice causes blood vessels to contract, decreasing blood flow to the site and increasing edema and swelling.

Answer:

FRACTURE

What Went Wrong?

A fracture is the separation of bone. The degree of the separation depends on the strength of the bone and energy of events that caused the fracture. Fractures are classified in four categories:
 ◑ Complete: The bone separates into two distinct parts.
 ◑ Incomplete: The bone does not separate into two distinct parts.
 ◑ Closed (simple): The bone does not break the skin.
 ◑ Open (compound): The bone breaks the skin.

There are three types of fractures:
 ◑ **Hairline:** An incomplete fracture.
 ◑ **Greenstick:** An incomplete fracture where the bone is partially broken resulting in the bone bending like a broken green stick.
 ◑ **Comminuted:** A complete fracture where the bone is broken into several fragments.

 Nursing alert **Fractures heal faster in children than in adults because children have a thick vascular periosteum, resulting in increased blood flow to the fracture site.**

Signs and Symptoms
 ◑ Pain
 ◑ Deformity
 ◑ Edema

- Crepitus
- Reduced range of motion
- Unable to bear weight on the injured bone

Test Results

- Radiograph: Confirms the fracture and confirms realignment of the surface area of the bone.
- Decreased hematocrit may indicate blood loss either from the injury or from surgical reduction of the fracture, if performed. This might result in low hemoglobin and reduced oxygenation of blood, which might inhibit tissue repair.

Treatment

- Closed reduction realigns the surface area of the bone by manipulating the bones or by applying **traction** to encourage healing.
- Open reduction is a surgical procedure performed when a closed reduction is not possible or when repair must be made to torn muscle and ligaments to encourage healing. Pins, screws, plates, or rods might be used to realign the bone.
- Immobilize the bone to prevent further injury and to keep the bone realigned.
- Apply traction to realign bones, reduce muscle spasms, and to immobilize:
  - Skin traction: Adhesive material, straps, or foam boot are used to pull the surface of the skin to cause traction on the bone. Types of skin traction are
    - Buck extension: For knee immobilization
    - Bryant traction: For hip dysplasia and fractured femur for children <3 years of age and weighing <17.5 kg
    - Russell traction: For fractures of the femur and lower legs
  - Skeletal traction: Pins, wires, and tongs are surgically placed in the bone applying direct traction to the bone. Types of skeletal traction are
    - Skeletal cervical traction (Crutchfield tongs): For cervical spine injuries.
    - Halo traction: For immobilizing the head and neck following a cervical injury.
    - 90/90 femoral traction: For femur or tibia fractures.
    - Dunlop (sidearm) traction: For humerus fractures where the arm is suspended.
    - External fixators: Pins or wires are transfixed percutaneously to the extremity.
- Provide adequate fluid to increase hydration and prevent renal calculi (rare condition for children).

○ Attach a sequential pneumatic compression device to the patient's legs when the patient is not mobile to prevent stasis of blood in the legs and to prevent emboli from developing.

Nursing Intervention

○ Assess the impact of the fracture on the child's growth. Fractures to a child's epiphysis might impede the child's growth.

○ Frequently assess circulation in the affected limb to ensure that edema following a fracture does not restrict blood flow to the limb.

○ Assess for nerve compression syndrome—pain, tingling, and numbness.

○ ④ Assess for compartment syndrome as a result of increased pressure from edema—pain, pallor, pulselessness, paresthesia, and paralysis.

○ Assess for osteomyelitis, which is an infection that might result from an open fracture or from surgery to reduce a fracture. Signs are irritability, abrupt fever, lethargy, pain, and warmth.

○ Assess for pulmonary embolism resulting from a fat, air, or blood emboli that occur within the first 24 hours following a fracture. Adolescents are at the greatest risk. Signs are sudden, severe dyspnea and chest pain.

○ Traction care:
  • Assess the position and placement of bandages and straps.
  • Assess neurovascular status.
  • Treat pain.
  • Assess the patient's psychological response to the treatment.
  • Assess the pin sites for infection, inflammation, and bleeding.
  • Clean the pin site if ordered with a cotton-tipped sterile applicator soaked with normal saline or saline/hydrogen peroxide solution. Apply antibacterial ointment if ordered.

○ Minimize immobility by performing range-of-motion exercises and ambulate when possible to prevent loss of muscle strength, impaired joint mobility, and venous stasis and increased bone catabolism.

○ Teach the patient and parents about the fracture and treatment.

Nursing alert **Open or remove the cast immediately at the first signs of compartment syndrome to prevent tissue damage and necrosis. Elevate the head of bed, administer oxygen to the patient, and notify the health-care provider at the first signs of pulmonary embolism.**

HIP DYSPLASIA

What Went Wrong?

Hip dysplasia occurs as a result of abnormal development of the hips during fetal development. There are three categories of hips dysplasia:

- Acetabular dysplasia (preluxation): The acetabulum is shallow and dish shaped rather than the normal cup shape, indicating delayed acetabular development. This is the mildest form of hip dysplasia.
- Subluxation: Incomplete dislocation of the femoral head from the acetabulum. This is the most common form of hip dysplasia.
- Dislocation: The femoral head loses contact with the acetabulum. This is the most serious form of hip dysplasia.

Signs and Symptoms

- Asymmetry of gluteal and thigh folds due to the dislocation
- Shortened femur due to the dislocation
- Unequal knee lengths when knees are flexed due to the dislocation

Test Results

- Positive Ortolani test administered from birth to 4 weeks of age due to the dislocation
- Positive Barlow test due to the dislocation
- Limited hip abduction due to the dislocation

Treatment

- Newborn to 6 months of age:
  - Place the patient in a **Pavlik harness** for 3 to 5 months. Legs are flexed and knees fall outward to place the hips in proper alignment.
- Six to 18 months of age:
  - Place the patient in a hip spica cast for 2 to 4 months following surgical realignment of hips. The hip spica cast immobilizes the legs and knees and holds the hips in proper alignment.
- Older than 18 months of age:
  - An osteotomy might be performed to align the femoral head with the hips.

Nursing Intervention

- Assess the patient for restricted movement and wide perineum and unequal gluteal and thigh folds.
- Assess the patient for limp or unequal gait.
- If the patient is in a Pavlik harness:
  - Examine the skin under the harness three times a day for redness and skin integrity.
  - Don't apply lotions or powder to the skin.
  - Place an undershirt between the skin and the harness.
  - Place the diaper under the harness straps.
  - Massage the skin once a day to stimulate circulation.

- Ask the health-care provider if the harness can be removed for daily sponge bathing.
- Teach the parents how to use the harness and care for the patient. Explain the benefits of the harness and that it is temporary.

◑ If the patient is in a hip spica cast:
- Assess for **compartment syndrome** and nerve compression syndrome.
- Make sure that the cast near the perineum is clean of fecal matter and urine.
- Teach the parents how to care for the patient who is in a hip spica cast. Explain the benefits of the cast and that it is temporary.

ROUTINE CHECKUP 3

Why place an undershirt between the skin and the Pavlik harness?
a. To keep the skin moist
b. To prevent infection caused by pins of the Pavlik harness
c. To prevent skin abrasions and irritation by the harness
d. To keep the skin clean

Answer:

OSTEOGENESIS IMPERFECTA

What Went Wrong?

Osteogenesis imperfecta is a genetic bone disease characterized by bones fracturing easily without any obvious cause. There are four classifications of osteogenesis imperfecta:

- ◑ Type I (most common): Bones fracture easily before puberty.
- ◑ Type II (most severe): Severe bone deformity and numerous fractures resulting in respiratory problems at or shortly after birth resulting in death.
- ◑ Type III: Fractures present at birth and may have healed.
- ◑ Type IV: Fractures are greater than type I and occur before puberty.

Signs and Symptoms

- ◑ Easy bruising
- ◑ Hyperextensible ligaments
- ◑ Epistaxis

- Blue sclera
- Fractures occurring for no obvious reason
- Short statue in all but type I

Test Results

- Radiograph: Shows fractures or healed fractures

Treatments

- No known cure
- Physical therapy to strengthen muscles and prevent osteoporosis

Nursing Interventions

- Handle patients gently to prevent fractures and bruising.
- Teach the parents how to care for the patient.

TORTICOLLIS

What Went Wrong?

The sternocleidomastoid muscle is damaged from intrauterine malposition of the fetus in or from birth trauma resulting in unusual contraction of the sternocleidomastoid muscle causing the head to bend toward the affected muscle. Torticollis can also occur from trauma not related to birth.

Signs and Symptoms

- Neck is flexed toward the affected sternocleidomastoid muscle.

Test Results

- Decreased range of motion of the head to the unaffected sternocleidomastoid muscle

Treatments

- Low-impact neck stretching exercise to strengthen the neck.
- Apply heat to encourage healing.
- Frequent shiatsu massages to relieve tension caused by the contracting muscle.

Nursing Interventions

- Provide support to the patient's neck and head.
- Teach the parents how to care for the patient.

SCOLIOSIS

What Went Wrong?

Scoliosis is the lateral curvature of the spine (see Fig. 13-2). The cause is unknown. There are three types of scoliosis:

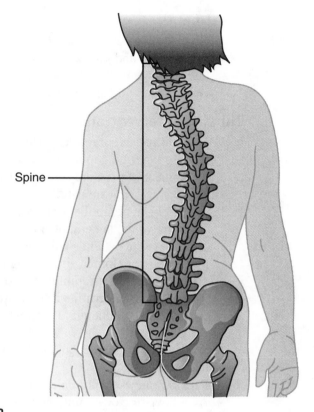

Spine

FIGURE 13-2

- Dextroscoliosis: Curvature on the right side
- Levoscoliosis: Curvature on the left side
- **6** Rotoscoliosis: Pronounced rotation of the vertebrae

Signs and Symptoms

- Rib hump
- Asymmetric rib cage
- Visible curvature of the spine
- Uneven shoulder
- Uneven pelvis

Test Results

- Radiograph: Shows abnormal curvature of the spine
- Computed tomography (CT) scan: Shows abnormal curvature of the spine
- Magnetic resonance imaging (MRI): Shows abnormal curvature of the spine

Treatments

- ◑ Up to 20-degree curvature: Exercise to enhance muscle tone and posture.
- ◑ Between 20 and 40 degree curvature: Apply a brace to maintain curvature.
- ◑ Greater than 40 degree curvature: Spinal fusion surgery.

Nursing Interventions

- ◑ If spinal fusion surgery is performed:
  - • Use log rolling to reposition the child every 2 hours to inhibit development of pressure sores and to adequately inflate lungs.
  - • Monitor vital signs following surgery.
  - • Apply antiembolism stockings while the patient is on bed rest. Remove the antiembolism stocking for 1 hour three times a day.
  - • Assess the patient's pain level.
  - • Assess for Homan sign for signs of an embolism.
  - • Measure the circumference of the calf frequently if the calf is swollen to determine if there are changes to the swelling.
  - • Assess for ischemia: Pain, pallor, pulselessness, paresthesia, paralysis.
- ◑ Support the back, feet, and knees with pillows when the patient lies on the side.
- ◑ Perform range-of-motion exercises to maintain muscle tone.
- ◑ Avoid twisting or turning the spine when moving the patient.
- ◑ Explain that spinal fusion surgery stabilizes the spine by inserting wires and rods into the spine to align the spine permanently.
- ◑ Teach the parents the importance of performing ordered exercises and the need for the patient to wear the brace.

SLIPPED CAPITAL FEMORAL EPIPHYSIS

What Went Wrong?

The upper end of the femur becomes dislocated during the onset of puberty due to weakness of the epiphysis and a growth spurt. There are four types of slipped capital femoral epiphysis:

- ◑ Acute: Caused by trauma.
- ◑ Chronic: Caused by a growth spurt.
- ◑ Stable: The patient can walk.
- ◑ Unstable: The patient is unable to walk.

Signs and Symptoms

- ◑ Visible limp.
- ◑ Groin pain.
- ◑ Knee, hip, or thigh pain.
- ◑ Patient holds hip in the external rotation while at rest.

Test Results
- Radiograph: Dislocation displayed on radiography

Treatments
- Traction prior to surgery to immobilize the femur
- Surgical realignment using threaded screws to stabilize the joint

Nursing Interventions
- Range-of-motion exercise following surgery to maintain muscle tone
- Traction care:
  - Assess the position and placement of bandages and straps.
  - Assess neurovascular status.
  - Treat pain.
  - Assess the patient's psychological response to the treatment.
  - Assess the pin sites for infection, inflammation, and bleeding.
  - Clean the pin site if ordered with a cotton-tipped sterile applicator soaked with normal saline or a saline/hydrogen peroxide solution. Apply antibacterial ointment if ordered.
- Teach the patient and parents about the dislocation and treatment.

OSTEOMYELITIS

What Went Wrong?
Osteomyelitis is an infection of the bone or bone marrow commonly caused by *Staphylococcus aureus* bacteria related to a skin infection, otitis media, or an upper respiratory infection.

Signs and Symptoms
- Irritability
- Abrupt fever
- Lethargy
- Pain
- Warmth
- Rapid pulse
- Swelling over affected area

Test Results
- Increased white blood cell count.
- Culture and sensitivity test to identify the bacteria and antibiotic.

Treatments
- Prolonged intravenous antibiotic therapy using nafcillin or clindamycin
- Physical therapy to restore muscle tone once the infection is reduced

Nursing Interventions

- ◑ Monitor hematologic, renal, and hepatic laboratory tests for signs of toxicity from long-term intravenous antibiotic therapy.
- ◑ Monitor for ototoxic side effects.
- ◑ Support the infected area when repositioning the patient.
- ◑ Avoid weightbearing on the infected area until healed.
- ◑ Keep the patient on bed rest.
- ◑ Assess for ischemia—pain, pallor, pulselessness, paresthesia, paralysis.
- ◑ Teach the patient and parents about the disorder and treatment.

✔ ROUTINE CHECKUP 4

1. Why is there an increase in the white blood cell count?
   a. White blood cells increase as part of the inflammation process to attack the bacteria that is causing the infection.
   b. The infection disrupts the bone marrow's production of white blood cells.
   c. This is in response to antibiotic treatment of the disorder.
   d. The increased white blood cell count is the result of production of immature white blood cells.

Answer:

JUVENILE RHEUMATOID ARTHRITIS

What Went Wrong?

 Juvenile rheumatoid arthritis (JRA) is an autoimmune disease that causes chronic inflammation of connective tissue and joints resulting in swelling, pain, and limited motion that occurs <16 years of age. The synovial membrane becomes inflamed, called synovitis, resulting in increased fluid, lymphocytes, and plasma in the joint, which causes the joint to swell and become joint effused. The joint can erode and deform over time resulting in bone loss, osteoporosis, subluxation, and ankylosis. There are two peak ages of onset—between 1 and 3 years and between 8 and 10 years of age.

There are three types of JRA:

- ◑ Oligoarticular: This affects fewer than five joints and might exhibit inflammation of the iris without joint symptoms.
- ◑ Polyarticular: This affects the small joints of the hands and weightbearing joints.
- ◑ Systemic: This affects the entire body resulting in high fever that suddenly drops to normal. A rash may appear and then suddenly disappear.

Signs and Symptoms

- Irritability
- Poor appetite
- Mild growth delay
- Tires easily
- Changes in gait
- Poor weight gain
- High fever
- Rash
- Flex position at rest

Test Results

- Increased erythrocyte sedimentation rate (ESR)
- Positive rheumatoid factor (RF) in serum
- Positive immunoglobulin (Ig)G and IgM present in serum
- Positive antinuclear antibodies (ANA) in serum
- Low hemoglobin

Treatments

- Administer nonsteroidal antiinflammatory drugs (NSAIDs) such as ibuprofen and naproxen for pain relief. It can take 3 weeks for antiinflammatory response to occur.
- Administer slow-acting antirheumatic drugs (SAARDS) such as methotrexate, sulfasalazine, and hydroxychloroquine to suppress the autoimmune response.
- Administer steroids if other treatments fail. Steroids reduce inflammation but have adverse side effects with long-term use.
- Administer etanercept (Enbrel) if NSAIDs and SAARDS fail. Etanercept blocks the binding of tumor necrosis factor with cell surface receptors, thus reducing inflammation.
- Physical therapy to ensure safety ambulation.

Nursing alert **Monitor the patient for signs of infection because antiinflammatory medication suppresses the immune system.**

Nursing Interventions

- Perform range-of-motion exercise on the affected joint to maintain joint mobilization.
- Encourage nonweight bearing activities to strengthen muscles.
- Use splints and braces to reduce flexion and minimize pain.
- Monitor renal and hepatic labs to detect adverse reaction to long use of NSAIDs.
- Apply warm compresses on joints when sleeping to prevent viscous that results in stiffness.

- Increase foods high in iron.
- Increase fluids if the patient has a fever to prevent dehydration.
- Encourage self-care and normal independent activities of daily life.
- No restrictions on daily activity.
- Teach the parent:
  - To give the patient a warm bath when awaking to reduce stiffness
  - To avoid the patient remaining in a fixed flexion position
  - That the patient should sleep 8 to 10 hours at a time to avoid fatigue. Avoid naps because this inactivity results in stiffness.
  - That the patient should alternate between active and quiet activities to avoid fatigue.

EWING SARCOMA

What Went Wrong?

Ewing sarcoma is cancer of the bone that stems from primitive nerve cells and is related to chromosomal abnormalities. Ewing sarcoma metastasizes to bone marrow, other bones, and the lungs.

Nursing alert **Ewing sarcoma is commonly misdiagnosed as a sports injury.**

Signs and Symptoms

- Awakening at night with pain at the site of the tumor
- Weight loss
- Swelling at the site
- A limp, if the legs are affected
- Difficulty breathing, if ribs are affected

Test Results

- Radiograph: Tumor present
- CT scan: Tumor present
- Bone marrow biopsy
- Positive serology study for Ewing sarcoma cells

Treatment

- Surgical removal of the tumor without amputation
- Chemotherapy to kill the Ewing sarcoma cells

Nursing Interventions

- Enable the child to make choices about daily care to give the child a sense of control.
- Teach the parents and the child about the disorder and treatment.
- Encourage the child to continue normal activities of daily living as possible, including interaction with the child's friends.

LEGG-CALVÉ-PERTHES DISEASE

What Went Wrong?

Legg-Calvé-Perthes disease is a necrosis of the femoral head that occurs in children between 2 and 12 years of age caused by a decreased blood supply to the femoral head. This disease is self-limiting, and the child will fully recover after the disease has run its course.

There are three stages of Legg-Calvé-Perthes disease:

- Avascular: Blood supply to the head of the femur is interrupted within 1 year.
- Revascularization: Creeping substitution occurs where connective and vascular tissue enter the necrotic bone causing live noncalcified bone to replace the necrotic tissue.
- Healing: The bone ossifies over 3 years.

Signs and Symptoms

- Painless limp
- Pin in the knee during activity
- Pain in the groin
- Pain in the anterior thigh

Test Results

- Radiograph: Shows decreased bone mass, ossification centers, and possibly subchondral fracture.

Treatment

- Legg-Calvé-Perthes disease is self-limiting.
- Physical therapy to restore range of motion.
- Administer analgesic to reduce pain.

Nursing Interventions

- Perform range-of-motion activities to maintain normal motion of the joint.
- Teach the patient how to use crutches.
- Explain to the parents and the patient that the disease is self-limiting and that the patient will fully recover once the disease has run its course.

TALIPES (CLUBFOOT)

What Went Wrong?

A clubfoot is a congenital deformity that occurs in utero due to adverse effects of medication, infection, trauma, or genetic trait resulting in contracture of soft tissue and abnormal development of a joint and muscles.

Signs and Symptoms

- Usually position or forming of one or both feet

Test Results

- ◐ Radiograph: Talus is superimposed and the metatarsal is ladder-like.

Treatment

- ◐ Splint the foot in the realigned position in the adduction position and then cast the foot for 2 weeks.
- ◐ Remove the cast and realign in the heel inversion position and then cast the foot for 2 weeks.
- ◐ Remove the cast and realign in the flexion of the ankle position and then cast the foot for 2 weeks.
- ◐ Apply an ongoing night brace once the cast is removed.
- ◐ If casting does not permanently realign the foot, corrective surgery is performed.
- ◐ 🔒 Special shoes containing adjustable bars are worn to realign the foot as a noncasting and nonsurgical intervention.

Nursing Interventions

- ◐ If the foot is in a cast:
  - Elevate the affected foot on pillows.
  - Assess for ischemia: Pain, pallor, pulselessness, paresthesia, paralysis every 2 hours.
  - Teach parents how to assess for ischemia and how to exercise the affected foot at home.
- ◐ Explain to parents the importance of wearing corrective shoes.

CONCLUSION

The musculoskeletal system provides the framework, protection, and movement for the body through the interconnectivity of bones, muscles, tendons, ligaments, and fascia. It is also the repository for calcium and phosphorus and the site where red blood cells are produced.

Soft tissue injuries are the most common musculoskeletal system disorder because children are exposed to activities that might result in sprains, strains, and contusions. These activities can also lead to fractures. Fractures can also be caused by osteogenesis imperfecta where fractures occur for no obvious reason.

Osteogenesis imperfecta is one of a number of disorders that affect the musculoskeletal system. Some disorders are congenital, such as clubfoot or hip dysplasia, where there is abnormal development of the hip and torticollis where the sternocleidomastoid muscle is damaged from intrauterine malposition of the fetus in or from birth trauma. Ewing sarcoma is cancer of the bone that is related to chromosomal abnormalities.

Children are also susceptible to scoliosis, which is the lateral curvature of the spine, and osteomyelitis in which the *Staphylococcus aureus* bacteria infects the bone. Some children <16 years of age develop juvenile rheumatoid arthritis, an autoimmune disease that causes chronic inflammation of connective tissue and joints resulting in swelling, pain, and limited motion.

Two other disorders that affect children are a slipped capital femoral epiphysis and Legg-Calvé-Perthes disease. A combination of a weak epiphysis and a growth spurt can cause a slipped capital femoral epiphysis where the upper end of the femur is dislocated. Legg-Calvé-Perthes disease is self-limiting. Disruption of the blood supply to the femoral head results in necrosis.

? FINAL CHECKUP

1. **What is a fracture where the bone is partially broken and bending called?**
   a. Hairline fracture
   b. Comminuted fracture
   c. Greenstick fracture
   d. Complete fracture

2. **What causes compartment syndrome?**
   a. Edema at the site of the fracture
   b. Infection
   c. Osteomyelitis
   d. Nerve damage

3. **What might you conclude if you notice a wide perineum and unequal gluteal and thigh folds when assessing a newborn?**
   a. Osteogenesis imperfecta
   b. Torticollis
   c. Scoliosis
   d. Hip dysplasia

4. **Following an upper respiratory infection, the 3-year-old becomes irritable and lethargic. He has an abrupt fever and swelling and warmth near his knee. What would you suspect?**
   a. Otitis media
   b. Ototoxic
   c. Legg-Calvé-Perthes
   d. Osteomyelitis

5. The health-care provider diagnosed a child with Legg-Calvé-Perthes disease. The parents expressed their concern to you that their child's leg will be amputated. How should you respond?
    a. It is too soon to determine if amputation is necessary.
    b. No amputation is necessary because the child will make a full recovery once the disease runs its course.
    c. The health-care provider is the best person to talk to you about amputation.
    d. Not all children who have the disease require amputation.

6. The parents of a child who has been diagnosed with juvenile rheumatoid arthritis calls you complaining that there is no improvement with their son's pain after a week of taking naproxen. How would you respond?
    a. I'll mention this to your health-care provider.
    b. You should switch to ibuprofen.
    c. It can take 3 weeks before you see pain relief when taking naproxen.
    d. Naproxen takes 2 weeks to work in children.

7. A child of short stature for his age is taken to the Emergency Department for a fractured arm. This is the second fracture that the child received this year. Both the child and parents say they have no idea how the fracture occurred. You notice that the child has a bluish sclera. What do you suspect?
    a. Greenstick fracture
    b. Child abuse
    c. Osteogenesis imperfecta
    d. Torticollis

8. An 8-year-old Little Leaguer was taken to the Emergency Department in January complaining that he was awakened by pain above his knee. There is slight swelling at the site. What would you suspect?
    a. A sports injury
    b. Talipes
    c. Juvenile rheumatoid arthritis
    d. Ewing sarcoma

9. A 10-year-old is brought to the Emergency Department following an automobile accident. You notice a contusion on her outer left thigh. What should you do?
    a. Bring the crash cart to the bedside.
    b. Encircle the area of the contusion and write the date and time outside the contusion so you can assess if bleeding has stopped or is continuing.
    c. Suspect child abuse.
    d. Notify the health-care provider immediately.

10. **A 2-month-old is diagnosed with hip dysplasia. The parent asks you how long will the child be in the hip spica cast. How should you respond?**
   a. Not longer than 4 months.
   b. The child will be placed in a Pavlik harness for 3 to 5 months.
   c. Following the osteotomy, the child remains in a cast for 5 months.
   d. Between 2 and 4 months.

ANSWERS

Routine checkup 1
   1. d. Cartilage does not contain blood vessels that are required for healing.

Routine checkup 2
   1. b

Routine checkup 3
   1. c

Routine checkup 4
   1. a

Final checkup

1. c	2. a	3. d	4. d
5. b	6. c	7. c	8. d
9. b	10. b		

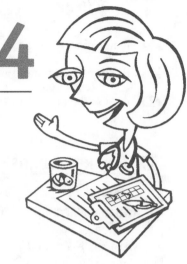

CHAPTER 14

Infectious and Communicable Conditions

Learning Objectives

At the end of the chapter, the student will be able to

1. Understand the stages of infection.

2. Identify signs of diphtheria.

3. Know the interventions for pertussis.

4. Explain the treatment for pertussis.

5. Care for a patient who is diagnosed with tetanus.

6. Assess a patient who has fifth disease.

7. Teach families about the mumps.

8. Intervene with a patient who has poliomyelitis.

9. Describe the incubation period for roseola infantum.

10. Discuss the transmission of rubella.

11. Recognize when a patient diagnosed with rubeola is contagious.

12 Determine who can visit a patient who has varicella.

13 Respond to a patient who has anaphylaxis.

14 Assess the signs and symptoms of mononucleosis.

 KEY WORDS

Allergen	Flora	Naturally acquired passive
Artificially acquired active	Forescheimer spots	immunity
immunity	Incubation period	Papules
Artificially acquired passive	Kernig sign	Parotitis
immunity	Koplik spots	Pathogen
Brudzinski sign	Macules	Prodromal
Contact isolation	Myalgias	Toxoids
Droplet isolation	Natural immunity	Urticaria
Endotoxins	Naturally acquired active	Vesicles
Exotoxins	immunity	

OVERVIEW

Normal functioning of the immune system protects the body against the invasion of outside microorganisms referred to as a **pathogen.** Two of the most common pathogens are bacteria and viruses. An infection occurs when there is a successful invasion of the host by a pathogen (antigen). However, for this to happen, each link in the chain of infection must be intact.

CHAIN OF INFECTION

The chain of infection describes the elements that must be in place for the infection to occur. These elements are

- Pathogen: Sufficient number of microorganisms strong enough to enter and survive the body.
- Reservoir: The proper environment within the body to prosper must include oxygen, water, food, and the best pH balance and temperature.
- Portal of exit: The pathogen must be able to exit its existing environment. For example, the pathogen must be able to leave the respiratory tract, gastrointestinal (GI) tract, or skin of its present host to infect another host.
- Mode of transmission: There must be a way for the pathogen to move from one host to another such as by air droplets, water, or contact.
- Portal of entry: The pathogen must be able to enter the new host such as through a break in the skin or via the respiratory tract.

◐ Susceptible host: The host's immune system must be weak and unable to define against the invading pathogen. A person who is very young or very old or who has a low white blood cell count or is taking antiinflammatory medication typically has a weakened immune system.

STAGES OF INFECTION

The infectious process begins once the pathogen has successfully invaded the host. There are four stages of the infectious process:

◐ **Incubation period:** This is the interval between the invasion and when the first symptoms appear.

◐ **Prodromal:** This is the interval between the appearance of nonspecific symptoms (e.g., I feel like I'm coming down with something) to when specific symptoms appear (e.g., starting to feel warm and having a headache).

◐ Illness: This is when symptoms for a specific type of infection occur (e.g., fever, chills, headache, running nose).

◐ Convalescence: This is the interval when the specific systems abate (i.e., starting to feel better but not yet back to normal).

A GOOD DEFENSE

The immune system protects the body using one of five methods:

◐ **Natural immunity:** The immune system recognizes the pathogen as a foreign cell that attacks and destroys the pathogen using nonpathogen-specific phagocytic action.

◐ **Naturally acquired active immunity:** The immune system develops **antibodies** to a pathogen once the pathogen infected the host previously. Antibodies then attack and destroy subsequent invasion by the pathogen.

◐ **Naturally acquired passive immunity:** Antibodies for specific pathogens are passed from mother to fetus and protect the fetus for approximately 6 months after birth until the infant's own immune system matures.

◐ **Artificially acquired active immunity:** A low potent or dead portion of the pathogen is introduced to the host in a vaccine causing the immune system to develop antibodies against the pathogen. Artificially acquired active immunity develops antibodies that last years or an entire lifetime.

◐ **Artificially acquired passive immunity:** The host is administered antibodies from a different host in the form of immunoglobulin such as gammaglobulin or convalescent serum globulin. Artificially acquired passive immunity provides short-term protection and does not encourage the host's immune system to develop antibodies against the pathogen.

THE DEFENDERS

Lymphocytes are the primary cells of the immune system. Lymphocytes are divided into B cells and T cells.

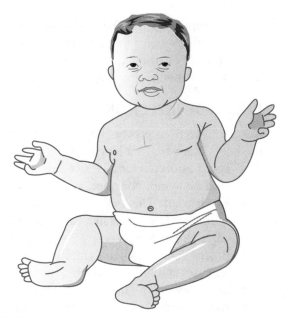

FIGURE 14-1

- B cells: Provide a humoral immune response because they produce an antigen-specific antibody.
- T cells: Provide a cellular immune response. Mature T cells are composed of CD4 and CD8 cells. CD8 cells are responsible for destroying foreign and viral inhabited cells, and they suppress immunologic functions. CD4 cells, also known as helper T cells, stimulate immune functions, such as B cells and macrophages. A macrophage is a cell whose functions include ingesting foreign or invading cells.

VACCINATIONS

There are three types of vaccinations:

- Live, attenuated: This vaccination contains a weakened pathogen.
- Inactivated: This vaccination contains portions of a dead pathogen.
- **Toxoids:** A microorganism itself might not cause an infection, but toxin released by the microorganism might cause the infection. Toxoids are vaccines that are a defense against the toxin.

Visit the American Academy of Pediatrics Web site (www.cispimmunize.org) for the recommended immunization schedule for children.

Common reactions to a vaccination are: swelling, redness, and pain at the injection site and fever of <102°F and fussiness.

Severe reactions to a vaccination that require emergency care are fever >102°F, anaphylaxis, and persistent crying for >2 hours.

Nursing alert **Children who are taking corticosteroids for >2 weeks or who have a weak immune system should not be administered live, attenuated vaccination. Don't administer the measles vaccine together with the tuberculin purified protein derivative test because this might cause a false-negative test result.**

BACTERIA

Bacteria adhere to mucosal surface or epithelial cells and produce proteins that disrupt cell function or destroy cells walls. There are two types of proteins that can be produced:

- **Exotoxins:** Protein is released during cell growth and is affected by antibiotics.
- **Endotoxins:** Protein is released when the bacteria decomposes and are not affected by antibiotics.

Flora consists of bacteria within the body that isn't harmful under normal circumstance and in some situations helps the body in digestion and in restraining the growth of harmful microorganism.

VIRUSES

A virus is a tiny microorganism that must invade a cell in order to reproduce. Once inside the cell, the virus modifies the cell's normal function to propagate the virus. Antibiotics are ineffective against a virus; however, the health-care provider may prescribe prophylactic antibiotics because a virus infection may weaken the patient's immune system, creating an environment for bacteria to prosper. A health-care provider may proscribe antiviral medication to fight the virus.

DIPHTHERIA

What Went Wrong?

Diphtheria is a bacterial infection typically of the larynx, tonsils, and nasopharynx that is caused by *Corynebacterium diphtheria*. The bacterium is transmitted by contact with discharge from a skin lesion or discharge from the nasal passages, pharynx, or eye between 2 and 4 weeks following the onset of symptoms. Symptoms can take up to 7 days to appear. Diphtheria is preventable with a series of immunizations (DTaP) that begin at 2 months of age. An infant is protected for 6 months by passive immunity if the infant's mother has diphtheria antibodies.

 Nursing alert **Place the patient on droplet isolation. If lesions are present, place the patient on contact isolation.**

Signs and Symptoms

- Purulent rhinitis
- Cough

- Stridor
- Thick grayish green lesion on the pharynx and tonsils
- Pharyngitis
- Fever
- Malaise

Nursing alert **Lesions can obstruct the airway, especially in infants who have small airways. Removal of the lesion risks bleeding.**

Test Results

- Culture and sensitivity test: Positive for *C. diphtheria.*
- Serologic test: Identifies diphtheria toxin.

Treatment

- Administer diphtheria antitoxin.
- Administer antibiotic (Penicillin G, erythromycin) within 3 days of the onset of the symptoms.

Nursing alert **Assess if the patient is allergic to penicillin. If there is an allergic reaction, administer erythromycin.**

Nursing Intervention

- Place the child in droplet isolation to prevent transmission of the disease.
- Everyone must wear gowns, masks, and gloves when in contact with the patient.
- Place the child on contact isolation if lesions are present.
- Monitor for signs of airway obstruction.
- Maintain bed rest.
- Report the diagnoses to local health officials according to policy.
- Explain the disorder and treatment to the family and to the patient.

Nursing alert **Isolation precautions remain in effect until two consecutive negative nasopharyngeal cultures are received.**

HAEMOPHILUS INFLUENZAE TYPE B

What Went Wrong?

Haemophilus influenzae type B (Hib) is a bacterial infection caused by the *Coccobacillus H. influenza* bacteria, which is secondary to an upper respiratory viral infection. *Coccobacillus H. influenza* bacteria is normal flora in the upper respiratory tract that is restrained from infecting the body by the immune system. However, an upper respiratory viral infection weakens the immune system sufficiently for the *Coccobacillus H. influenza* bacteria to penetrate the mucosal tissue and enter the bloodstream.

Signs and Symptoms

Signs and symptoms depend on which part of the body becomes infected. Typically the infection results in bronchiolitis, epiglottiditis, meningitis, otitis media, or laryngotracheobronchitis.

Test Results

- ☉ Culture and sensitivity test: Positive for *Coccobacillus H. influenza.*
- ☉ Serologic test: Identifies *Coccobacillus H. influenza* toxin.

Treatment

- ☉ Administer antibiotic (ceftriaxone [Rocephin], cefotaxime [Calforan], chloramphenicol [Chloromycetin]).
- ☉ Administer rifampin (Rifadin) prophylatically to others who have been in close contact with the patient.

Nursing Intervention

- ☉ Place the child in droplet isolation to prevent transmission of the disease.
- ☉ Provide cool humidification.
- ☉ Explain the disorder and treatment to the family and to the patient.

 Nursing alert Isolation precautions remain in effect until after the first 24 hours of antibiotic treatment.

 ROUTINE CHECKUP 1

1. A parent of a child who has a fever and is coughing is brought to the Emergency Department (ED). You notice a lesion on the child's tonsil. What is your best response?
   a. Explain that the child probably has tonsillitis and will be fine in a couple of days following antibiotic treatment.
   b. Immediately place the child in droplet isolation until the child's condition is diagnosed.
   c. Show the parent and child to a gurney located in the main area of the ED.
   d. Show the parent and child to a gurney located in the main area of the ED and make sure the curtain is pulled.

Answer:

2. The mother of a child recently diagnosed with *Haemophilus influenzae* type B looked up this disorder on the Internet and learned that her other child also has the *Coccobacillus H. influenza* bacteria. She is concerned. What is your best response?

a. All of us have bacteria in our bodies called flora. Flora isn't harmful and is sometimes helpful. The bacteria that caused your child's infection are flora; however, your child's recent viral infection weakened your child's immune system enabling these bacteria to cause the infection.

b. All of us have bacteria in our bodies called flora. Flora isn't harmful and is sometimes helpful. The bacteria that caused your child's infection are flora; however, your child's recent viral infection weakened your child's immune system enabling these bacteria to cause the infection. Your other child didn't come down with the viral infection and therefore won't get this bacterial infection.

c. All of us have bacteria in our bodies called flora. Flora isn't harmful and is sometimes helpful. The bacteria that caused your child's infection are flora; however, your child's recent bacterial infection weakened your child's immune system enabling these bacteria to cause the infection. Your other child didn't come down with the viral infection and therefore didn't get this bacterial infection; however, you should talk to your health-care provider to determine if your child should be vaccinated against these bacteria.

Answer:

PERTUSSIS

What Went Wrong?

Pertussis in a bacterial infection caused typically by *Bordetella pertussis* but can also be caused by *B. parapertussis* or *B. bronchiseptica* that causes an upper respiratory tract infection resulting in an irritating cough that ends in high-pitched inspiratory whoop, which is why pertussis is commonly referred to as whooping cough. Pertussis occurs because the patient was in contact with contaminated respiratory droplets or in contact with items that become contaminated by respiratory droplets. Once exposed, the bacteria incubate for 3 to 12 days before symptoms appear. Children should be vaccinated (DTaP) against pertussis beginning at 2 months of age.

 Nursing alert The patient is contagious from a week after exposure to the bacteria through the first 7 days of antibiotic therapy.

Signs and Symptoms

- Nasal congestion
- Nonproductive cough
- Sneezing
- Watery eyes
- Low-grade fever
- Severe, irritable coughing spasms
- Whooping sound on inspiration

Test Results

- Culture and sensitive test: Identified *B. pertussis, B. parapertussis,* or *B. bronchiseptica*

Treatment

- Administer erythromycin for 14 days to kill the bacteria.
- Administer erythromycin prophylatically to others who have been in close contact with the patient.

Nursing alert **Administer cotrimoxazole (Bactrim) if the child is unable to tolerate erythromycin.**

Nursing Intervention

- Provide droplet isolation immediately.
- Everyone must wear gowns, masks, and gloves when in contact with the patient.
- Provide a quiet environment to avoid stimulants that might lead to coughing.
- Report the diagnoses to local health officials according to policy.
- Explain the disorder and treatment to the family and to the patient.

Nursing alert **Isolation precautions remain in effect until after day 7 of antibiotic treatment.**

✔ ROUTINE CHECKUP 2

1. A father brought his 7-year-old son to the ED complaining that his son was achy and has a slight fever and headaches. He said he was fine 4 weeks ago when they spent time in the family's woodland cabin. What is your best response?
   a. Look for a bull's-eye rash.
   b. Tell the father that the health-care provider will probably perform tests to determine if his son has Lyme disease.
   c. Tell the father that the son probably caught a cold and it will resolve within 10 days.
   d. Place the child in isolation immediately.

Answer:

2. A mother mentioned to you in passing that her daughter's best friend frequently goes into a coughing spasm and makes this strange sound after each cough. She thinks it must be allergies because nothing is coughed up. What is your best response?
   a. Has your daughter been vaccinated for whooping cough?
   b. Has your daughter's friend been vaccinated for whooping cough?
   c. Have you been vaccinated for whooping cough?
   d. Does your daughter have allergies?

Answer:

TETANUS

What Went Wrong?

Tetanus is a bacterial infection caused by the *Clostridium tetani* bacteria when the bacteria enters the body through an opening in the skin, causing muscles to tighten and become rigid especially in the mouth, making it difficult to breath and swallow. The incubation period can be up to 14 days before symptoms appear. The child should receive immunization to tetanus as part of the DTaP vaccination beginning at 2 months of age.

Nursing alert **The patient is alert and has full mental capacity while infected.**

Signs and Symptoms

- Lockjaw
- Stiff neck
- Facial muscle spasms
- Difficulty swallowing (dysphagia)
- Low-grade fever
- Sweating
- Sensitivity to external stimulation

Test Results

- Serum: Normal

Nursing alert **Diagnosis is based on symptoms and history and by ruling out neurologic disorders.**

Treatment

- ◐ Administer tetanus immune globulin to reverse tetanus toxin.
- ◐ Administer tetanus toxoid at an injection site different from the tetanus immune globulin.
- ◐ Administer antibiotic (penicillin G, metronidazole, erythromycin, tetracycline).
- ◐ Administer muscle relaxants.
- ◐ Debride the wound.

Nursing Intervention

- ◐ Place the patient in the intensive care unit to monitor cardiorespiratory function.
- ◐ Provide a quiet environment to reduce external stimuli.
- ◐ Limit touching and moving the patient to reduce external stimuli.
- ◐ Explain the disorder and treatment to the family and to the patient, remembering that the patient has full mental capacity.

Nursing alert **Keep rescue equipment nearby because all muscles might become rigid and disrupt the patient's cardiorespiratory function.**

FIFTH DISEASE

What Went Wrong?

Fifth disease is a viral infection caused by the human parvovirus B19 virus that is transmitted through infected blood and respiratory droplets. The incubation period is between 6 and 14 days after symptoms appear. The fifth disease is the fifth most common rash producing viral infection in children. The others are rubella, rubeola, roseola infantum, and varicella.

Signs and Symptoms

- ◐ Slapped-cheek-like rash on the face.
- ◐ Flat red spotted rash on the trunk and proximal extremities. The rash fades in the center of the rash.
- ◐ No rash on the palms and soles.
- ◐ Upper respiratory infection.
- ◐ Low-grade fever.
- ◐ Headache.

Test Results

- ◐ No tests

Nursing alert **Diagnosis is based on symptoms, history, and by ruling out other disorders.**

Treatment

No treatment. The infection is self-limiting.

Nursing Intervention

  ☾ Administer antipyretics (acetaminophen) to relieve fever.
  ☾ Soothing baths to relieve itching.
  ☾ Antipruritics to relieve itching.
  ☾ Explain the disorder and treatment to the family.

Nursing alert **There is no need to isolate the patient because the infection is no longer contagious when the rash appears.**

MUMPS

What Went Wrong?

Mumps, also known as **parotitis,** is a viral infection of the parotid glands and at times the sublingual or submaxillary glands caused by the paramyxovirus. The infection causes swollen glands and is spread by airborne droplets or contact with infected saliva. The infection can become systemic or can resolve without treatment or with treatment of symptoms alone. The disease is highly communicable, particularly immediately before and after swelling. The incubation period is between 12 and 25 days before the symptoms appears.

Signs and Symptoms

  ☾ Early signs:
    • **Prodromal phase** (early manifestation of disease to period of overt symptoms), initial 24 hours:
      ∘ Fever
      ∘ Headache
      ∘ Malaise
      ∘ Anorexia
      ∘ Neck pain
      ∘ Fever
    • Pain in jaw or ear increased with chewing
    • Dehydration may result if child refuses to drink
  ☾ Late signs:
    • Bilateral or unilateral enlargement of the parotid gland(s)
    • Painful parotid glands
    • Complications from infection may include
      ∘ Deafness (sensorineural)

- Encephalitis
- Myocarditis
- Meningitis
- Hepatitis
- Arthritis
- Epididymoorchitis
- Sterility

Test Results

- Serum: Elevated amylase due to enlarged parotid glands
- Complete blood count: Elevated white blood count (leukocytosis) and elevated lymphocytes (lymphocytosis)
- Culture to confirm involved organism
- Mumps titer may be performed to determine immunity

Treatment

- Prevention:
  - Encourage immunization—measles, mumps, and rubella (MMR) vaccine:
    - Initial immunization is given after 12 months of age.
    - Immunization is recommended for individuals born after 1957 who have not had the mumps or been immunized, or do not have titers showing immunity.
- Treatment:
  - Administer corticosteroids to reduce inflammation.
  - Administer NSAIDs to reduce inflammation.
  - Administer acetaminophen (Tylenol), ibuprofen (Advil), or naproxen sodium (Aleve) to relieve pain.
  - Maintain bed rest during the prodromal stage and while swelling present.
  - Isolate child and contaminated items from other children or adults, including used cups, plates, and utensils to prevent exposure to contaminated saliva.
  - Apply warm or cold compresses to neck, based on comfort and preference.
  - Provide support in the event of orchitis:
    - Warmth.
    - Local support with tight-fitting clothes.
  - Push fluids to prevent dehydration.
  - Hydration therapy, including intravenous fluid, if child dehydrates.

Nursing Intervention

- Droplet isolation, if hospitalized.
- Bed rest: Provide age-appropriate diversion activities.

- Soft diet with bland foods requiring minimal chewing.
- Warm or cool compresses on the swollen neck.
- Monitor for swollen testicles, which indicates complications of the disorder.
- Monitor for **Kernig sign** (unable to straighten legs at knees), which indicates complications of the disorder.
- Monitor for **Brudzinski sign** (flexion of the hips and knees when neck is flexed), which indicates complications of the disorder.
- Report the diagnoses to local health officials according to policy.
- Explain the disorder and treatment to the family.

Nursing alert Emphasize to the parents that anyone can be infected, adult or child, and sterility can result from infection.

Nursing alert The patient is contagious beginning 7 days before the swelling of the parotid gland and until 9 days after the swelling subsides.

POLIOMYELITIS

What Went Wrong?

Poliomyelitis is a viral infection by the polioviruses that is transmitted by contact with infected oropharyngeal secretions or infected stools resulting in a brief illness to paralysis. The incubation period is between 7 and 10 days before the symptoms appear. Children should be vaccinated (inactivated poliovirus vaccine [IPV]) beginning at 2 months of age.

There are three types of poliovirus:
- Type 1: *Brunhilde*
- Type 2: *Lansing*
- Type 3: *Leon*

Signs and Symptoms

- No symptoms
- Fever
- Headache
- Vomiting
- Nausea
- Pharyngitis
- Lethargy
- Muscle weakness
- Constipation
- Urine retention
- Paresthesia

Nursing alert **The patient may have no symptoms or a range of symptoms.**

Test Results
- ◗ Stool sample: Presence of the virus
- ◗ Serum: Elevated antibodies

 Nursing alert **Diagnosis is based on symptoms and history and by ruling out other disorders.**

Treatment
- ◗ No treatment except for symptomatic treatment

🕗 Nursing Intervention
- ◗ Place the child on droplet and contact isolation.
- ◗ Only those who have received the IPV vaccination are permitted to contact the patient.
- ◗ Monitor for skin breakdown.
- ◗ Monitor for demineralization.
- ◗ Monitor for pneumonia.
- ◗ Apply high-top sneakers to the patient to prevent contractures.
- ◗ Perform range-of-motion exercise.
- ◗ Report the diagnoses to local health officials according to policy.
- ◗ Explain the disorder and treatment to the family.

ROSEOLA INFANTUM

What Went Wrong?

🕘 Roseola infantum is a viral infection caused by the human herpes virus 6 and is suspected of being transmitted via oral viral shedding. Oral viral shedding is the process by which the virus can travel along the patient's nerves to the skin surface where the virus is transferred by contact with the skin. The incubation period is between 5 and 15 days before the symptoms appear.

Signs and Symptoms
- ◗ Rash beginning on the trunk and spreading to the extremities and face that resolves by the third day.
- ◗ Sudden fever between 103°F and 106°F that resolves within 4 days.

Test Results
- ◗ No tests

Treatment

- ◑ Roseola infantum is self-limiting.
- ◑ Administer acetaminophen (Tylenol) for fever.
- ◑ Administer intravenous (IV) fluids and electrolytes as ordered.

Nursing Intervention

- ◑ Monitor vital signs.
- ◑ Explain the disorder and treatment to the family.

Nursing alert **Monitor for febrile seizures.**

RUBELLA

What Went Wrong?

10. Rubella is a viral infection commonly called German measles and is caused by the rubella virus that is transmitted by airborne droplets, contact with contaminated items, or direct contact with an infected person. The incubation period is between 14 and 21 days.

Nursing alert **Only the nonpregnant should come in contact with the patient. Assume that a woman who is of childbearing age is pregnant because a woman in very early pregnancy may not know she is pregnant. Women of childbearing age should receive the rubella vaccine.**

Signs and Symptoms

- ◑ Early signs (first 5 days):
  - • Headache
  - • Fever
  - • Sore throat
  - • Pus containing (purulent) nasal drainage
  - • Malaise
  - • Swollen lymph nodes
- ◑ Late signs:
  - • Rash appears first on the face and then spreads to the trunk and legs.
  - • **Forescheimer spots** (small red flat spot on the soft palate).

Test Results

- ◑ Serum: Positive for rubella antibodies

Nursing alert **Diagnoses is usually made based on signs and symptoms.**

Treatment

- ◑ Rubella is self-limiting.
- ◑ Administer acetaminophen (Tylenol) for fever.

Nursing Intervention
- Place the child on droplet isolation if hospitalized.
- Report the diagnoses to local health officials according to policy.
- Explain the disorder and treatment to the family.

 Nursing alert **The patient is contagious beginning 1 week before a rash appears and until 4 days after the rash appears.**

RUBEOLA

What Went Wrong?
Rubeola, commonly called the measles, is a viral infection caused by the rubeola virus and is transmitted by airborne droplets or direct contact with contaminated items. The incubation period is from 8 to 12 days before the symptoms appear. The children should be vaccinated for rubeola (MMR) at 12 months of age.

Signs and Symptoms
- Early stage:
  - Malaise
  - Fever
  - Cough
  - Lethargy
  - Conjunctivitis
  - **Koplik spots** (gray specks with red halos in the buccal mucosa): 2 days before the rash appears on the body
  - Periorbital edema
- Later stage:
  - Red flat rash on the face and spreads to the trunk and extremities that disappears in 7 days
  - Severe cough
  - Swollen glands
  - Watery nose (rhinorrhea)

Test Results
- No tests

 Nursing alert **Diagnoses is usually made based on signs and symptoms.**

Treatment
- Rubeola is self-limiting.
- Administer acetaminophen (Tylenol) for fever.
- Administer antipruritic medication for itching.

Nursing Intervention

- ◐ Monitor vital signs.
- ◐ Increase fluids to reduce secretion viscosity.
- ◐ Provide cool mist from a vaporizer for inflamed mucous membranes.
- ◐ Place the child on droplet isolation if hospitalized.
- ◐ Report the diagnoses to local health officials according to policy.
- ◐ Explain the disorder and treatment to the family.

 Nursing alert **⚑** The patient is contagious beginning several days before a rash appears and until 5 days after the rash disappears.

VARICELLA

What Went Wrong?

Varicella, commonly called chickenpox, is a viral infection caused by the varicella zoster virus (VZV) that is transmitted by airborne droplets and by contact with lesions. The VZV is latent in the dorsal root ganglia and can become reactivated later in life as a herpes zoster infection, commonly called shingles. The incubation period is between 10 and 21 days before the symptoms appear. Children should receive the varicella vaccination beginning at 12 months of age.

 Nursing alert **⚑** Only the nonpregnant should come in contact with the patient. Assume that a female who is of childbearing age is pregnant because a woman in very early pregnancy may not know she is pregnant. Women of childbearing age should receive the rubella vaccine.

Signs and Symptoms

- ◐ Early signs:
  - Malaise
  - Fever
  - Anorexia
- ◐ Late signs:
  - Itchy rash of red **macules** begins on the face, scalp, or trunk.
  - Macules transform into small solid (not pus containing) elevation of the skin (**papules**).
  - Papules develop into clear sacs (**vesicles**) with a red base.
  - Vesicles break and scabs form a lesion.
  - Lesions are crusted over.

Test Results

- ◐ VZV antibody test: Positive

Nursing alert **Diagnoses is usually made based on signs and symptoms.**

Treatment
- Varicella is self-limiting.
- Administer acetaminophen (Tylenol) for fever.
- Administer antipruritic medication for itching.

Nursing Intervention
- Place the child on droplet and contact isolation if hospitalized.
- Provide oatmeal baths to soothe itching.
- Explain the disorder and treatment to the family. Tell the family not to use over-the-counter locations that contain antihistamines. Lotions such as calamine lotion and Aveeno are permissible to help soothe itching.

Nursing alert **The patient is contagious beginning 5 days before a rash appears and until all lesions are crusted over.**

ANAPHYLAXIS

What Went Wrong?
Anaphylaxis is the dilating of capillaries and contracting of smooth muscles in the respiratory tract caused by the release of histamines in response to an **allergen** resulting in respiratory distress, hives (**urticaria**), and edema.

Signs and Symptoms
- Shortness of breath due to swelling of the larynx
- Hypotension and shock due to generalized vasodilation
- Sneezing due to an allergen
- Anxiety secondary to difficulty in breathing
- Rales (crackles) heard in the lungs due to fluid in the lungs
- Wheezing (rhonchi) due to bronchospasm

Test Results
- Serum: Elevated tryptase levels from mast cells

Treatment
- Administer emergency medications:
  - Epinephrine to open airways and to reduce bronchospasm
  - Corticosteroids to reduce symptoms
  - Antihistamines to mitigate symptoms

◑ Administer circulatory volume expanders to treat hypotension caused by vasodilation:
  - Saline
  - Plasma
◑ Administer vasopressors to counteract vasodilation and to increase blood pressure:
  - Norepinephrine
  - Dopamine
◑ Oxygen therapy to support breathing.
◑ Insert endotracheal tube to maintain airways.
◑ Allergy skin testing to identify allergen.

Nursing Intervention

◑ Maintain airway to facilitate breathing.
◑ Monitor for hoarseness and difficulty breathing to check for symptoms of decreased respiration.
◑ Explain to the family to avoid exposure to allergens to prevent future occurrences and to seek medical help immediately if exposed to allergens to prevent anaphylaxis.

MONONUCLEOSIS

What Went Wrong?

Mononucleosis is a viral infection commonly caused by the Epstein-Barr virus but can also be caused by the cytomegalovirus and frequently secondary to a streptococcus bacterial infection that weakened the immune system. Mononucleousis is transmitted by contact.

14 Signs and Symptoms

◑ Malaise
◑ Fever
◑ Muscle ache (**myalgias**)
◑ Headache
◑ Sore throat

Test Results

◑ Heterophil antibody test: Positive
◑ Mono spot test: Positive

Treatment

◑ No treatment except for symptomatic treatment

Nursing Intervention
- Adequate rest
- Increase fluids
- Monitor vital signs

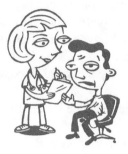

CASE STUDY

Six-year-old Martin Rivera presented in the ED with his parents at 8 AM. His mother reported that he has been lethargic and coughing. His mother said he had a temperature of 102.4°F during the overnight hours and he hasn't been feeling well for a week or so. She and her husband became concerned when his face began turning red.

Assessment data: Temperature 102.5°F. Periorbital edema. Conjunctivitis. Red flat rash on the child's face and faint the rash on his trunk. Severe coughing. Watery nose. Swollen lymph nodes. The parents are unsure about the child's vaccinations. No Forescheimer spots.

Interpretation: The rash on the face and a faint rash on the trunk are consistent with the rash starting on the face rather than the trunk and then spreading to the trunk. This probably rules out roseola infantum, which begins on the trunk. No Forescheimer spots rules out rubella, which also causes a rash on the face. Conjunctivitis, periorbital edema, a fever, lethargy, and coughing is consistent with rubeola. The fact that the parents are unsure of the child's vaccinations can lead to the supposition that the child might not have received all his vaccinations.

Nursing intervention: Place the child on droplet isolation. Expect the health-care provider to order acetaminophen for fever and antipruritic medication for itching. Administer fluids to reduce secretion viscosity and provide cool mist from a vaporizer for inflamed mucous membranes. Explain the disorder and treatment to the family and child and explain to the family that other children at home should be vaccinated for rubeola and other communicable diseases. Also tell the parents that child will be contagious for 5 days after the rash disappears and that the rash should disappear in about 7 days. Report the diagnoses to local health officials according to policy.

Evaluation: Assess the child's temperature and how well the antipruritic medication is relieving the itching. Monitor the rash to determine if the skin is opened from the child scratching.

CONCLUSION

The immune system protects the body against invasion of microorganisms. Microorganisms that cause infection are called pathogens. Two of the most common are bacteria and viruses. The chain of infection must be followed in order for the pathogen to infect the body. Infection follows four stages beginning with the incubation period and progressing to the convalescence period.

The immune system uses five methods to protect the body: natural immunity, naturally acquired active immunity, naturally acquired passive immunity, artificially acquired active immunity, and artificially acquired passive immunity.

A person can become immune by receiving a vaccination. The vaccination can be live attenuated, inactivated, or toxoids.

Bacterial infections include diphtheria, *Haemophilus influenzae* type B, Lyme disease, pertussis, and tetanus. Viral infections include fifth disease, mumps, roseola infantum, poliomyelitis, rubella, rubeola, varicella, and mononucleosis.

 FINAL CHECKUP

1. **The health-care provider orders a live attenuated vaccine to be administered to a 3-year-old. What question should you ask before administering the vaccination?**
   a. Has the child been taking corticosteroids for the past 2 weeks?
   b. Can the child sit still when you give the injection?
   c. Has the child ever received an injection before?
   d. Is the parent able to hold the child when the injection is administered?

2. **A mother calls you saying that her 1-month-old daughter was exposed to a child who has diphtheria. What is your best response?**
   a. Bring your child immediately to the ED.
   b. Get your child vaccinated immediately.
   c. If you were vaccinated for diphtheria and you gave birth to your daughter, then your daughter is protected the first 6 months of her life by your antibodies.
   d. Don't be concerned. Diphtheria is not contagious.

3. **The health-care provider orders penicillin G for a child who has been diagnosed with tetanus. The child's mother tells you that the child is allergic to penicillin. What should you expect the health-care provider to order?**
   a. Erythromycin
   b. Acetaminophen
   c. Antipruitics
   d. NSAIDs

4. **A father of a 4-year-old boy diagnosed with roseola infantum questions you why the health-care provider didn't order antibiotics. What is your best response?**
   a. There is no cure for roseola infantum.
   b. Roseola infantum is a viral infection and bacterial is used to treat bacterial infections.
   c. Roseola infantum is self-limiting.
   d. I'll mention this to the health-care provider.

5. **A parent is amazed how the health-care provider, who diagnosed her daughter as having rubeola, predicted that her daughter would develop a rash in a couple of days. How would you explain this prediction?**
   a. Rubeola is going around the area.
   b. The health-care provider noticed periorbital edema, which precedes the rash by 4 days.
   c. The health-care provider noticed a red flat rash in the buccal mucosa of the patient's mouth, which appears 2 days before the rash appears on the patient's face.
   d. The health-care provider probably noticed Koplik spots, which appear 2 days before the rash appears.

6. **A child was rushed to the ED having difficulty breathing with hypotension and shock after eating a peanut butter and jelly sandwich. The parents ask what might have gone wrong. What is your best response?**
   a. The child aspirated the sandwich.
   b. The child experienced anaphylaxis as a result of a response by the immune system to an allergen, which is likely to be peanuts.
   c. The child has pneumonia.
   d. The child experienced food poisoning.

7. **A parent of a child who is diagnosed with mumps asks if she can send her child to child care because it seems that his parotid glands are no longer swollen. What is your best response?**
   a. Yes, he is no longer contagious.
   b. No, not until he is examined by the health-care provider.
   c. No, he remains contagious for 9 days after the swelling of the parotid glands subsides.
   d. Yes, as long as no other child at the child-care center is infected.

8. **A new ED nurse wants to call the hospital's child protection team to investigate a child who had a red slapped mark on his cheek. His mother brought him in with a headache and a low-grade fever and he has slight wheezing on inspiration. How would you respond?**
   a. Ask the nurse if he assessed the child's trunk for a flat red spotted rash.
   b. Tell the nurse to call the police first.
   c. Tell the nurse not to leave the child alone with the parent.
   d. Tell the nurse to let the health-care provider make that determination.

9. **Amy, a 9-year-old girl, is showing signs and symptoms of the mumps. What would be appropriate family and client teaching?**
   a. You can send your child back to school immediately after the swelling subsides.
   b. Your child is not contagious until we note the swelling is fully present.
   c. Symptoms may not be noted until 12 or more days after exposure.
   d. There is no danger of complications from the mumps, so don't worry.

10. **Why would a health-care provider order antibiotics for a child who has a viral infection?**
   a. Antibiotics can slow the progression of some viruses.
   b. The viral infection might weaken the immune system, enabling bacteria to infect the body. Antibiotics are administered as a prophylactic.
   c. Antibiotics increase the effectiveness of antiviral medications.
   d. Question the order.

ANSWERS

Routine checkup 1
   1. b
   2. c

Routine checkup 2
   1. b
   2. a

Final checkup

1. a	2. c	3. a	4. b
5. d	6. b	7. c	8. a
9. c	10. b		

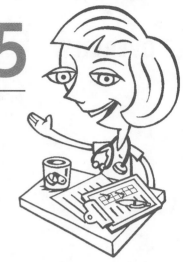

CHAPTER 15

Integumentary Conditions

Learning Objectives

At the end of the chapter, the student will be able to

1 Using appropriate terms, describe skin lesions and other skin conditions.

2 Assess a child with an integumentary condition.

3 Discuss the common treatment plan for a child with a skin condition.

4 Discuss the nursing implications when caring for a child with a skin condition.

5 Determine the care needs of a child and family with a skin condition.

 KEY WORDS

Bulla	Nodule	Pustule
Cyst	Papule	Vesicle
Erythema	Patch	Wheal
Lanugo	Plaque	
Macule	Pruritus	

OVERVIEW

The skin serves multiple purposes and is important for maintenance of health and well-being and also impacts physical appearance and self-esteem. Skin serves as a protective covering; a barrier against mechanical, thermal, radiant, and chemical trauma. Key anatomic aspects related to skin include the following:

- Skin is resistant to penetration by microorganisms, dirt, and other substances.
- The skin plays a role in heat regulation by permitting heat loss or retention.
- The skin is a sensory organ with nerve endings that transmit touch, pain, and temperature.
- The skin has two layers—the epidermis (outer) and the dermis (inner).
- The dermis is primarily connective tissue and thus is affected by collagen diseases.
- 🔔 Hair grows on the skin at different lengths; hair follicles are developed fully at birth, the presence of **lanugo** (fine body hair) indicates premature birth because it usually disappears by full-term birth.
- Subcutaneous tissues are under the dermis and provide a cushion for the underlying musculature.
- Sebaceous glands produce sebum (a fatty substance) that increases the water resistance of the skin.
- Sweat glands are present in areas of the body and function to assist in release of heat, fluid, and some electrolytes. Sweat glands located in the axilla, areola of the breast, and anal areas are not active during infancy and childhood, but they become mature at puberty.

SKIN LESIONS/DERMATITIS

🔔 What Went Wrong?

More than half of dermatologic problems are types of dermatitis (inflammation of the dermis) from various causes. Irritation results in inter- and intracellular swelling and infiltration of the dermis and epidermis with vascular dilation and cellular infiltration around blood vessels. The type of lesion produced depends on where and how the response settles in and on the skin. Skin lesions vary in nature and can result from a multitude of injuries from abrasion to penetrating wound to infection, among other factors. Lesions can be primary resulting from an initial insult, or secondary resulting from healing or additional breakdown of the original involved area. Primary lesions may be classified in the following ways:

- **Bulla:** Vesicle >1 cm in diameter (larger blister)
- **Cyst:** Palpable, elevated, encapsulated liquid or semisolid filled lesion with distinct borders (e.g., sebaceous cyst)

- **Macule:** A flat, nonpalpable brown, red, purple, white, or tan area with a distinct regular border less than a centimeter in diameter
- **Nodule:** A 1- to 2-cm elevated, firm, palpable mass deep in the dermis, with a distinct border
- **Patch:** A flat nonpalpable irregular shaped macule that is >1 cm in diameter
- **Papule:** A firm, elevated palpable brown, red, purple, white, or tan area with a distinct regular border less than a centimeter in diameter(such as warts)
- **Plaque:** A firm, elevated flat rough superficial papule >1 cm in diameter; may be joined (e.g., psoriasis or seborrhea)
- **Pustule:** Elevated, superficial, distinct, purulent fluid-filled lesion (acne, impetigo)
- **Vesicle:** Elevated, superficial, distinct, serous fluid-filled lesion <1 cm in diameter (blister)
- **Wheal:** Solid, elevated area of edema with irregular shape, varied changing diameters with lighter center, pale pink in color (e.g., insect bites)

Causes vary with type of lesion but could include physical irritant such as chemical, allergic, traumatic, or infectious assault. Lesion can progress from smaller single lesion to larger or combined lesions. Secondary lesions occur with healing, additional trauma such as scratching, or infection to the site. Secondary lesion types include

- Scale: Elevated keratinized (hardened) cells, flaky, irregular thick or thin, dry or oily lesion, various size and tan, silver or white in color (e.g., psoriasis)
- Crust: Slightly elevated, dried blood, serum, or purulent exudates, various sizes, brown, red, black, tan, or pale in color (eczema or scab)
- Lichenification: Thickened epidermis, bolder skin markings caused by rubbing or irritation (chronic dermatitis)

🔑 Signs and Symptom

- History may reveal recent infection (measles) or allergic sensitivity (contact dermatitis or drug rash).
- Physical assessment should reveal the distribution, size, shape, and arrangement of the lesions.
- Itching (**pruritus**), mild to severe, is a common symptom with some lesions.
- Other sensations may be reported such as stinging, burning, or crawling.
- Pain or tenderness may be noted with some lesions due to pressure on or irritation of nerve endings.
- Some lesions appear in association with contact with or ingestion of substances to which the client is allergic.

- Primary or secondary lesion types may be present depending on duration of the condition prior to the physical examination.
- Paresthesia (burning or numbness) or anesthesia (absence of sensation) may be reported depending on extent of nerve disruption.

2 Test Results

- Studies are needed to rule out collagen disease or immunodeficiency disease.
- Microscopic examination.
- Cultures.
- Biopsy (skin scraping).
- Cell diagnosis (cytodiagnosis).
- Patch testing.
- Wood light examination.
- Allergic skin testing.
- Blood testing: Complete blood count, sedimentation rate.

3 Treatments

- Dressings are applied for the following reasons:
  - Provides a healing environment with moist gauze
  - Protects wound from infections
  - Provides compression to reduce bleeding or swelling
  - Facilitates the application of medication
  - Absorbs drainage
  - Debrides necrotic tissue
  - Controls odor
  - Reduces pain
- Topical ointment may be applied to relieve local discomfort, reduce swelling, or prevent or resolve infection (such as calamine lotion for poison ivy contact).
- Pain medication or antihistamine to relieve discomfort or irritation.
- Topical therapies: Cautery or cryosurgery (wart removal), electrodesiccation, ultraviolet therapy, laser therapy, acne therapy (chemical peel).
- Systemic medication such as antibiotic for infection or corticosteroid to reduce inflammation.

4 Nursing Interventions

- Apply topical treatments and give medications as ordered and monitor for side effects.
- Monitor for healing or lack of healing and report findings as indicated so treatment can be changed if needed.

Nursing alert Prolonged administration of corticosteroids can temporarily suppress growth, so developmental assessments should be performed regularly.

◑ Teach parents and child to avoid skin irritants such as poison ivy, oak, or sumac and any objects or clothing that touched these plants.
◑ 🔑 Teach child and parents how to care for skin and lesions:
  • Specify amount and frequency of ointment application; stress that extra ointment or increased frequency could increase systemic levels in children so prescribed schedule should be adhered to.
  • Caution parents to use clean gauze or applicator for each area being cleaned to avoid spread of debris.
  • Teach parents and child about lesion relative to method of spread and anticipated time for healing because visible skin lesions may cause distress due to concern about appearance and self-esteem concerns as well as concerns that lesion may be contagious.

WOUNDS

🔑 What Went Wrong?

Wounds are disruptions of the skin integrity that result in a normal or abnormal tissue repair response by the body. All wounds can be classified as acute or chronic:

◑ Acute wounds heal within an expected, usual time frame without complication:
  • Abrasions are superficial rubbing or scraping off of epidermis (and portions into the dermis); most common wound of childhood.
◑ Chronic wounds require a prolonged time for healing or involve additional problems such as infection or poor circulation (such as burn injury).
◑ Generally healing occurs by primary, secondary, or tertiary intention:
  • Primary intention involves a clean cut with healing occurring in all layers of the wound; margins (edges) join without complication; minimal scar.
  • Secondary intention happens with ulcer or cut with jagged edges that do not meet smoothly or do not meet; debris with cells and exudates gather and debridement may be needed to remove. Large scar may be noted.
  • Tertiary intention involves delayed closure of wound with great risk of infection; wound may be sutured after infection present; large deep scar results.

🔑 Signs and Symptoms

◑ Wound appearance depends on type and degree of skin and other tissue disruption and stage of healing.
◑ Initially, wound may be red and swollen due to inflammation with blood and cells of immunity moving to site for healing (phase I healing).
◑ During the second stage of healing, a collagen mesh begins to form and appearance is red and shiny with thin layer of epithelial cells; bleeds easily if traumatized.

◑ The third and fourth phases of healing involve wound contraction and maturation. A pink elevated scar with possible itching over time advances to a pale scar tissue (a child may develop more scar tissue than an adult).

◑ Signs of infection may include
  • **Erythema,** redness of the skin due to inflammation, particularly in the area around the wound
  • Edema
  • Purulent drainage (exudates)
  • Pain
  • Increased temperature (systemic and warmth at site)

❸ Test Results

◑ Wound size measurement with tape or caliper may be performed to assess healing.

◑ Wound culture may be done to determine organism in infection.

❹ Treatments

◑ Healing is promoted by good nutrition, circulation, and avoidance of irritants, including antiseptics such as Neosporin or Bacitracin or Betadine (povidone-iodine).

Nursing alert **Povidone-iodine should be avoided with open wounds and in children with thyroid or renal conditions because it is absorbed into the bloodstream of small children.**

◑ Pain relief medication.

◑ Dressings may applied for the following reasons:
  • Provides a healing environment with moist gauze
  • Protects wound from infections
  • Provides compression to reduce bleeding or swelling
  • Facilitates the application of medication
  • Absorbs drainage
  • Debrides necrotic tissue
  • Controls odor
  • Reduces pain

❹ Nursing Interventions

◑ Use sterile technique to avoid introduction of organisms into clean wound.

◑ ❺ Teach child and parents how to care for skin and wound(s):
  • Specify frequency of dressing change and medication application; stress that extra ointment or increased frequency could damage

wound or increase systemic levels in children so prescribed schedule should be followed.
- Caution parents to use clean gauze or applicator for each area being cleaned to avoid spread of debris.
- Teach parents and child proper hygiene to avoid wound contamination or spread of infection from wound.
- Discuss signs of side effects from medication and signs of wound healing complications that should be reported immediately.
- Discuss acceptable coverings that allow for decreased wound visibility without trauma or excess pressure on site because visible skin lesions may cause distress for child or adolescent and impact self-esteem around peers.

ROUTINE CHECKUP 1

1. The nurse would describe a lesion that is a flat brown mole <1 cm in diameter noted on a client's body as a _____.

Answer:

2. A toddler has a deep laceration contaminated with dirt and sand. Before closing the wound, the nurse should irrigate with:
   a. Povidone-iodine
   b. Alcohol
   c. Sterile saline
   d. Hydrogen peroxide

Answer:

PSORIASIS

What Went Wrong?

Psoriasis is a skin overgrowth and flaking of unknown origin that may be triggered by stress and has a possible hereditary association. Seldom occurs in children <6 years of age.

Signs and Symptoms

- Red skin patches with coarse scales over extremities and trunk, scalp, and face
- Pruritus (itching)

Test Results

- History and physical examination reveal skin flakes and possible itching.

Treatment

- Sunlight or ultraviolet light exposure
- Topical corticosteroids
- Psoralen-ultraviolet A (PUVA)
- Tar ointment
- Trihydroxy-anthracene
- Emollients to relieve dry skin
- Keratolytic agents to remove skin overgrowth
- Humidifier to increase moisture

Nursing Interventions

- Instruct client and family to follow measures to maintain moisture for skin.
- Explain that psoriasis is not contagious and cannot be transferred from person to person.

SCABIES

What Went Wrong?

Infestation by scabies mite occurs after exposure and an impregnated female scabies mite deposits eggs in the epidermis of the skin.

Signs and Symptoms

- Pruritus from the inflammatory response.
- Deep scratches from the itching.
- Maculopapular lesions in involved areas.
- Infants have eczema-like lesions as well as papules or vesicles.
- Lesions may be located on hands and wrists (child <2 years of age) or feet and ankles (child >2 years of age).

Nursing alert **A child who is mentally challenged or has difficulty communicating may not be able to explain the discomfort; thus examination of the skin and anticipatory treatment for itching may be needed.**

Test Results

- Microscopic examination of a scraping from the lesion

Treatment

- Treatment with a scabicide (permethrin 5% cream [Elimite]).
- Ivermectin, an oral medication, may be given if topical medication is not effective (for children >5 years of age).
- Antibiotics may be given for secondary infections.
- Members of the family who have been exposed may need to be treated.

Nursing Interventions

- Apply cream to all skin surfaces being careful to use gloves.
- Teach family and older child/adolescent the importance of following the prescribed regimen:
  - Avoid applying cream after hot bath and avoid contact with eyes.
  - Leave cream on skin for full 8 to 14 hours.
  - Apply cream under nails.
  - Explain that itching may persist after mites are killed because skin is still raw and needs to heal.
  - All clothes and bed linens must be washed in hot water and dried at high-heat settings.

LYME DISEASE (TICK BITE)

What Went Wrong?

This tick-borne condition is caused by a spirochete (*Borrelia burgdorferi*) that enters the bloodstream through tick saliva and feces when the victim is bitten by a deer tick. The tick must feed for up to 72 hours to transmit the bacteria. Although most will remove the tick within this time frame, some will be unaware of the bite.

Signs and Symptoms

- Bull's-eye rash (erythema migrans) at the site of the bite for 3 weeks following the bite.
- In stage I, from 3 days to a month after bite:
  - May note a small erythematous papule that progresses to larger raised bordered lesion (erythema chronicum migrans [ECM]) commonly found in the axilla, thigh, or groin.
  - May report warmth, burning, or itching at the site of lesion.
  - Multiple small secondary lesions may be noted on body except palms and soles.
  - Systemic symptoms may be noted such as fatigue, anorexia, fever, headache, stiff neck, malaise, lymphadenopathy, splenomegaly, conjunctivitis, sore throat, abdominal pain, and cough.
  - Generalized aches.
- Stage II occurs 2 to 11 weeks following stage I lesion and involves neurologic, cardiac, and musculoskeletal symptoms:
  - Headache is an early symptom.
  - Later symptoms include cranial nerve palsy, peripheral radiculoneuritis, or meningoencephalitis.
  - Cardiac symptoms may include atrioventricular heart block, syncope, palpitations, chest pain, dyspnea, and bradycardia.
- Stage III is a late stage with musculoskeletal discomfort:
  - Tendon, muscle, and synovia pain that develops months to years after initial bite.

• Chronic arthritis with occasional joint swelling, particularly knees with exacerbations and remissions.
• Deafness, keratitis, or encephalopathy may be noted in late stages.

➌ Test Results

◐ History and physical data is supportive of the diagnosis.
◐ Serum: Elevated IgM antibody.
◐ Lyme titers: *B. burgdorferi* present.
◐ Enzyme-linked immunosorbent assay (ELISA): Identifies antibodies to *B. burgdorferi*.
◐ Western blot test: Identifies antibodies to *B. burgdorferi*.
◐ Serologic testing (results could be inaccurate; useful in late stages):
  • By indirect immunofluorescence (IFA)
  • By enzyme immunoassay (EIA)

➍ Treatments

◐ A vaccine can be given against Lyme disease for high-risk persons.
◐ Administer corticosteroids to reduce inflammation.
◐ Maintain fluid and electrolyte balance to prevent seizures.
◐ Antibiotics often prevent development of stage II:
  • Doxycycline (Vibramycin) or amoxicillin (Amoxil), for children >8 years of age.
  • Amoxicillin (Amoxil) or penicillin for children <8 years of age.
  • Cefuroxime (Ceftin) or erythromycin (E-Mycin) if child is allergic to penicillin.
  • Tetracycline (Sumycin).
  • Administer ceftriaxone IM or IV.

Nursing alert Avoid administering tetracycline (Sumycin) in children <8 years of age because this medication discolors the teeth.

➎ Nursing Interventions

◐ Assess closely for ticks on skin.
◐ Monitor for nodules or other symptoms of Lyme disease.
◐ Assess closely for risk factors for tick bite and Lyme disease:
  • History of time in high tick areas (northeastern and north central United States)
◐ Educate parents and children regarding the condition and the protective measures to avoid tick bite:
  • Wear light-colored long-sleeved shirts and pants.
  • Avoid grass and shrubbery; walk in clear trails.
  • Use appropriate insect repellant.
  • Inspect pets and maintain flea and tick collar or treatments.

- Check bare skin for ticks, including neck, armpits, scalp, and groin area.
- Remove any ticks, being careful to get all portions of the tick:
  - Grasp tick close to skin with tweezers, trying not to squeeze or crush the tick.
  - Pull tick in a steady motion, straighten up with steady pressure.
  - Use a sterile needle to remove any remaining parts and then clean the site.
  - Wash hands with soap and disinfectant immediately after removing the tick.

Impetigo

What Went Wrong?

Impetigo is a superficial skin infection caused most often by *Staphylococcus aureus*. Children who come in contact with infectious persons are at highest risk for spread of the infection. Commonly found in toddlers or preschoolers.

Signs and Symptoms

- May begin with red macule that becomes a vesicular lesion.
- Bullous lesions may be noted in neonatal form.
- Lesions found on body surface, usually trunk, extremities, face, perineum, or buttocks.
- Lesions vary in size from millimeters to several centimeters.
- Lesions often spread peripherally from one skin area to another without precautions.
- Lesions rupture easily and leave a red moist eroded area.
- Minimal crusting in neonates.
- Honey-colored crusting may be noted in older infants and children.
- May be noted in addition to eczema.
- Pruritus (itching) often noted.

Test Results

Culture may be performed and commonly reveals *S. aureus* infection.

Treatment

- Isolation until treatment instituted
- Systemic antibiotics: Oral or intravenous if severe lesion
- Topical bactericidal ointment such as mupirocin (Bactroban)
- Burrow solution (1:20 solution) compress to skin to remove crusts, debris

Nursing Intervention

- Teach child and family the importance of handwashing and not touching lesions to minimize the spread of infection to other areas of the body or to other persons.

◐ Explain that lesions often heal without scaring if no secondary infection occurs.

    ◐ Teach child and family to apply ointment and compress as ordered.

ROUTINE CHECKUP 2

1. Impetigo, without secondary infection, ordinarily results in which of the following?
   a. No scarring
   b. Keloid scars
   c. Atrophic scars
   d. Depressed scars

Answer:

2. Explain why Lyme disease is not a contagious from one child to another.

Answer:

BURN INJURY

🔺 What Went Wrong?

Burns are injuries to the skin caused by heat, friction, radiation, chemicals, or electricity. Damage to skin varies based on intensity of exposure (degree of heat, radiation, etc.), length of exposure, and source of burn. Burns may be described based on level of penetration ranging from superficial burn (first degree) impacting the epidermis to a deeper burn (second degree/partial thickness) impacting the dermis to a severe burn (third degree/full thickness) that penetrates through all layers of skin to the underlying subcutaneous tissue/fat. The most severe fourth-degree burns, also called full thickness, involve underlying muscle, fascia, and bone. Burns are also categorized by the amount of surface area impacted with children experiencing greater distress than adults with the same percentage of surface area damage.

    Children <10 years of age most commonly experience flame injury from playing with fire (such as playing with matches or cigarette lighters) or scald injury (burn from hot liquid) secondary to hot water in bathtub by error or due to child abuse. Adolescents commonly experience flame or electrical burn injury secondary to high-risk behavior such as dealing with fireworks or climbing utility poles.

Signs and Symptoms

- First-degree burns:
  - Pain due to nerve-ending irritation; worse with touch
  - Erythema (redness)
- Second-degree burns:
  - Pain from damaged epidermis and dermis
  - Red clear fluid-filled blisters
- Third-degree burns:
  - Color ranges from red to tan, white, charred brown, or black with a dry leathery appearance.
  - Absence of sensation.
  - Incapable of regenerating skin.
- Fourth-degree burns:
  - Brown, black charred muscle, fascia, and bone visible.
  - Wound is dry, dull, and leathery in appearance.

Nursing alert **While the burn injury appears most acute, additional injury, such as smoke inhalation resulting in airway constriction or wounds resulting in excessive bleeding, may be life threatening and need immediate attention.**

Test Results

- Body surface area determination is critical in determining treatment.
- A rule of 9's measure may be used with specific percentages of surface area designated for body part involved.

Nursing alert **Pediatric scales vary based on the age of the infant or child. Consider child size as well. If a 7-year-old is small and the size of a 5-year-old, use the scale for the smaller child.**

- Pulse oximetry: Measures oxygen saturation to determine oxygenation problem due to damage to airways or lungs from smoke or superheated air.
- Pulmonary function tests: Determine lung damage that may impair respiration.

Treatments

- Immediate:
  - Stop the burning.
    - Remove the source:
      - Flame—cover and smother the fire.
      - Hot liquid/chemical—apply cool water to dilute.

- For electrical burn—turn off power or use wood or nonconductive material to separate child from electricity.
  ○ Apply cool water.

Nursing alert **Do not use ice!**

- Cover the wound with a clean cloth.
- Remove burned clothing to remove heat and clear the wound for covering.
- Remove jewelry, particularly rings, which restrict circulation with edema.
○ Assess for airway and breathing and provide rescue breathing if indicated.
○ Keep victim warm.
○ Follow-up management:
  - Begin intravenous therapy (for burns ≥15 to 20% total body surface area [TBSA]).
  - Fluid volume lost from open wound is replaced using formula to calculate.
  - Maintain fluid infusion to keep urine output at 30 mL/hour or more [1 to 2 mL/kg in children weighing <66 pounds (30 kg)].
○ Maintain stable airway (intubate if signs of respiratory distress noted, drowsiness, tachypnea, shortness of breath, wheezing, decreased oxygen levels).
○ Begin oxygen therapy.
○ Pain management:
  - Analgesia, particularly prior to dressing change
  - Fentanyl and midazolam (Versed)
  - Patient-controlled analgesia (PCA) for older child
○ Burn wound care:
  - Clean wound with ordered cleanser.
  - Dress wound with antimicrobial ointment and gauze:
    ○ Acticoat
    ○ Adaptic/Aquaphor
    ○ Scarlet red
    ○ Xeroflo
    ○ Xeroform
    ○ Silver nitrate 0.5% ($AgNO_3$)
    ○ Silver sulfadiazine 1.0%
    ○ Mafenide acetate 10% (Sulfamylon)
    ○ Bacitracin
  - Occlusive dressing (hydrocolloid) if ordered to promote proper healing.
  - Debride wound with hydrotherapy (soak in tub) or dressing change that strips away dead skin and secretions.

- Cover site with biologic or synthetic skin coverings, or artificial skin (Integra) prior to permanent skin graft.
- Skin grafts: Allografts from other person (homografts), xenografts (heterografts) pigskin, or autografts from another part of the client's body.

Nursing Interventions

- Monitor and record strict intake and output to maintain fluid volume and prevent fluid overload.
- Assess nutrition status and supplement with snacks as indicated.
- Monitor for signs of paralytic ileus (absent bowel sounds).
- Monitor for signs of infection and report.
- Prevent hypothermia: Reduce heat loss, minimize exposure to drafts with dressings and items such as warming blankets, radiant warmer, and heat shields.
- Provide pain medication as needed for comfort, particularly before wound care.
- If skin graft surgery is performed, assist through operative process:
  - Prepare donor graft site prior to surgery.
  - Monitor both donor and graft site for infection.
- Provide support to child and family:
  - Explain all procedures.
  - Emphasize the need to maintain sterile procedure to prevent infection.
  - Include family as much in care as possible:
    ○ Teach caregiver to change dressing as ordered.
    ○ Instruct caregiver to monitor for signs of infection.
- Monitor growth and development and support continued progress for the child or adolescent.
- Support child and family through concerns about appearance and possible plastic surgery in future.
- Discuss preventive measures to avoid future burn injury.

? FINAL CHECKUP

1. The nurse would record the name of an elevated circumscribed skin lesion that is <1 cm in diameter and filled with serous fluid noted on her client as which type of lesion?
   a. Cyst
   b. Papule
   c. Pustule
   d. Vesicle

2. **When giving instructions to a parent whose child has scabies, what should the school nurse include?**
   a. Treat all family members if symptoms develop.
   b. Be prepared for symptoms to last 2 to 3 weeks.
   c. Carefully treat only those areas where there is a rash.
   d. Notify practitioner so an antibiotic can be prescribed.

3. **Fluid replacement should be determined by which most reliable guide for an infant with burns?**
   a. Absence of thirst
   b. Decreased hematocrit level
   c. Increased serous drainage from burn wound
   d. Urinary output of 1 to 2 mL/kg of body weight per hour

4. **What condition does not require family teaching regarding control of the spread of disease to the caregiver or another child?**
   a. Impetigo
   b. Lyme disease
   c. Scabies
   d. Pustules

5. **A nurse working in a pediatric burn unit is caring for a 10-year-old client with full-thickness burns over 25% of the body. The laboratory tests ordered to assess the client's fluid and electrolyte balance are reviewed. Which laboratory value should the nurse report to the physician immediately?**
   a. Arterial pH: 7.4
   b. Hematocrit: 42%
   c. Serum sodium: 137mEq/L
   d. Serum potassium: 6.8 mEq/L

6. **The nurse can explain to a family that Lyme disease is which of the following?**
   a. An nonpreventable condition that affects some children
   b. Easily treated with oral antibiotics in stages I, II, and III
   c. Caused by a spirochete that enters the skin through a tick bite
   d. The result of ingesting soil containing the mycotic spores that cause the disease

7. **What finding might indicate a need for additional fluids therapy for a small child with burn injury?**
   a. Absence of thirst
   b. Elevated hematocrit
   c. Decreased burn wound drainage
   d. Urinary output 5 mL/kg of body weight per hour

8. **What type of healing occurs with a surgical wound with minimal scarring?**
   a. Healing by fourth-degree intention
   b. Healing by tertiary intention
   c. Healing by secondary intention
   d. Healing by primary intention

9. **A child with an open wound might receive wound care with which of the following solutions?**
   a. Normal saline flush
   b. Povidone iodine liquid
   c. Alcohol
   d. Acetaminophen solution

10. **A family of a child with psoriasis is most likely to encounter what problems?**
    a. Difficulty keeping the skin dry enough to avoid the condition
    b. Problems preventing other children from catching the condition
    c. Concern with facial lesions causing permanent disfigurement from the condition
    d. Inability to block exposure to sunlight that results in a worsening of the condition

ANSWERS

Routine checkup 1
   1. Macule
   2. c

Routine checkup 2
   1. a
   2. Lyme disease is spread through the saliva from a tick and is not transmitted from person to person.

Final checkup

1. d	2. b	3. d	4. b
5. d	6. c	7. b	8. d
9. a	10. c		

Final Exam

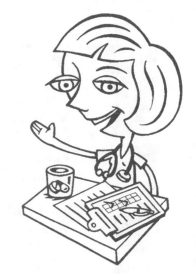

? FINAL CHECKUP

1. **Trey, 11 years old, has been classified as belonging to a high-risk population. Which of the following are indicators for this?**
   a. Trey's father has been unemployed for over a year.
   b. Trey has a nutritional preference for candy.
   c. Trey's 15-year-old sister is dating and unmarried.
   d. All of the above.

2. **Nurses working with high-risk pediatric clients should do which of the following?**
   a. Address community resource needs prior to discharge
   b. Perform community assessment to identify factors that may contribute to child's illness
   c. Coordinate with community agencies to provide comprehensive care to clients and their families
   d. All of the above

3. **Nurses working with diverse populations should do which of the following?**
   a. Support cultural norms as long as they do not interfere with medical care
   b. Discourage cultural rituals and taboos that involve idols or other objects
   c. Seek to actively remove the child from the cultural environment
   d. None of the above

4. **The caseworker, Mrs. McDonald, informed the nurse that all African American children are usually overweight. What does her comment show?**
   a. Open communication between the caregiver and community support
   b. Cultural preference
   c. Stereotyping
   d. b and c only

5. **Which of the following are examples of cultural norms?**
   a. Nuclear families consist of a father, mother, and children.
   b. Only the grandmother can decide what type of care the child is allowed to receive.
   c. Male members of the family must be addressed with regard to patient care.
   d. All of the above.

6. **Lilly, age 7, is being raised by her 19-year-old twin siblings and her aunt. When she is admitted in renal failure the nurse should quickly determine what issue?**
   a. What type of house Lilly lives in
   b. How far the home is from the hospital
   c. Who can assist Lilly with her daily bath?
   d. Who is Lilly's legal custodial guardian?

7. **Growth and development can be categorized in which of these ways?**
   a. Cognitive
   b. Physical
   c. Spiritual
   d. a and b

8. **Sue was born in 1999. What is her chronological age in 2009?**
   a. Based on her physical size
   b. Dependent on her adaptive capabilities
   c. Ten years old
   d. Undetermined

9. **An assessment of a child's language and social skills and her emotional development are typically part of which of these categories?**
   a. Oral stage assessment
   b. Growth and development charting
   c. Sensory assessment
   d. All of the above

10. **A growth and development plan for 2-year-old Timmy might include which of the following?**
    a. Teaching him using simple one- and two-word phrases
    b. Creating activities with colorful materials he can touch and play with
    c. Allowing him to hold his own bottle
    d. Encouraging his efforts to crawl

11. **Which of these are three of the leading growth and development theorists?**
    a. Jung, Freud, and Mendelson
    b. Piaget, Jung, and Erickson
    c. Freud, Erickson, and Piaget
    d. None of the above

12. **Freudian theory is based on which of the following?**
    a. Ego
    b. Id
    c. Superego
    d. All of the above

13. **Coordination of physical experiences such as touch with visual experiences is the basis of what age/stage of development?**
    a. 6 months, oral
    b. 2 years, sensorimotor
    c. 18 months, social
    d. None of the above

14. **The early childhood stage of development is associated with which of these characteristics?**
    a. Bladder control
    b. Conscience development
    c. Short attention spans
    d. All of the above

15. **Beth is 6 years old. She is bed-wetting, sucking her thumb, and reluctant to be away from her mother. Her developmental stage is associated with what chronological age group?**
    a. 2 to 4 years
    b. 18 months
    c. 6 to 12 months
    d. 0 to 6 months

16. **In the anal stage of development, what nursing intervention is a primary focus?**
    a. Teaching handwashing
    b. Providing puzzles for play
    c. Building self-esteem
    d. None of the above

17. **Which of the following are possible signs of developmental delays in a 2- to 6-year-old child?**
    a. Weight gain of 5 pounds in a year
    b. Inability to hop on one foot
    c. Friendliness to strangers
    d. All of the above

18. **When assessing the growth and development of a school-aged child, which of the following might be noted?**
    a. Appearance of larger more adult-like teeth
    b. Peer groups lack importance
    c. Inability to express ideas with word or sentences
    d. b and c

19. **Erikson's theory of development for the school-aged child includes which of the following key nursing care initiatives?**
    a. Encourage individual play
    b. Protect against accidental injury
    c. Discourage questions regarding sex
    d. a and c

20. **What is a learning disability characterized by letter reversals and writing difficulties called?**
    a. Enuresis
    b. Dyslexia
    c. Dysgraphia
    d. b and c

21. **Enuresis can be caused by which of the following?**
    a. Physiological developmental delays
    b. Social developmental delays
    c. Neuromotor developmental delays
    d. All of the above

22. **Liz is moody, developing acne and experiencing menstruation. Most of the time she stays in her room and talks on the phone. What is her likely age?**
    a. 6 to 8 years
    b. 7 to 10 years
    c. 13 to 18 years
    d. None of the above

23. **Lori, age 16, has been eating and sleeping poorly for months; and recently she gave away her prize collection of Barbie dolls. How would you describe her?**
    a. Bored
    b. Suicidal
    c. Hyperactive
    d. Anorexic

24. **Age-appropriate care includes which of the following?**
    a. A knowledge and consideration of a child's developmental stage
    b. A recognition that illness does not impact a child's growth and development
    c. An understanding that teaching seldom reduces injury in children
    d. All of the above

25. **It is important that a child with acute streptococcal pharyngitis be treated with antibiotics to prevent which of these conditions?**
    a. Osteogenic sarcoma
    b. Diabetes insipidus
    c. Nephrotic syndrome
    d. Scarlet fever

26. **What condition might be suspected if a child presents with a chronic cough, no retractions, but diffuse wheezing during the expiratory phase of respiration?**
    a. Asthma
    b. Pneumonia
    c. Croup
    d. Foreign body aspiration

27. **An assessment of a child with cancer includes but is not limited to which of the following?**
    a. Symptomatic assessment
    b. Physical assessment
    c. Diagnostic assessment
    d. All of the above

28. **A plan of care for a child with cancer should include which of the following?**
    a. Avoiding pain medication
    b. Stabilization of nutritional intake
    c. Encouraging focus on changes in the body
    d. All of the above

29. **When explaining cancer treatment protocol to parents, which of these responses is appropriate?**
    a. Child should be included in teaching as age permits.
    b. Parents should be told to continue with regular immunizations.
    c. Parents should be encouraged to give aspirin to the child for pain.
    d. b and c only.

30. **Hair loss, constipation, and numbness of the extremities may all result from the effects of which of these situations?**
    a. Dietary deficits due to anorexia
    b. Neurotoxic chemotherapy agents
    c. Mucosal ulcerations
    d. Pain medication given by patient-controlled analgesia (PCA)

31. **The priority care need(s) of families of newly diagnosed children with cancer include which of the following?**
    a. Encouraging weight loss during chemotherapy
    b. Referral for grief counseling to prepare for death
    c. Maintaining activity within the child's tolerance
    d. All of the above

32. **Which therapy uses radiation to kill cancerous cells?**
    a. Chemotherapy
    b. Radiotherapy
    c. Aromatherapy
    d. Laser therapy

33. **Immobility, particularly after surgery, can result in which most potentially life-threatening complication?**
    a. Urinary stasis
    b. Deep vein thrombosis
    c. Pressure ulcer
    d. Muscle atrophy

34. **An oncology nurse is planning care for a client who is scheduled to receive chemotherapy. When developing the plan of care for this client, which nursing diagnosis should have the highest priority?**
    a. Alteration in family processes
    b. Self-esteem disturbance
    c. Potential for infection
    d. Impaired skin integrity

35. **A woman who was diagnosed with gestational diabetes mellitus tells you she is prepared to take insulin injections for the rest of her life. What is your best response?**
    a. You'll need to balance your diet with appropriate amounts of insulin.
    b. It is good that you are prepared to deal with your disorder.
    c. You will recover following pregnancy.
    d. You will recover following pregnancy; however, you are at risk for developing type 2 diabetes mellitus later in life.

36. **A child arrived in the ED with fruity smell, constant urination, hyperventilation, agitation, and sluggishness. What is your best response?**
    a. Administer short-acting insulin
    b. Administer long-acting insulin
    c. Administer a glucagon injection
    d. Administered 4 ounces of fruit juice

37. **The mother of a child who has been diagnosed with Cushing syndrome asks why her child has developed a moon face. What is your best response?**
    a. Because the child has a sleep disturbance.
    b. Your child has gained weight.
    c. Excess cortisol production.
    d. Because of delayed wound healing.

38. **Parent of a 1-month-old diagnosed with congenital hypothyroidism tells you that she wants to hold off treatment for a few months to see if the child will outgrow this disorder. What is your best response?**
    a. You should discuss this approach with your health-care provider.
    b. That's fine but the child must begin treatment within 6 months.
    c. Treatment must begin within 3 months of age to ensure normal development.
    d. I'll inform the health-care provider about your decision.

39. A patient being treated for galactosemia is concerned that her son still vomits and has diarrhea although she stopped giving him milk. What is your best response?

    a. He probably has a viral infection.

    b. Is he eating cakes, cookies, or pies?

    c. Ask your health-care provider to change your son's diet.

    d. Is he drinking soda?

40. A mother of a child diagnosed with Graves disease asks why her son sweats so much. What is your best response?

    a. Graves disease is caused by an abnormally low amount of thyroid hormone. The thyroid controls the body's metabolism. Too much thyroid hormone decreases the metabolic rate, which among other signs increases sweat production.

    b. Graves disease is caused by an abnormally low amount of thyroid hormone. The thyroid controls the body's metabolism. Too much thyroid hormone increases the metabolic rate, which among other signs increases sweat production.

    c. Graves disease is caused by an abnormally high amount of thyroid hormone. The thyroid controls the body's metabolism. Too much thyroid hormone increases the metabolic rate, which among other signs increases sweat production.

    d. Excess thyroid hormone raises the metabolic rate.

41. A parent of a child who is diagnosed and being treated for galactosemia asks why her child has a skin rash, diarrhea, and is lethargic. What is your best response?

    a. These are signs of phenylalanine deficiency caused by too much phenylalanine in the diet. Let's ask the health-care provider to adjust your child's diet.

    b. These are signs of phenylalanine deficiency.

    c. These are signs of phenylalanine deficiency caused by too little phenylalanine in the diet. Let's ask the health-care provider to adjust your child's diet.

    d. Has your child received all his vaccinations?

42. A parent whose child has recently returned from surgery to treat Graves disease tells you that her son's cheek twitches every time she kisses him on the cheek. What is your best response?

    a. This is a muscle spasm and a sign of low calcium, which occurs sometimes following surgery. I'll notify the health-care provider immediately.

    b. This is a sign of low calcium, which occurs sometimes following surgery. I'll notify the health-care provider immediately.

    c. This is a muscle spasm and a sign of low calcium, which occurs sometimes following surgery. I'll notify the health-care provider immediately. The health-care provider is likely to adjust your son's medication.

    d. This is the Chvostek sign, which occurs sometimes following surgery. I'll notify the health-care provider immediately.

43. **A 2-year-old arrives in the ED with rapid rise in body temperature of 102.2°F that is increasing. What should you prepare for?**
    a. Febrile seizure presenting as an akinetic seizure
    b. Febrile seizure presenting as an atonic seizure
    c. Febrile seizure presenting as a tonic-clonic seizure
    d. Epilepticus seizure presenting as a tonic-clonic seizure

44. **A parent of a child who is diagnosed with meningitis asks why her child is experiencing nausea and vomiting. What is your best response?**
    a. Nausea and vomiting is due to increased intracranial pressure.
    b. The membrane that surrounds the brain is inflamed. The inflammation is causing an increased pressure on the brain inducing nausea and vomiting.
    c. The membrane that surrounds the brain is inflamed. The inflammation is causing an increased pressure on the brain inducing nausea and vomiting. Don't worry. Your child will be walking out of here by the end of the week.
    d. Nausea and vomiting is due to increased intracranial pressure. Don't worry. Your child will be walking out of here by the end of the week.

45. **The mother of a child diagnosed with encephalitis tells you that the health-care provider said there was demyelination of the nerve fibers. She looks puzzled. What is your best response?**
    a. Think of nerves as an electrical cord. And like an electrical cord, nerves are contained within insulation to prevent interference with nerve impulses. The insulation around the nerve is called myelin. In encephalitis, portions of the myelin are removed by the infection, which is called demyelination. The body replaces the myelin once the infection resolves.
    b. Think of nerves as an electrical cord. And like an electrical cord, nerves are contained within an insulation to prevent interference with nerve impulses. The insulation around the nerve is called myelin. In encephalitis, portions of the myelin are removed by the infection, which is called demyelination.
    c. Nerves are contained within insulation to prevent interference with nerve impulses. The insulation around the nerve is called demyelination. The body replaces the myelin once the infection resolves.
    d. Nerves are contained within an insulation to prevent interference with nerve impulses. The insulation around the nerve is called myelination. The body replaces the myelin once the infection resolves.

46. **What influences the recovery of a child who has Reye syndrome?**
    a. Recovery is related to the child's age.
    b. Recovery is related to secondary disorders.
    c. Recovery is related to the quantity of aspirin taken by the child.
    d. Recovery is related to the degree of cerebral edema.

47. **The parent of a 10-year-old said her son experienced an upset stomach with the flu so she has been giving him Pepto-Bismol and it seems to work fine. She made certain to mention that she gave him acetaminophen rather than aspirin. What is your best response?**
    a. Don't give him too much Pepto-Bismol because it will constipate him.
    b. Don't give him Pepto-Bismol because it contains aspirin.
    c. Don't give him Pepto-Bismol because it contains aspirin. A viral infection and aspirin are linked to Reye syndrome.
    d. Don't give him Pepto-Bismol. Give him the children's Pepto-Bismol because it contains the right dose for a child.

48. **You are in the delivery room and you notice a newborn with a tuft of hair in the sacral area. What disorder should you suspect?**
    a. Spinal bifida cystica meningocele
    b. Spinal bifida occulta
    c. Spinal bifida cystica myelomeningocele
    d. Anencephaly

49. **A 4-year-old over the past few weeks lost the ability to speak and he is showing slowing mental activity in addition to personality changes. The health-care provider suspects that the child has a brain tumor. Where might this tumor be located?**
    a. Occipital lobe
    b. Parietal lobe
    c. Frontal lobe
    d. Temporal lobe

50. **When entering the room of a 5-year-old who has cerebral palsy, you overhear the family speaking about placing the child in a home for the mentally disabled. What is your best response?**
    a. Tell the family that the case manager will help them find the right home.
    b. Asks if you might have a word with the family in the conference room. Tell them that the child has normal intelligence regardless of his uncontrollable movements.
    c. Tell the family that the social worker will help them find the right home.
    d. Tell them that the child has normal intelligence regardless of his uncontrollable movements.

51. **The parent of a child who is diagnosed with Hirschsprung disease is concerned that following surgery her son will be stool incontinent. What is your best response?**
    a. This is age related and your son will grow out of it.
    b. This is an adverse side effect of Hirschsprung disease.
    c. This is an adverse side effect of the surgery.
    d. Return of anal sphincter control and complete continence can take months to develop.

52. **Which of the following conditions would you find in a child who is diagnosed with pyloric stenosis?**
    a. Metabolic acidosis
    b. Metabolic alkalosis
    c. Respiratory acidosis
    d. Respiratory alkalosis

53. **Why would you give a pacifier to an infant who had surgery for a tracheoesophageal fistula?**
    a. Keeps the infant quiet.
    b. Soothes the infant.
    c. Sucking the pacifier helps prepare the infant for speech.
    d. The pacifier trains the infant to suck for nourishment.

54. **A father of a boy diagnosed with ulcerative colitis wonders why his son is anemic. What is your best response?**
    a. The youngster is eating too much junk food.
    b. You are not providing a proper diet.
    c. Chronic bloody diarrhea as a result of ulcerative colitis causes a decrease in hemoglobin, which causes the anemic condition.
    d. Chronic bloody vomiting as a result of ulcerative colitis causes a decrease in hemoglobin, which causes the anemic condition.

55. **Which of the following conditions would be found in a child who is diagnosed with ulcerative colitis?**
    a. Metabolic acidosis
    b. Metabolic alkalosis
    c. Respiratory acidosis
    d. Respiratory alkalosis

56. **A father of a boy diagnosed with ulcerative colitis asks why he must keep a stool diary for his son. What is your best response?**
    a. To identify irritating foods that exacerbate ulcerative colitis
    b. To measure the child's output volume accurately
    c. To estimate the amount of water in the stool
    d. To identify if your son is taking his medication

57. **The mother of a child who is diagnosed with volvulus wonders what could have caused this disorder. What is your best response?**
    a. Ingesting a foreign substance
    b. Ingesting too much starch
    c. Ingesting too much sugar
    d. Not ingesting enough water

58. **The mother of a child who underwent an appendectomy asks why her daughter must wait until bowel sounds return before she can have food. What is your best response?**

   a. Before giving your daughter any food we must be sure that the food can move through her intestine.

   b. Bowel sounds are the result of muscles in the intestine contracting. This is necessary for food to move through the intestine. The anesthetic from the appendectomy slows muscle contractions of the intestine. Muscle contractions will return when the anesthetic wears off and bowel sounds return.

   c. Before giving your daughter any food we must be sure that the food can move through her intestine. This happens by muscles in the intestine contracting, which causes bowel sounds to occur. The anesthetic from the appendectomy slows muscle contractions of the intestine. Muscle contractions will return when the anesthetic wears off. We'll know when this happens when the bowel sounds return.

   d. The anesthetic reduces peristalsis and therefore food can't pass through the intestine until bowel sounds return.

59. **What would you do if you received an order to administer Kayexalate to a child who has glomerulonephritis?**

   a. Question the order because the child's kidneys are not functionally normally.

   b. Administer the medication as order.

   c. Assess the child's potassium level before administering the medication.

   d. Administer the medication only if the child's potassium level is low; otherwise there is a risk of cardiac arrest.

60. **A parent of a child who is recently diagnosed with a kidney disorder asks you why the health-care provider tests her son's blood urea nitrogen (BUN) and creatinine. What is your best response?**

   a. The health-care provider measures BUN and creatinine to determine if your son's kidneys are working. BUN and creatinine are waste products in the blood and removed from the blood by the kidneys. If the kidneys are functioning, then the BUN and creatinine levels in the blood are normal. If they are not functioning, then these levels are abnormal.

   b. The health-care provider measures BUN and creatinine to determine if your son's kidneys are working.

   c. I'll ask your health-care provider to explain these tests.

   d. The health-care provider orders these and other tests to determine your son's health.

61. **The mother of a child who has been diagnosed with nephrotic syndrome asks why you are administering Albuminar to her son. What is your best response?**

    a. Albumin is released by the kidneys into the urine resulting in decreased albumin in blood because the glomerular filtration membrane is injured causing a fluid switch and edema because of the decreased albumin in the blood. Albuminar replaces the albumin.

    b. Your son is experiencing a fluid imbalance caused by nephrotic syndrome. Your son's kidneys are releasing a chemical called albumin that helps maintain fluid balance. Albuminar is a replacement for albumin and restores fluid balance.

    c. It is best that you ask your health-care provider to explain the medication.

    d. I'll ask a more experienced nurse to explain once I administer the medication.

62. **A new nurse is about to palpate a child who has Wilms tumor. What is your best response?**

    a. Always observe the site before palpating.

    b. Don't palpate the site of the tumor. Palpation can rupture the tumor capsule resulting in the tumor metastasizing quickly.

    c. Always explain the procedure to the patient.

    d. Review the disorder before visiting the patient.

63. **A mother of an 8-year-old is curious why her daughter has frequent urinary tract infections. What is your best response?**

    a. You probably want to remind your daughter about proper hygiene when toileting because a urinary tract infection is commonly caused by *Escherichia coli* entering the urinary tract. *E. coli* is found in stool.

    b. Mention this to the health-care provider.

    c. Urinary tract infection is commonly caused when *E. coli* enters the urinary tract.

    d. Your child has a kidney infection.

64. **The parents of a recently diagnosed child with Wilms tumor asks for a definition of stage III of the disorder? What is your best response?**

    a. The tumor has metastasized to lymph nodes and the abdomen.

    b. The tumor is contained in one kidney.

    c. The tumor has metastasized to the bone, liver, lung, and brain.

    d. The tumor has metastasized to both kidneys.

65. **A parent of a child who is diagnosed with chronic renal failure asks why this condition seemed to develop so suddenly. What is your best response?**

    a. It is best that you ask your health-care provider.

    b. The symptoms usually go unnoticed because they resemble a simple head cold.

    c. The symptoms were there but you didn't notice them.

    d. Chronic renal failure is asymptomatic until kidney function declines 20% at which time the child becomes lethargic and fatigued.

66. **The health-care provider ordered amoxicillin, phenazopyridine, and aceta-minophen for a child diagnosed with pyelonephritis. What is your best response?**
    a. Question the order for acetaminophen because it causes an adverse reaction with amoxicillin.
    b. Question the order for amoxicillin.
    c. Tell the child and the family that phenazopyridine causes orange-colored urine.
    d. Question the order for phenazopyridine because it causes an adverse reaction with amoxicillin.

67. **A mother brings her 9-year-old boy to the ED with an ankle injury. She tells you he broke his ankle. What is your best response?**
    a. Suspect child abuse.
    b. Assess for compartment syndrome.
    c. Most ankle injuries in children are sprains; however, the health-care provider typically orders a radiograph to rule out a fracture.
    d. Prepare to move the child to the ICU as a result of Compartment syndrome.

68. **The parents of a 1-year-old diagnosed with type I osteogenesis imperfecta didn't fully understand the nature of the disorder. What is your best response?**
    a. Your health-care provider is the best one to explain this to you.
    b. Type I, the most common, occurs when there is severe bone deformity and numerous fractures resulting in respiratory problems at or shortly after birth.
    c. Type I, the most common, occurs because bones fracture easily before puberty.
    d. Type I, the most common, occurs when fractures present at birth healed.

69. **The parent of a child diagnosed with Legg-Calvé-Perthes disease is fearful that her child will have a limp for the rest of his life. What is your best response?**
    a. Your child's body will adjust for the limp.
    b. Your child will partially recover after the disease has run its course.
    c. Your child will fully recover after the disease has run its course.
    d. Surgery can be performed to minimize the limp.

70. **Parents of a child who is diagnosed with talipes ask how this disorder is treated. What is your best response?**
    a. A splint, cast, or special shoes might be applied and possible surgery.
    b. A 10-day antibiotic therapy will return child to normal.
    c. Your child will fully recover after the disorder has run its course.
    d. A daily routine of range-of-motion exercises is a common treatment for this disorder.

71. **Parents of a child who was diagnosed with polyarticular juvenile rheumatoid arthritis wonder how this differs from juvenile rheumatoid arthritis. How should you respond?**
    a. This is a type of juvenile rheumatoid arthritis that affects fewer than five joints and might exhibit inflammation of the iris without joint symptoms.
    b. This is a type of juvenile rheumatoid arthritis that affects the entire body resulting in high fevers that suddenly drop to normal.
    c. This is a type of juvenile rheumatoid arthritis that has a rash that suddenly appears and disappears.
    d. This is a type of juvenile rheumatoid arthritis that affects the small joints of the hands and weight-bearing joints.

72. **How should you care for a child who has scoliosis?**
    a. Support the back, feet, and knees with pillows when the patient lies on the side.
    b. Avoid twisting or turning the spine when moving the child.
    c. Perform range-of-motion exercises to maintain muscle tone.
    d. All of the above.

73. **Parents of a child diagnosed with torticollis asked what caused this disorder. What is your best response?**
    a. Viral infection
    b. Bacterial infection
    c. Intrauterine malposition
    d. Fungal infection

74. **A child who has a cast on his left arm complains about pain and being unable to move his fingers on his left hand. You notice that the left hand is pale and you are unable to detect a pulse. What is your best response?**
    a. Open the cast immediately per protocol.
    b. Call the health-care provider immediately.
    c. Assess if the child can move fingers on his right hand.
    d. Assess if the child can move his legs.

75. **You have been assigned to care for an infant diagnosed with diphtheria. What must be monitored?**
    a. Reverse isolation procedures.
    b. That the infant doesn't scratch scabs on the sites of the rash.
    c. The child's airway. Lesion can obstruct the airway especially in infants.
    d. That the infant's legs are kept at a 30-degree angle.

76. **The health-care provider orders you to administer penicillin G to a child who has been diagnosed with diphtheria. What is your best response?**
    a. Question the order because diphtheria is a viral infection.
    b. Administer the medication.
    c. Assess if the child is allergic to penicillin.
    d. Administer the medication because diphtheria is a bacterial infection.

77. **The health-care provider orders Sumycin for a 6-year-old who has been diagnosed with Lyme disease. What is your best response?**
    a. Question the order because Sumycin will permanently stain the child's teeth.
    b. Administer the medication.
    c. Question the order because you expected the health-care provider to order tetracycline.
    d. Question the order because Lyme disease is a viral infection.

78. **What would you expect the health-care provider to order if a child diagnosed with pertussis is unable to tolerate erythromycin?**
    a. Penicillin G
    b. Sumycin
    c. Bactrim
    d. Tetracycline

79. **Why is a child diagnosed with tetanus placed in the ICU?**
    a. To prevent transmitting tetanus to other children.
    b. To limit the spreading of the *Clostridium tetani* bacterium.
    c. To monitor cardiorespiratory function because muscles tightening the mouth make it difficult to breathe and swallow.
    d. To protect the child from seizures.

80. **A mother of a 3-year-old called saying she noticed a small red flat spot on the roof of her child's mouth. What is your best response?**
    a. Bring the child to the ED immediately.
    b. Bring the child to the health-care provider immediately.
    c. Ask the woman if she is pregnant.
    d. Tell her to mention this to her health-care provider during her next scheduled appointment.

81. **A parent of a child who is diagnosed with rubeola asks if she can send her child to child care tomorrow since the rash disappeared 2 days ago. What is your best response?**
    a. Yes, he is no longer contagious.
    b. No, not until she is examined by the health-care provider.
    c. No, he remains contagious for 5 days after the rash subsides.
    d. Yes, as long as no other child at the child-care center is infected.

82. **Father of 7-year-old who is diagnosed with the measles tells his son that he will be fine after taking an antibiotic for 10 days. How would you respond?**
    a. The measles is a viral infection. Antibiotics are prescribed for bacterial infections and won't have any therapeutic effect on the measles virus.
    b. The measles is self-limiting.
    c. The treatment for the measles is to let it run its course.
    d. The treatment for the measles is to let it run its course and treat the symptoms of the infection.

83. **A hydrocolloid occlusive dressing is applied to a large abrasion. The dressing was applied for what primary purpose?**
    a. To deliver vitamin E to the wound
    b. Improves the appearance of the wound
    c. Provides a moist environment for healing
    d. Promotes mechanical friction to remove abrasion

84. **What physiological process results in edema form as a result of a burn?**
    a. Capillary vasoconstriction
    b. Reduced capillary permeability
    c. Hydrostatic pressure in the capillaries
    d. Increased capillary permeability

85. **What systemic response is involved with severe burns in a child?**
    a. Acute metabolic alkalosis
    b. Decreased metabolic rate
    c. Abrupt drop in cardiac output
    d. Increased renal plasma flow

86. **What should the nurse suspect and prepare for if a child is admitted with extensive burns with burns on the lips and singed nasal hairs?**
    a. An inhalation injury
    b. A hot-water scald
    c. An electrical burn
    d. A chemical burn

87. **What is the primary intended impact of a high-protein diet for the child with major burns?**
    a. To promote weight gain
    b. To improve the child's appetite
    c. To minimize muscle breakdown
    d. To avoid stress-induced hyperglycemia

88. **Prior to burn wound debridement, Fentanyl and midazolam (Versed) are given. What is the primary reason for this action?**
    a. Facilitate healing
    b. Provide pain relief
    c. Minimize risk of infection
    d. Decrease amount of debridement needed

89. **Nursing actions related to the application of biologic or synthetic skin coverings for a child with partial-thickness burns of both legs include which of the following?**
    a. Immobilize legs to prevent movement
    b. Observe burn area for signs of infection
    c. Monitor closely for signs of cardiovascular shock
    d. Assess dressings for indications of tissue overgrowth

90. **A mother rushed her daughter to the ED claiming they were in the woods today for the first time in years and she thinks her daughter contracted Lyme disease. What is your best response?**
    a. Tell me how it makes you feel that your daughter may have deer tick bites.
    b. Bring your daughter back in 3 days and we can tell if the bacterium that causes Lyme disease was transmitted to your daughter.
    c. Let's examine your daughter for deer tick bites. It takes up to 72 hours before the bacterium that causes Lyme disease is transmitted to your daughter.
    d. It is unlikely your daughter has the bacterium that causes Lyme disease unless she has been in contact with a child or adult who is infected with Lyme disease.

91. **A clinic nurse assesses a 1-year-old and notes small moist, circular eruptions on the child's arms. The nurse knows that further investigation is needed because the lesions could be a sign of what condition? Choose all that apply.**
    a. Impetigo
    b. Ringworm
    c. Cigarette burns
    d. Eczema

92. **A pediatric client, who has been treated for anemia, has a hemoglobin level of 11.2 g/dL, down from an earlier finding of 12.2 g/dL. Which intervention by the nurse is most appropriate?**
    a. Notify the physician to get orders for a blood transfusion.
    b. Advise the client to remain on bed rest.
    c. Instruct the client on a diet that is high in iron.
    d. Assess the client for symptoms of anemia.

93. **Which laboratory test should a nurse monitor to determine if a client is responding to the administration of iron for iron deficiency anemia?**
    a. Eosinophils
    b. Monocytes
    c. Reticulocytes
    d. Lymphocytes

94. **The nurse would record which name to most accurately describe an elevated, superficial, distinct, purulent fluid-filled lesion?**
    a. Cyst
    b. Papule
    c. Pustule
    d. Vesicle

95. **Baby boy Johnson is a newborn who is experiences hypoxia and cyanosis. The most likely diagnosis is a congenital heart defect caused by what type of shunt?**
    a. Right-to-left
    b. Left-to-right
    c. Pulmonary infection
    d. Dilated pulmonary artery

96. **Which description would best support a newborn suspected of having coarctation of the aorta?**
    a. Cyanosis
    b. Bulging carotid arteries
    c. Cool arms
    d. Weak or absent femoral pulses

97. **What is the name of the structure between the aorta and pulmonary artery in fetal circulation?**
    a. Foramen ovale
    b. Mitral value
    c. Ductus arteriosus
    d. Foramen magnum

98. **Baby Alice was born weeks ago and now presents with poor feeding, fatigue, dyspnea, and a murmur. She is diagnosed with a patent ductus arteriosus. How would you describe the alteration?**
    a. Increased cardiac output
    b. Right-to-left shunt
    c. Left-to-right shunt
    d. Increased systemic blood flow

99. **Jason arrives to his physician for his 8-week-old well-baby check. The examination reveals a murmur, and the electrocardiogram (ECG) reveals a large ventricular septal defect. Left untreated, this defect will result in which of the following conditions?**
    a. Pulmonary hypertension
    b. Cyanosis
    c. Pulmonary stenosis
    d. Right ventricular atrophy

100. **Congestive heart failure precipitated by a ventricular septal defect in a 6-month-old is likely to produce which of the following?**
   a. Failure to thrive and periorbital edema
   b. Dependent edema to the hands and feet
   c. Weight loss and jaundice
   d. Flat neck veins and decreased urinary output

ANSWERS

1. a	2. d	3. a	4. c
5. c	6. d	7. d	8. c
9. b	10. b	11. c	12. d
13. b	14. d	15. c	16. a
17. b	18. d	19. b	20. b
21. d	22. a	23. b	24. a
25. d	26. a	27. d	28. b
29. a	30. b	31. b	32. b
33. b	34. c	35. d	36. a
37. c	38. c	39. b	40. c
41. c	42. c	43. c	44. b
45. a	46. d	47. c	48. b
49. c	50. b	51. d	52. b
53. c	54. c	55. a	56. a
57. a	58. c	59. c	60. a
61. b	62. b	63. a	64. a
65. d	66. c	67. c	68. c
69. c	70. a	71. d	72. d
73. c	74. a	75. c	76. c
77. a	78. c	79. c	80. b
81. c	82. a	83. c	84. d
85. c	86. a	87. c	88. b
89. b	90. c	91. a and c	92. c
93. c	94. c	95. a	96. d
97. c	98. c	99. a	100. a

Index

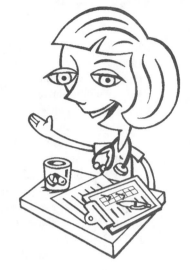